Pediatric Neurologic Physical Therapy
Second Edition

CLINICS IN PHYSICAL THERAPY

EDITORIAL BOARD

Pediatric Neurologic Physical Therapy

Second Edition

Edited by
Suzann K. Campbell, Ph.D., P.T., F.A.P.T.A.

Professor
Department of Physical Therapy
College of Associated Health Professions
University of Illinois at Chicago
Chicago, Illinois

CHURCHILL LIVINGSTONE
New York, Edinburgh, London, Melbourne, Tokyo

Library of Congress Cataloging-in-Publication Data
Pediatric neurologic physical therapy / edited by Suzann K. Campbell.
— 2nd ed.
    p.   cm. — (Clinics in physical therapy)
    Includes bibliographical references and index.
    ISBN 0-443-08764-4
    1. Pediatric neurology. 2. Physical therapy for children.
    I. Campbell, Suzann K. II. Series.
    [DNLM: 1. Nervous System Diseases—in infancy & childhood.
    2. Nervous System Diseases—therapy. 3. Physical Therapy—in
    infancy & childhood.   WS 340 P3685]
    RJ486.P32 1991
    618.92'8'0462—dc20
    DNLM/DLC
    for Library of Congress   91-13667
                                                              CIP

Second Edition © Churchill Livingstone Inc. 1991
First Edition © Churchill Livingstone Inc. 1984

Distributed in the United Kingdom by Churchill Livingstone, Robert Stevenson House, 1–3 Baxter's Place, Leith Walk, Edinburgh EH1 3AF, and by associated companies, branches, and representatives throughout the world.

Accurate indications, adverse reactions, and dosage schedules for drugs are provided in this book, but it is possible that they may change. The reader is urged to review the package information data of the manufacturers of the medications mentioned.

The Publishers have made every effort to trace the copyright holders for borrowed material. If they have inadvertently overlooked any, they will be pleased to make the necessary arrangements at the first opportunity.

Acquisitions Editor: *Leslie Burgess*
Copy Editor: *Christina Joslin*
Production Designer: *Marci Jordan*
Production Supervisor: *Jeanine Furino*

P02855

Printed in the United States of America

First published in 1991   7 6 5 4 3 2 1

To Dick, my mentor and friend—the second time around

Contributors

Jack Berndt, P.T.
Physical Therapist, Madison Metropolitan School District, Madison, Wisconsin

Jocelyn Blaskey, M.S., P.T.
Senior Clinician, Department of Adult Orthopedics and Pediatrics, Rancho Los Amigos Medical Center, Downey, California

Suzann K. Campbell, Ph.D., P.T., F.A.P.T.A.
Professor, Department of Physical Therapy, College of Associated Health Professions, University of Illinois at Chicago, Chicago, Illinois

Ann Falconer, M.A., P.T.
Physical Therapist, Madison Metropolitan School District, Madison, Wisconsin

Linda Fetters, Ph.D., P.T.
Assistant Professor, Department of Physical Therapy, Sargent College of Allied Health Professions, Boston University, Boston, Massachusetts

June Bridgford Garber, P.T., M.A.C.T.
Assistant Professor, Division of Physical Therapy, Emory University School of Medicine, Atlanta, Georgia

Susan R. Harris, Ph.D., P.T., F.A.P.T.A.
Associate Professor, School of Rehabilitation Medicine, University of British Columbia, Vancouver, British Columbia, Canada; Adjunct Associate Professor, Department of Orthopedic Surgery and Rehabilitation, Hahnemann University, Philadelphia, Pennsylvania

Thubi H.A. Kolobe, M.S., P.T.
Senior Research Specialist, Department of Physical Therapy, University of Illinois at Chicago, Chicago, Illinois; Doctoral Candidate, Department of Physical Therapy, Hahnemann University, Philadelphia, Pennsylvania

Karen Yundt Lunnen, M.S., P.T.
Physical Therapy Consultant, Developmental Evaluation Center, School of Education and Psychology, Western Carolina University, Cullowhee, North Carolina; Director, Rehabilitation Services, C.J. Harris Hospital, Sylva, North Carolina

Alice M. Shea, P.T., Sc.D.
Adjunct Associate Professor, Department of Physical Therapy, Sargent College of Allied Health Professions, Boston University; Associate for Research and Continuing Education, Department of Physical Therapy, and Physical Therapist, Down Syndrome Program, Developmental Evaluation Center, Children's Hospital, Boston, Massachusetts

Roberta B. Shepherd, Dip.Phty., M.Ed., Ed.D., F.A.C.P.
Associate Professor, School of Physiotherapy, Cumberland College of Health Sciences, University of Sydney, New South Wales, Australia

Thomas J. Stengel, M.S., P.T.
Executive Director, Intervention with Parents and Children Together, Inc.,Baltimore, Maryland

Irma J. Wilhelm, M.S., P.T.
Research Associate Professor, Division of Physical Therapy, Department of Medical Allied Health Professions, University of North Carolina at Chapel Hill School of Medicine, Chapel Hill, North Carolina

Janet M. Wilson, M.A.C.T., P.T.
Adjunct Associate Professor, Division of Physical Therapy, Department of Medical Allied Health Professions, University of North Carolina at Chapel Hill School of Medicine, Chapel Hill, North Carolina; Private Practice, Hillsborough, North Carolina

Preface

Preparation of this new edition of a successful book provides the opportunity to correct the weaknesses of the original edition, include new material, and update each section. Feedback from readers of the first edition is used in adding new case histories and photographs to many sections of the book. Some material has been deleted because more detailed treatments of those subjects have since been published elsewhere. Each chapter is updated with new research findings from the literature and innovations developed in clinical practice.

The first three chapters present theoretical and research-based information to guide the practice of physical therapy in the management of neurologic disorders. Chapter 1 presents a summary of new information on pathology and kinesiologic dysfunction in central nervous system disorders. This new information will provide a better understanding of the underlying pathophysiology. Following this summary is a new chapter summarizing the theory and practical application of current information on motor development and on the learning of motor skills in a functional context. Chapter 3 presents information on formal tests that clinicians will find useful in assessing developmental dysfunction.

Chapters 4 through 10 present information on specific neurologic conditions, with updates from the research laboratory and the clinical setting. The book ends with two new chapters addressing physical therapy in the community settings of the public school and early intervention programs. The introduction of new federal legislation, Public Law 94-142 and Public Law 99-457, has presented physical therapists with the opportunity to test the advantages of moving away from the medical model of "fixing" the problems of a disabled child. Today's service delivery models emphasize family-centered and community-based approaches to ameliorating and managing potentially handicapping physical disabilities in order to maximize a child's ability to function successfully in his or her unique environment. The chapters on school-based practice and family-focused early intervention should help therapists understand and contribute to the development of these models for practice.

Whatever the problem, our purpose has always been to facilitate the maximum attainment of each child's potential and be ever mindful that our patients are *children*, with special needs for fun, play, and love, and that parents and other professionals are partners in our enterprise. As with the first edition, the primary purpose of this book is to bring to the practicing pediatric specialist in physical therapy the most current information on management of typical problems in pediatric neurology.

Suzann K. Campbell, Ph.D., P.T., F.A.P.T.A.

Acknowledgments

During the time that this edition was being compiled, my work was supported by the Bureau of Maternal and Child Health Care Delivery and Assistance, the Agency for Health Care Policy and Research, the National Institutes of Health, and the Foundation for Physical Therapy. I am very grateful for the support of these agencies, but, most of all, I want to acknowledge the help of the many friends and colleagues who made this work possible by their professional and personal support. Special thanks are owed to Thubi Kolobe, Beth Osten, Gay Girolami, Judy Anderson, Russ Carter, Linda Fetters, Irma Wilhelm, Nancy Thoresen, and Wendy Phillips. I particularly want to thank Dick Campbell, Dan Corcos, Martha Piper, Helene Larin, and Susan Harris for their special contributions, which stimulated my thoughts and directed me to challenging new information.

Contents

1 | Central Nervous System Dysfunction in Children

Suzann K. Campbell

The treatment of pediatric patients with neurologic dysfunction is both an exciting challenge and a frustrating dilemma for the physical therapist. The problems are so complex, so enigmatic, we barely understand the simplest facts about the neuromuscular dysfunction we treat. Still, helping a child to function better so that he or she can participate fully in life is a joyous undertaking.

The first purpose of this introductory chapter is to review selected information from the literature on brain dysfunction in children (primarily spastic cerebral palsy because this is the most frequently encountered subject of research), including the effects of lesions at various ages; the etiology, neuropathology, and pathokinesiology of central nervous system (CNS) dysfunction; and recovery following injury to the developing nervous system. The second purpose is to propose a model for assessing and studying the effects of physical therapy on children with CNS dysfunction.

THE VARYING PICTURE OF SENSORIMOTOR DYSFUNCTION WITH AGE

The clinical literature provides evidence that the effects on sensorimotor function of a brain lesion in the exceptionally premature infant differ from those in the full-term infant,[1-5] and that the 5-year-old trauma victim presents yet another picture.[6] Differing etiologies and sites of injury may be factors accounting for significant variance, but the clinical outcome varies primarily because the insult is inflicted on brains that are tremendously different in structure and physiology. Indeed, the brain of the very premature infant may resemble that of the full-term infant less than the full-term infant's brain resembles the

1

adult brain.[2] Even similar lesions may produce strikingly different results at different chronologic ages.

Prenatal brain damage may be roughly separated into events during the first half of gestation versus later events.[7] Early interference with brain development leads to disorders of cell production and migration, such as microcephalies and lissencephalies. These may be largely related to genetic defects, teratogens, or infections such as cytomegalovirus. Perfusion failures caused by placental, embolic, and other factors are more common in the second half of gestation and lead to conditions such as hydranencephaly, destructive microcephalies, and periventricular leukomalacia.

It is not accidental that the incidence of spastic diplegia is greater among survivors of extreme prematurity than in full-term babies who experience asphyxia.[2,3] Cerebral convolutions first appear in the fetal human brain during the fifth month of gestation and continue to develop into the first postnatal year.[8] During the sixth and seventh months of gestation, the cerebral cortex remains largely underdeveloped with smooth surfaces quite uncharacteristic of the full-term brain with its many cerebral cortical convolutions.[2] The blood supply of the fetal brain is directed toward the most metabolically active parts; thus, the area of germinal matrix near the caudate nucleus and the periventricular area are especially vulnerable in the preterm infant.[1-3] Prenatal perfusion failure in the newborn of less than 32 weeks' gestation is likely to cause damage to tracts in the periventricular area of the internal capsule, including those axons projecting to motoneurons to the lower extremities and trunk, resulting in the typical outcome of spastic diplegia. Relative sparing of intellect is typical, although perceptual problems are not uncommon.

New information suggests that prenatal ischemia and hypoxia were often present, leading to periventricular leukomalacia visualized postnatally as echodensities on ultrasound examination.[3] This finding is an accurate predictor of risk for cerebral palsy (CP). Postnatal hemorrhage may contribute to the production of additional brain damage, but is probably not the primary source of disability.[4,5]

This type of neuropathology is rarely seen in the full-term child who has been asphyxiated.[1,2,4] The more likely area of vulnerability is the now highly developed cerebral cortex, with resultant spastic quadriplegia or, if more localized, hemiplegia. The basal ganglia and brain stem nuclei are also highly metabolically active; if the basal ganglia are damaged by lack of blood supply and oxygen, athetosis results. Prenatal etiologies are often implicated, complicated by problems during labor and delivery.

Two critical factors in the production of CNS dysfunction have received recent attention. One is the study of cerebral blood flow regulation, especially the concept of loss of autoregulation of arterial pressure in the presence of hypoxia.[9,10] Loss of autoregulation exposes the fragile cerebral vessels to large changes in systemic blood pressure that may result from many conditions, such as maternal shock, infant resuscitation, and volume expansion. A second important area of research is that of metabolic factors resulting from hypoxic–ischemic effects that may compound the damage, such as activation of glutamate receptors allowing calcium ion influx into cells. This event results in cell death that may be preventable if glutamate receptors are blocked.[11] These new research findings hold out renewed hope for the possibility of preventing or diminishing the effects of hypoxic-ischemic events on the developing brain.

In research on monkeys, Goldman-Rakic[12] demonstrated that prenatal injury to a localized area of cerebral cortex results in widespread changes in the configuration of brain convolutions, corresponding to those areas of cerebral cortex that normally receive input from the damaged areas during the final weeks of gestation. On the other hand, the subcortical areas normally projecting to the now damaged cortex were more normal in neuronal structure than expected, presumably because their projections were directed to new sites. These results were not seen in postnatally damaged infant animals whose brains showed little signs of reorganization of connections. If the same is true in humans, early CNS damage may create abnormal function in areas far removed from the initial insult; on the other hand, the ability of circuits to reorganize may provide a basis for ameliorating the effects of brain damage in the preterm infant, which would not be possible in those with later injury.

In the preschool-age child, the cerebral hemispheres have become increasingly specialized, individualized, and committed in function,[13,14] with resulting effects on muscle tone, cognition, and language that differ from those in children experiencing prenatal insults.[6] Chapters 4, 8, and 10 on the high-risk infant, head trauma, and CP further clarify some of the ways in which these patients differ from each other.

Musculoskeletal Changes with Age and Sensorimotor Dysfunction

Movement coordination is clearly affected by the disruption in neural circuits produced by a brain lesion; however, little attention has been paid to the fact that the musculoskeletal system is undergoing developmental changes in the early months and years of life as well. A prenatal or perinatal brain injury results in an abnormal nervous system attempting to direct the growth and development of muscles that are largely composed of slowly contracting fibers[15-17] but are genetically programmed to gradually differentiate into at least three types of fibers specialized in their endurance and force production properties.[18] These properties of individual muscle fibers can be varied, within certain limits, in accordance with the task demands of exercise.[19] Because brain injury affects the coordination, force, speed, and duration of movement and therefore the quality of exercise engaged in by the individual, it is possible, although unproven, that abnormalities in muscle fiber development are produced secondarily by brain dysfunction.

In the older child, brain damage will also create movement problems, but these difficulties will be imposed on a muscular system unlike that of the newborn who has only begun to move against the force of gravity. Nevertheless, muscular dysfunction is likely to occur in the older child as well. In addition to the possible pathologic effects of abnormal patterns of posture and movement on individual muscle fibers, such as abnormal hypertrophy in some and atrophy in others,[20] developing contracture in a muscle increases its stiffness (unit change in force per unit change in length) and may contribute to increasing spasticity.[21] Thus, spasticity may be more than just a primary problem in the nervous system, for muscle stiffness is determined not only by the neural components of the neuromuscular system, but also by the passive viscoelastic properties of muscle and connective tissue. Berger and colleagues, for example, have demonstrated that restraint of ankle movement during gait is often related to the development of passive tension in the Achilles tendon of a relatively inactive muscle rather than to a hyperactive stretch reflex.[22]

Tardieu and colleagues believe that equinus contracture can develop for at least two reasons[23,24]: overuse of a hyperactive muscle or failure of muscle tissue to demonstrate the plasticity needed to add sarcomeres to keep up with skeletal growth. Because the effects of "inhibitive" casting are likely to be based primarily on the ability of muscle to lengthen when held in a stretched position, not on tone reduction, treatment effectiveness may be limited in children with reduced muscle plasticity. The Tardieu research group also postulated that prevention of contractures requires that a muscle at risk must be stretched for 6 to 7 hours per day.[25] Because prevention of contractures and deformities is held by a majority of physicians to be an important outcome of physical therapy for CP, more study of this issue is urgently needed.[26]

Other effects on the muscular system derive from general poverty of movement. Muscular atrophy and disuse weakness are inevitable results of lack of exercise, and stretch weakness is likely to develop in muscles that are excessively elongated for prolonged periods by overactive antagonists.[27]

A major question in the management of CP must be whether reduction of force output in spasticity syndromes is amenable to remediation. Olney suggests that poor power output of the ankle plantar flexors is the most important deficit in the gait of children with spastic CP, but whether this problem can be positively affected by physical therapy has not been systematically studied.[28] A case study on the effects of a weight-training program suggests that strength can be increased in adults with CP, with accompanying increases in range of motion, but further research is needed.[29]

Inactivity and abnormal muscle physiology undoubtedly can have negative effects on the development of the skeletal system, although the effects may once again vary with the age and plasticity of the bones. The deforming forces of contractured muscle are well known to physical therapists, and prevention of bony deformities is a major goal of physical therapy for the client with CNS dysfunction. Indeed, physical therapy that aids muscles to work in normal ranges and with more normal force, and the repetition afforded by active exercise in the overload range, may be our most important contributions to the health and habilitation or rehabilitation of children with sensorimotor dysfunction.

Pathokinesiology

The complexity of the outcome of brain lesions in childhood is also re-vealed by new studies of patterns of muscular activity recorded by electro-myography (EMG). These studies demonstrate the inadequacy of many of our clinical methods, including supposedly differential tests for individual muscle function and observational analysis of muscle dysfunction underlying individual patterns of movement coordination. They also bring into question the maxim that abnormal tone is the *major* problem that must be treated to improve move-ment in the child with CP.

Electromyographic studies of children with CP have revealed that clini-cally similar patterns of movement can be produced by several different pat-terns of muscular activity.[30-33] Chong and colleagues,[30] for example, identified three types of abnormal patterns of muscle activity during gait characterized by abnormal medial rotation at the hip. These patterns included (1) activation of hip adductor and medial rotator muscles at the normal time during the gait cycle, but phasically prolonged medial hamstring activity so that muscular force creating medial rotation was applied at an inappropriate point in the cycle; (2) on–off patterning of phasic muscle activity, but with no relationship to gait cycle; and (3) mass turning on and off at the same time of all muscles used in gait, leading to a stumplike progression pattern. Knutsson[34] reported that the latter pattern was the most common in patients with CP; however, Chong and associates[30] reported the first pattern to be most frequent in children with abnormal medial rotation.

Orthopedists have made a major point of the finding that clinically similar patterns, such as the presence of medial rotation of the hip during gait, can be produced by different patterns of muscle activation that are not identifiable with visual observation. This finding has made EMG a powerful tool for making decisions regarding orthopedic surgery. Offending muscles are identified by EMG recordings during locomotion.[30-33] If the suspect muscle is overactive during its normal place in the gait cycle, it can be lengthened. If a muscle acts at the wrong point in the gait cycle, it might be considered for transplantation. In the situation in which numerous muscles work together to produce a dys-functional pattern, surgery is unlikely to be successful. One can only guess that the future holds similar promise for physical therapists that EMG analysis, combined with kinematic and kinetic information, might lead to differential treatments depending on the pattern of dysfunction present. A challenge for the future must be the introduction of more sophisticated quantitative assess-ment into the typical clinical environment and the establishment of patient profiles of dysfunction.

Three types of restraint of movement are found in patients with spastic-ity.[34] One is the result of activation of tonic stretch reflexes by muscle stretch. The forces produced by stretch reflex activation are weak relative to normal forces of muscle used to restrain movement; however, they occur at the wrong point in a cycle of movement. Restraint of movement by stretch reflex activation may *or may not* appear in the patient with strong stretch reflex activity on passive motion; therefore, assessment of tone during passive manipulation is not highly predictive of ability to control voluntary movement.

A second type of restraint is mechanical. This type of restraint is caused by an increase in passive tension resulting from stretch of a hypoextensible muscle that is unable to lengthen adequately when muscles on the opposite side of a joint are actively contracting.[22] Two-joint muscles, such as hamstrings and gastrocnemius, are likely to be major offenders.

Most common, indeed almost diagnostic, of CP of either the spastic or hypertonic athetoid type is pathologic coactivation of muscles when reciprocal inhibition should occur during voluntary movement.[34–36] Abnormal restraint of movement occurs because muscles outbalance the action of each other. Abnormal reciprocal innervation through spinal circuits, rather than spasticity, is then a cause of disrupted voluntary control, contributing to delayed initiation of movement.[35,36]

Abnormal timing of muscle activation occurs in a number of different ways that are characteristic of the incoordination problem in spasticity syndromes. Nashner and colleagues have shown that even when the correct synergic pattern of muscle activation was chosen for responding to a perturbation of standing balance, abnormal timing of muscle contraction (proximal muscle before distal synergist) created a destabilizing response.[37] Activation of postural setting muscles for voluntary activity may also be poorly timed or absent, and the widespread activation of muscles in abnormal synergic patterns creates internally generated forces that must then be contended with to prevent postural instability. The use of inappropriate coordinative structures in poorly timed sequences of activity is thus the major hallmark of movement dysfunction in spasticity syndromes. Ability to isolate movement (dissociation) to individual joints is severely impaired.

These findings suggest that most patients would have difficulty coordinating movement even if muscle tone and reflexes were normal.[35] Spasticity is only one of the symptoms of a CNS lesion. It is one of the positive symptoms, along with clonus, disinhibition of primitive reflexes, and increased size of reflexogenic zones.[35,38,39] Spasticity is defined as "a motor disorder characterized by a velocity-dependent increase in tonic stretch reflexes ('muscle tone') with exaggerated tendon jerks, resulting from hyperexcitability of the stretch reflex, as one component of the upper motoneuron syndrome."[40] Negative symptoms, such as paresis, inadequate force production opposed by cocontraction, delayed initiation of movement, and inappropriate postural set for activity of prime movers may be far more significant in producing dysfunction and difficult to improve with therapy. Indeed, this has been the case with some patients in controlled studies of the effect of orally administered baclofen on cerebral or spinal spasticity and voluntary movement in which tone was decreased by the drug without notable improvement in function.[41] The findings of a consensus conference on effects of physical therapy on movement dysfunction in CP indicated that little evidence exists that abnormal tone and reflexes can be permanently inhibited by physical therapy.[42] Results such as these should be taken into account when attempting to develop a theory for treatment of CNS dysfunction.

The many signs of movement dysfunction in CP result in movement that is inefficient and metabolically costly. Average heart rates of 164 beats/min are associated with activities such as walking that normally cause only minor increases above resting levels.[43] Endurance for physical activity appears to be reduced in children with CNS dysfunction, except those with hemiplegia.[44] In a longitudinal study by Lundberg, most values related to work capacity did not appear to deteriorate in the teenage years, but youngsters with spastic diplegia demonstrated a decrease in net mechanical efficiency of movement over time.[44] Lundberg speculated that low physical activity resulted in insufficient intensity of stimulation for neuromuscular function, which may have increased spasticity and lowered net mechanical efficiency. These data suggest that fitness programs for adolescents with CP might be useful in maintaining or improving physical work capacity. My own observations of physical endurance in adolescents with CP suggest that relatively undemanding physical function tests lasting more than 1 or 2 hours result in significant fatigue and reduced ability to perform. One wonders whether such individuals will be able to enter the work force with sufficient endurance to function for an 8-hour day.

The causes of poor work capacity have been inadequately studied but may include the presence of low muscle mass, the metabolic demands of overcoming mechanical restraint of movement, low cardiovascular fitness from lack of exercise and inadequate physical training, and inability of the motor control system to control force output. Whether the coordinative structures selected by the abnormal motor control system produce movement that is as efficient as can be expected is a topic of debate. The important question for physical therapists, of course, is whether therapy can improve efficiency of motor control or only provides compensatory measures, such as powered mobility or assistive devices, to reduce demands on the system.

Overall Effects of Treatment

Given the multitude of problems influencing movement in clients with CNS dysfunction, it is understandable that the theoretic foundations of treatment are unclear regarding the expected outcomes of intervention. The existing research literature documents the effects (only moderate) of physical therapy on the rate of motor development,[45] but study of many other potential outcomes is needed. The design of future studies should be guided by the results of the Consensus Conference on the Efficacy of Physical Therapy in the Management of Movement Dysfunction in Cerebral Palsy.[42] Physical therapists concluded that effects on postural control and alignment, prevention of contractures and deformities, efficiency and endurance, functional independence, and family functioning are important outcomes in need of study. Physicians agree that these outcomes are important and express especially high degrees of belief in the value of physical therapy in helping parents to manage disability and cope with the emotional aspects of having a disabled child.[26] Physicians also believe that physical therapy helps children to profit from educational experiences in school.

RECOVERY OF FUNCTION FOLLOWING BRAIN INJURY

As Blaskey suggests (Ch. 8), the therapist probably does not produce recovery in a patient with neurologic damage, but rather takes advantage of the recovery and maturation that are occurring, directing energy into the most functional paths to encourage maximal use of returning and developing functions. Recovery of function following nervous system injury is not well understood. Animal studies are the primary source of information, because very few natural history studies of the recovery of function in humans are available in the literature, and almost no studies of quantitative changes across time in neurologic functions following lesions have been done. Although species differences must be kept firmly in mind, the animal studies suggest that several variables are important in determining extent of recovery, including site and extent of lesion, whether lesions were staged, age at time of lesion, and pre- and postlesion experience and training.[46,47]

The effects of each of these variables in recovery are complex and poorly understood. For example, young age is no longer considered to be the significant advantage suggested by early studies.[47,48] Careful reanalysis of some of the data suggests that delayed deficits appeared in animals lesioned at young ages and that few differences between immature- and adult-lesioned animals were evident when tests were made several years postlesion rather than only immediately after damage. Indeed, the period of shock that follows any nervous system lesion may have an effect on maturation of the nervous system that irreversibly compounds the damage caused by the lesion. Such an effect is suggested by the work of Myklebust and colleagues,[49] who reported that stretch of the soleus muscle produces a reciprocal *excitation*, rather than the expected inhibition, in the antagonist tibialis anterior muscle only in patients who suffered perinatal injury and not in adult-injured subjects. This finding suggests that either abnormal circuits were formed in the immature spinal cord as a result of cerebral injury or that primitive spinal cord circuits that should have regressed or been altered during early development failed to do so. One of the prime areas of dysfunction affecting movement in children with CNS dysfunction is the aberrant spread of excitation to many muscles from afferent stimulation of sensory receptors,[38] making the production of isolated movements difficult or impossible. The interaction, therefore, between the course of maturation and the attempts of the nervous system to compensate for damage may alter the usual regressions and transformations of neural circuitry,[50] the normal decrease with maturation of dependence on sensory cues,[51] and the ability to use flexible combinations of sensory modalities in coping with postural and environmental demands.[50,52] The stimulus-bound nature of movement in CNS dysfunction results.

Numerous theories, not necessarily mutually exclusive, exist regarding recovery of function after brain damage.[52,53] These are summarized in the following sections.

Diaschisis. Diaschisis suggests that return of function following brain damage occurs as the nervous system recovers from a period of shock, having widespread effects on areas of the brain not directly damaged by the lesion. As diaschisis resolves, some previously lost functions reappear.

Equipotentiality/Vicariation. Equipotentiality and vicariation refer to the idea that undamaged parts of the nervous system have the potential to take over functions previously subserved by damaged areas. Equipotentiality specifically refers to assumption of control by undamaged parts of the same neural system; the size of the lesion would be important in determining whether sparing or recovery of function would occur. Vicariation refers to takeover by other parts of the nervous system. Age is an important variable in this theory because the degree to which vicariation can occur appears to depend to a great extent on how committed to other functions a potential substitute area is at the time of damage. During early development, an uncommitted area may easily substitute for the damaged one; however, the substitute area's commitment may mean a consequent impairment in performance of its own intended function at the appointed time, resulting in the delayed appearance of deficits.[54] Takeover of language functions by the right hemisphere in early left hemisphere-damaged children, for example, is postulated to decrease overall intellectual functioning as a cost of vicariation.[6]

Reorganization of Circuits. Regrowth of damaged axons or sprouting of undamaged axons to assume vacated synaptic sites has been demonstrated to occur under some conditions in the CNS of experimental animals.[55] Goldman-Rakic[12] has also demonstrated significant redirection of fiber projections in the cerebral cortical development of prenatally brain-damaged primates. Although theories involving establishment of new circuits are under investigation and are frequently suggested as underlying the effects of treatment of CNS dysfunction, actual analysis of the effects on behavior of such nervous system remodeling are rare. The effects may more often be harmful and responsible for aberrant behavior rather than necessarily beneficial and responsible for recovery. Great caution is warranted in using these types of theories as possible rationale for treatment effects when no firm evidence is available to support this supposition.

Supersensitivity. Target neurons of the damaged system develop supersensitivity to remaining neurotransmitter molecules, thus enhancing their ability to function in a deprived state and producing a degree of recovery. This response to damage could obviously provide a molecular basis for vicariation or equipotentiality.

Compensation. The theory of compensation suggests that rather than true recovery occurring, the functions damaged by the nervous system lesion are taken over by other circuits that accomplish the same goal but by different means, such as using a different sensory system to guide performance. This means that the function is not really recovered, although defects may be extremely subtle, but rather compensated for with varying degrees of abnormality in achieving the performance goal. LeVere and LeVere[56] believe that compensation is the critical process: as soon as damage occurs, compensations begin to develop as the organism struggles to function with an inadequate system. If these compensations are relatively effective in helping the individual to meet its goals, recovery of the original function may actually be retarded or prevented. These investigators suggest that the aim of early intervention after brain damage must be to prevent the establishment of compensatory mechanisms and to force the organism to use the function that may be present but temporarily suppressed. In support of this argument, LeVere and LeVere cite studies of monkeys with deafferented limbs whose normal limbs were restrained, demonstrating that this intervention could produce significant recovery of function in the deafferented limb, which did not occur if the animal was allowed to compensate for the useless limb by use of undamaged parts. Although the theory of LeVere and LeVere does not take into account the maturational forces directing change in the developing nervous system, their ideas are commensurate with several of the major approaches to early management of CNS dysfunction in children. Preventing the development of compensatory patterns of movement by early treatment may in turn prevent or limit the development of spasticity, which may itself be a compensation engaged in by the nervous system for the inadequate force production generated by a defective CNS. This is a generally accepted goal of neurodevelopmental treatment.

A THEORETIC MODEL FOR THE EFFECTS OF CENTRAL NERVOUS SYSTEM DYSFUNCTION IN CHILDHOOD

I believe that it is time to develop a model for the effects of CNS dysfunction based on *clinical* observations and *human* experimentation with subjects with neurologic dysfunction and to abandon outdated neurophysiologic theories of a stimulus–response nature. These theories neglect many important factors involved in the response of the nervous system to injury and exercise, some of which I have tried to describe in this chapter. The results of the II Step Conference on motor control and motor learning suggest that therapists are ready for this to occur because the switch to a new theoretic paradigm has the potential to improve patient outcomes.[57]

I would like to present here a model for the effects of CNS dysfunction in the immature organism that can be used to develop a set of testable hypotheses regarding the efficacy of treatment of neurologic dysfunction in children. Lest this model be used to provide yet another rationale for the effects of treatment, I hasten to emphasize that it is a theoretic model with a set of resulting hypotheses, one or more of which are likely to be proved wrong by research. We must avoid perpetuating what are mere hypotheses by accepting them as truth and not subjecting them to experimental tests. I encourage and challenge clinicians to test, support, or refute the hypotheses presented.

The model I propose suggests that a CNS lesion in childhood of the type that typically produces spastic CP syndromes results in three primary problems: abnormal movement, deprivation and compensatory reactions in sensory systems, and disturbed patterns of social interaction. Each of these major areas of deficit results in typical outcomes if no intervention is undertaken. The signs of motor dysfunction vary with age because the neuromusculoskeletal system response to CNS damage varies with age, previous experience, and compensatory reactions to primary deficits.

In general, however, abnormal movement in spasticity syndromes is characterized by increased latency of movement onset, poor temporal and spatial organization of coordinative structures (muscles and joints), poor force production by prime movers, inadequate postural set, and decreased speed of movement, all at least partially related to the presence of abnormal amounts of cocontraction in antagonists opposing prime movers and the use of abnormal muscle synergies. These problems eventually result in compensatory responses, including increasingly abnormal postural tone, stretch weakness in muscles antagonistic to hypertonic muscles, loss of extensibility in hypertonic muscles, compensatory postural responses, contractures, and skeletal deformities. Functional results include poor endurance and motivation for movement, poor growth, lack of adequate exercise for cardiovascular fitness, and poor work capacity. Overuse syndromes related to repetitive activity of hypertonic muscles are also possible effects.

Sensory deprivation is experienced because of lack of opportunity to move and because of possible damage to sensory circuits and compensatory reactions to feedback from poorly coordinated movement. These problems result in impaired sensory processing, perceptual motor dysfunction, and deviant cognitive development. At the spinal level, impaired processing of sensory inputs has been documented and several theories exist regarding how it develops.[38,49,58] The effects on motor control include the production of abnormal synergies of movement and increased postural tone. Drugs such as intrathecally administered baclofen[59] and neurosurgery such as selective posterior rhizotomy[60] are under study because of their potential ability to interrupt the effects of such abnormal processing of sensory information at the spinal cord level. Improved function has been suggested to follow, but to date is insufficiently documented by controlled clinical trials. Whether physical therapy alone can produce such effects is unknown; however, augmented sensory feedback and functional electrical stimulation have potential usefulness in this area if long-term effects can be demonstrated.[61-65]

Finally, abnormal social interaction is engendered by poor ability to signal emotions and intent, difficulty expressing body and vocal language, and, perhaps, autonomic instability, resulting in frustration, lowered motivation, and impaired cognitive development. These effects will limit quality of life, community integration, and functional independence.

If this model is an accurate reflection of the problems created by CNS dysfunction in children, the following hypotheses regarding the effects of physical therapy might be tested by research:

1. Important effects of therapy are related to the well-documented (in animals and human adults) general effects of exercise, including prevention of disuse atrophy, promotion of normal posture preventing the development of stretch weakness and deformities, and improvement of strength and endurance for physical activity which are also thought to contribute to a subjective sense of well-being and self-esteem.

2. More normal patterns of muscular coordination result from improving force production, decreasing latency of movement initiation, increasing speed of movement, improving postural set for movement, and decreasing the amount of abnormal cocontraction in groups of muscles, including prime movers. The result is improved mechanical efficiency of movement.

3. Abnormal compensatory patterns, including development of abnormal tone and assumption of abnormal postures, can be prevented if the above effects occur.

4. Primary and secondary sensory deprivation and lack of social interaction can be decreased by providing the opportunity for more normal movement accompanied by increased endurance for physical activity.

5. The opportunity to be successful in movement performance leads to increased motivation to move and decreased frustration when doing so, with resulting improvement in self-confidence and self-esteem, and improved ability to learn.

6. If all of the outcomes listed above occur in combination with the contributions of other professional disciplines and the family, there will be improved functional independence, community integration, and overall quality of life.

Considered from this perspective, what would an assessment strategy look like? The International Classification of Impairment, Disability, and Handicap (ICIDH)[66] defines a hierarchy of levels of physical dysfunction: impairments (organ and system level), disabilities (functional/organism level), and handicaps (social role level). Examples of constructs to assess in the area of abnormal movement, as categorized within the ICIDH framework, are shown in Table 1-1.

Clinical data base collection in these and other areas to provide a comprehensive picture of impairment, disability, and handicap, as well as family management of disability, would be an important contribution to the literature on CP. Especially important is a taxonomy of patient profiles based on clusters of impairments that would be useful in evaluation of the efficacy of various treatment approaches for each defined profile of involvement. Important questions that could be answered with such a data base are as follows:

1. Can motor control be improved in CP, or does therapy only provide compensatory strategies that are better than those chosen by the abnormal

Table 1-1. Constructs to Assess in the Area of Abnormal Movement

Impairment	Disability	Handicap
Mechanical	Reaching	Play
Force production	Grasping	Mobility
Hypoextensibility	Creeping	School integration and
Posture	Walking	performance
Coordination	Motor milestones	Community
Hemiparesis, etc (abnormal synergies)	attainment	integration
EMG (synergies)	Need for assistive	Employability
Involuntary movement	devices	
Endurance/efficiency	Functional independence	
Fatigue		
Speed		
Repetitions		
Step test/VO$_2$ maximum		
Mental retardation		
Sensory deficits		

motor control system (i.e., can we treat underlying impairment or only disability)?

2. Can secondary problems, such as contractures and deformities, be prevented or reduced with physical therapy or assistive devices? If so, does this result in improved functional abilities, mechanical efficiency, or endurance for productive activities?

3. Is there an age range in which prevention and amelioration of impairment are most effective? Is there an age beyond which improvement in impairment should be abandoned as a goal and only methods to compensate for disability be instituted?

Each question needs to be answered for every type of CP patient defined by profiles of impairment and severity.

At the least, we need to develop systematic data collection and recording methods that will be more productive for program evaluation. At present, from typical records of children under treatment, it is almost impossible to tell the age at which they attained important motor milestones, the history of progressive development (or amelioration) of contractures, the limits of functional mobility, and so on. If we had such records, effectiveness research would be possible.

Research designed to test the hypotheses and answer the questions listed above would require a new look at measurement tools. Research outcome measures might be extended to include EMG analysis of patterns of muscular coordination during gait and other activities, posture, endurance, muscle biopsies, quality, and extent of social interaction, self-esteem, perceptual, functional, and cognitive abilities. Because exercise and other intervention effects are typically specific to the type of experience provided,[19,46] we must direct our efforts, as Shepherd and Harris and Shea suggest (Chs. 5 and 6), toward finding successful means for treating the specific problems that children with neurologic dysfunction have (e.g., genu recurvatum during stance phase of gait, lack of scapular muscle cocontraction during reaching into space, and head posture characterized by excessive upper cervical and capital extension). This problem-solving approach to documenting treatment effectiveness focuses on the specific abnormalities of the child with CNS dysfunction. It may free us to consider new treatment adjuncts such as augmented sensory feedback[61–65] and functional electrical stimulation.[34] Lest critics suggest that this would mean a return to technique-oriented approaches to management of children's problems, I hasten to add that this type of treatment planning and clinical research need not preclude consideration of the whole child in the overall plan of management. Indeed, the effects of treatment are likely to be related to numerous factors, such as age at time of injury, site of lesion, severity and type of involvement, intellectual potential, home environment, age at initiation of treatment, and other variables that should be considered in the analysis of outcome, as well as in the planning of a management program.

The challenge for the future of physical therapy is to develop our potential as a scientific, as well as compassionate, clinical field. To do this we need testable theories, quantitative analysis of movement dysfunction, common terminology, creative scholars and clinicians with well-educated minds, and motivation to demonstrate accountability for our methods to clients and the public. I hope that the chapters that follow will be a source of knowledge and a prod to further investigation for all who read them.

REFERENCES

1. Hill A, Volpe JJ: Seizures, hypoxic-ischemic brain injury, and intraventricular hemorrhage in the newborn. Ann Neurol 10:109, 1981
2. Pape K, Wigglesworth JS: Haemorrhage, Ischaemia and the Perinatal Brain. Clinics in Developmental Medicine, No. 69/70. JB Lippincott, Philadelphia, 1979
3. Stewart AL, Reynolds EOR, Hope PL et al: Probability of neurodevelopmental disorders estimated from ultrasound appearance of brains of very preterm infants. Dev Med Child Neurol 29:3, 1987
4. Ment LR, Duncan CC, Ehrenkranz RA: Intraventricular hemorrhage of the preterm neonate. Semin Perinatol 11:132, 1987
5. Ment LR, Duncan CC, Ehrenkranz RA: Perinatal cerebral infarction. Semin Perinatol 11:142, 1987
6. Woods BT, Teuber H-L: Early onset of complementary specialization of cerebral hemispheres in man. Trans Am Neurol Assoc 98:113, 1973
7. Evrard P, de Saint-Georges P, Kadhim HJ et al: Pathology of prenatal encephalopathies. p. 153. In French JH, Harel S, Casaer P (eds): Child Neurology and Developmental Disabilities. Paul H Brookes, Baltimore, 1989
8. Richman DP, Stewart RM, Hutchinson JW et al: Mechanical model of brain convolutional development. Science 189:18, 1975
9. Stewart WB: Blood flow and metabolism in the developing brain. Semin Perinatol 11:112, 1987
10. Wladimiroff JWA, van Bel F: Fetal and neonatal cerebral blood flow. Semin Perinatol 11:335, 1987

11. Johnston MV: Symposium on Frontiers of Research in Developmental Disabilities. 44th Annual Meeting of the American Academy for Cerebral Palsy and Developmental Medicine, Orlando, FL, October 4, 1990
12. Goldman-Rakic PS: Morphological consequences of prenatal injury to the primate brain. Prog Brain Res 53:3, 1980
13. Buser P: Higher functions of the nervous system. Annu Rev Physiol 38:217, 1976
14. Galaburda AM, LeMay M, Kemper TL et al: Right-left asymmetries in the brain. Science 199:852, 1978
15. Spielholz NI: Skeletal muscle: a review of its development in vivo and in vitro. Phys Ther 62:1757, 1982
16. Slaton D: Muscle fiber types and their development in the human fetus. Phys Occup Ther Pediatr 1:47, 1981
17. Kelly AM, Rubinstein NA: Why are fetal muscles slow? Nature 288:266, 1980
18. English AWM, Wolf SL: The motor unit: anatomy and physiology. Phys Ther 62:1763, 1982
19. Rose SJ, Rothstein JM: Muscle mutability: part I. General concepts and adaptations to altered patterns of use. Phys Ther 62:1773, 1982
20. Castle ME, Reyman TA, Schneider M: Pathology of spastic muscle in cerebral palsy. Clin Orthop 142:223, 1979
21. Perry J: Rehabilitation of spasticity. p. 87. In Feldman RG, Young RR, Koella WP (eds): Spasticity: Disordered Motor Control. Year Book Medical Publishers, Chicago, 1980
22. Berger W, Quintern J, Dietz V: Pathophysiology of gait in children with cerebral palsy. Electroencephalogr Clin Neurophysiol 53:538, 1982
23. Tardieu C, Huet de la Tour E, Bret MD et al: Muscle hypoextensibility in children with cerebral palsy, parts I and II. Arch Phys Med Rehabil 63:97, 1982
24. Tardieu G, Tardieu C: Cerebral palsy—mechanical evaluation and conservative correction of limb joint contractures. Clin Orthop Rel Res 219:63, 1987
25. Tardieu C, Lespargot A, Tabary C et al: For how long must the soleus muscle be stretched each day to prevent contracture? Devel Med Child Neurol 30:3, 1988
26. Campbell SK, Anderson J, Gardner HG: Physicians' beliefs in the efficacy of physical therapy in the management of cerebral palsy. Pediatr Phys Ther 2(3):169, 1990
27. Gossman MR, Sahrmann SA, Rose SJ: Review of length-associated changes in muscle: experimental evidence and clinical implications. Phys Ther 62:1799, 1982
28. Olney SJ: New Developments in the Biomechanics of Gait in Children With Cerebral Palsy. Topics in Pediatrics Lesson 1. American Physical Therapy Association, Alexandria, VA, 1989
29. Horvat M: Progressive resistance training program on an individual with spastic cerebral palsy. Am Corrective Ther J 41:7, 1987
30. Chong KC, Vojnic CD, Quanbury AO et al: The assessment of the internal rotation gait in cerebral palsy—an electromyographic gait analysis. Clin Orthop 132:145, 1978
31. Perry J, Hoffer MM: Preoperative and postoperative dynamic electromyography as an aid in planning tendon transfers in children with cerebral palsy. J Bone Joint Surg 59A:531, 1977
32. Perry J, Hoffer MM, Antonelli D et al: Electromyography before and after surgery for hip deformity in children with cerebral palsy: a comparison of clinical and electromyographic findings. J Bone Joint Surg 58A:201, 1976
33. Perry J, Hoffer MM, Giovan P et al: Gait analysis of the triceps surae in cerebral palsy. A preoperative and postoperative clinical and electromyographic study. J Bone Joint Surg 56A:511, 1974

34. Knutsson E: Restraint of spastic muscles in different types of movement. p. 123. In Feldman RG. Young RR, Koella WP (eds): Spasticity: Disordered Motor Control. Year Book Medical Publishers, Chicago, 1980
35. Milner-Brown HS, Penn RD: Pathophysiological mechanisms in cerebral palsy. J Neurol Neurosurg Psychiatr 42:606, 1979
36. Neilson PD: Voluntary control of arm movement in athetotic patients. J Neurol Neurosurg Psychiatr 37:162, 1974
37. Nashner LM, Shumway-Cook A, Marin O: Stance posture control in select groups of children with cerebral palsy: deficits in sensory organization and muscular coordination. Exp Brain Res 49:393, 1983
38. Barolat-Romana G, David R: Neurophysiological mechanisms in abnormal reflex activities in cerebral palsy and spinal spasticity. J Neurol Neurosurg Psychiatr 42:333, 1980
39. Lance JW: The control of muscle tone, reflexes and movement: Robert Wartenberg lecture. Neurology 30:1303, 1980
40. Lance JW: Symposium synopsis. p. 485. In Feldman RG, Young RR, Koella WP (eds): Spasticity: Disordered Motor Control. Year Book Medical Publishers, Chicago, 1980
41. Hattab JR: Review of European clinical trials with baclofen. p. 71. In Feldman RG, Young RR, Koella WP (eds): Spasticity: Disordered Motor Control. Year Book Medical Publishers, Chicago, 1980
42. Campbell SK (guest ed): Proceedings of the consensus conference on the efficacy of physical therapy in the management of movement dysfunction in cerebral palsy. Pediatr Phys Ther 2(3): 1990
43. Rose J, Medeiros JM, Parker R: Energy cost index as an estimate of energy expenditure of cerebral-palsied children during assisted ambulation. Dev Med Child Neurol 27:485, 1985
44. Lundberg A: Longitudinal study of physical working capacity of young people with spastic cerebral palsy. Dev Med Child Neurol 26:328, 1984
45. Ottenbacher KJ, Biocca Z, DeCremer G et al: Quantitative analysis of the effectiveness of pediatric therapy: emphasis on the neurodevelopmental treatment approach. Phys Ther 66:1095, 1986
46. Herdman SJ: Effect of experience on recovery following CNS lesions. Phys Ther 63:51, 1983
47. Johnson D, Almli CR: Age, brain damage, and performance. p. 115. In Finger S (ed): Recovery From Brain Damage: Research and Theory. Plenum, New York, 1978
48. St James-Roberts I: Neurological plasticity, recovery from brain insult, and child development. Adv Child Dev Behav 14:253, 1979
49. Myklebust BM, Gottlieb GL, Penn RD et al: Reciprocal excitation of antagonistic muscles as a differentiating feature in spasticity. Ann Neurol 12:367, 1982
50. Prechtl HFR: Regressions and transformations during neurological development. p. 103. In Bever TG (ed): Regressions in Mental Development: Basic Phenomena and Theories. Lawrence Erlbaum Associates, Hillsdale, NJ, 1982
51. Broom DM: Behavioural plasticity in developing animals. p. 361. In Garrod DR, Feldman JD (eds): Development in the Nervous System. Cambridge University Press, New York, 1981
52. Nashner LM: Analysis of stance posture in humans. p. 527. In Towe AL, Luschei ES (eds): Handbook of Behavioral Neurobiology. Vol. 5: Motor Coordination. Plenum, New York, 1981

53. Laurence S, Stein DG: Recovery after brain damage and the concept of localization of function. p. 369. In Finger S (ed): Recovery From Brain Damage: Research and Theory. Plenum, New York, 1978
54. Goldman PS: An alternative to developmental plasticity: heterology of CNS structures in infants and adults. p. 149. In Stein DG, Rosen JJ, Butters N (eds): Plasticity and Recovery of Function in the Central Nervous System. Academic Press, San Diego, 1974
55. Marx JL: Regeneration in the central nervous system (Research News). Science 209:378, 1980
56. LeVere ND, LeVere TE: Recovery of function after brain damage: support for the compensation theory of the behavioral deficit. Physiol Psychol 10:165, 1982
57. Lister MJ (ed): Contemporary Concepts in Management of Motor Control Problems. Williams & Wilkins, Baltimore (in press)
58. Harrison A: Spastic cerebral palsy: possible spinal interneuronal contributions. Dev Med Child Neurol 30:769, 1988
59. Corcos DM: Strategies underlying the control of disordered movement. Phys Ther 71:36, 1991
60. Cioffi M, Gaebler-Spira DJ: Selective Posterior Rhizotomy and the Child With Cerebral Palsy. Topics in Pediatrics Lesson 10. American Physical Therapy Association, Alexandria, VA, 1990
61. Flodmark A: Augmented sensory feedback as an aid in gait training of the cerebral-palsied child. Dev Med Child Neurol 28:147, 1986
62. Laskas CA, Mullen SL, Nelson DL et al: Enhancement of two motor functions of the lower extremity in a child with spastic quadriplegia. Phys Ther 65:11, 1985
63. Neilson PD, McGaughey J: Self-regulation of spasm and spasticity in cerebral palsy. J Neurol Neurosurg Psychiatry 45:320, 1982
64. Seeger BR, Caudrey DJ: Biofeedback therapy to achieve symmetrical gait in children with hemiplegic cerebral palsy: long-term efficacy. Arch Phys Med Rehabil 64:160, 1983
65. Skrotzky K, Gallenstein JS, Osternig LR: Effects of electromyographic feedback training on motor control in spastic cerebral palsy. Phys Ther 58:547, 1978
66. World Health Organization: International Classification of Impairment, Disability, and Handicap. World Health Organization, Geneva, Switzerland, 1980

2 | Foundations for Therapeutic Intervention*

Linda Fetters

Physical therapy is guided by both implicit and explicit assumptions regarding child development. These assumptions, usually derived from models of development, affect our recommendations for young children. This chapter explores assumptions and conceptual models used in therapy, such as nonlinear models of development, ecologically valid environments for therapy, and the role of reflexive development in motor abilities. The chapter is intended to challenge and expand the conceptual knowledge necessary for therapeutic intervention.

MODELS OF DEVELOPMENT

Development as a Nonlinear Process

One assumption typically made about development is that it is linear or continuous, with each successive step depending on the previous one. The logical extension of this assumption is that events at an early point in development have consequences for later development. An example of this is the expectation that the infant who has sustained an insult at birth or in the early

---

* Portions of this chapter are from Topics in Pediatrics, In Touch Professional Development Series. Lesson 7, pp. 1–12. American Physical Therapy Association, Alexandria, VA, 1990, with permission.

prenatal period is likely to have developmental problems later in life. Although this is an intuitively appealing notion about development, it is not always an accurate one. The past two decades of research with high-risk infants provides more complex assumptions about development. For instance, the single best predictor of cognitive development is not the presence of a birth insult; rather, it remains the socioeconomic status of the infant's family.[1] While an insult at or before birth *may* have developmental consequences for an infant, it is also possible that the consequences may be minimal or nonexistent.

This tendency for *self-righting* is independent of intervention programs as therapists conceive of them. This does not mean that early intervention is not necessary or does not facilitate self-righting; it indicates only that the human organism tends toward adaptation and self-correction. The self-righting ability must be recognized and facilitated as we attempt to understand how and why it occurs. One important task for therapists is to work toward understanding when, for what purpose, and for whom intervention is essential. This understanding may require observation over time *without* specific intervention in order to understand the self-righting abilities of the family unit. For example, an infant may have suffered neonatal hypoxia. Developmental assessment at 3 months of age suggests delayed motor and affective development. Is it prudent or premature to suggest early intervention at this point? Assuming a self-righting tendency, early intervention would be premature. Family support, anticipatory guidance, and a scheduled reassessment in 2 months would be a prudent approach to focusing on family needs at this time. Suggestions can be given to the family, but more formal referral would wait for more definitive evaluation. The approach of frequent assessment gives families support, but does not prejudge the developmental outcome of the child.

Nonlinear models of child development characterize development as a dynamic process in which prediction is multifaceted and perhaps possible only within limited time spans. One of the most popular models of development resulting from the study of the high-risk infant is the *transactional* model,[1,2] a type of interactional model (distinguished from a simple interactional model discussed below) in which the participants, perhaps infant and parent, change as they develop. The important concept in this process is the development of the dyad, (that is, the infant as well as the parent). One feature of the transactional model is that both (or all) members of the interaction(s) change as a result of the interaction and the context in which it has occurred. This is different from thinking only of the infant as developing or changing. It means that all members of the interaction come to future interactions somewhat modified by the previous event.

A familiar clinical example is the spastic infant who is initially picked up by a parent. The infant's body may stiffen and thus communicate that physical contact is not desirable. The parent may experience this as rejection and may perhaps be less willing to embrace the infant again soon, or the physical act of picking up the infant may be altered in some way. The point is that the experience has altered the participants. These changed participants then experience future events and continue to change each other. The interaction may decrease the frequency of future physical interactions or modify them in ways that are not optimal for the infant or parent.

Contrasting the transactional model to the simpler interactional model may help to clarify how these two models differ. In a simple interactional model, the participants are viewed as remaining more constant. These constancies are brought to each varying interaction or situation, but the participant characteristics are seen as having stability over time. In a transactional model, the participants are viewed as flexible or changing as a result of each other and the context in which they interact. Although this may seem a bit of a word game, it means that we are constantly changing as a result of our experiences, rather than bringing the same abilities to each new situation. Change in participants as a result of experience fits with the nonlinear model of development and indicates that we cannot easily predict the future developmental course of an infant based on events at only one point in time. This nonlinear concept requires therapists to continually assess the abilities of children and their families. In addition, therapists change as a result of interactions and experiences. Families shape therapists in important and often unpredictable ways. The transactional model of development offers a fluid and changing picture in which prediction, if possible at all, is complex.

The transactional model is ideal for developing family focused intervention. Public Law 99-457 requires that families be included in developing the therapeutic plan for meeting their needs. The transactional model suggests that child change is not realistic *unless* the intervention is family focused.

Interaction as a Requirement for Normal Development

Interaction with the environment is essential for normal development, although the exact mechanisms for growth and development through environment–organism interaction are not at all clear. One interesting process, termed *experience-expectant* by Greenough and colleagues, suggests that the developing organism "expects" particular environmental events to occur at points within development.[3] These "expectations" are species-specific in that all members of a species would be genetically organized to take advantage of certain environmental stimuli that would normally be available to that species in order to produce certain abilities. This process enables the organism to develop advanced performance capabilities and uniqueness within the species.

The mechanism proposed for this experience-expectant process is the overproduction of synaptic connections within the nervous system.[3] Experiencing functional use allows only certain synapses to survive; the normal loss of synapses characterizes development shaped by experience. Consequently, experience that has both generic and individual components determines the final neuronal pattern for certain developmental competencies.

Development as a U-Shaped Function

Another nonlinear model or function (from the mathematic idea of a function) is referred to as the U-shaped function.[4] The U can be either right-side-up or inverted. When placed in the context of time, this type of function describes abilities that come and go as a natural part of the developmental process. Although the following examples are controversial in interpretation, they illustrate the meaning of the function.

Evidence exists that the newborn can direct arm movements toward a fixated target.[5-7] Although this movement is not functional in the way it will be at a later point in development, its presence provides evidence that the visual and motor systems have an initial linkage for performance. After the first 4 to 6 weeks of life, this "prereaching," as it has been described, is difficult to elicit and it seems to disappear. Sometime after the third or fourth month of age, infants begin to develop functional reach and grasp behaviors. This development initially has the characteristics of the newborn prereaching in that the arm is directed toward a fixated target but cannot yet grasp the target. Only as the infant matures is functional grasping evident. Thus, a newborn ability disappears and then reappears in a more mature and functional pattern.

Another example of this type of "disappearing-reappearing" function is automatic stepping and its relationship to later infant walking. Although the relationship of automatic walking (newborn stepping) to later walking is not completely clear, it has been hypothesized that newborn walking is a precursor to independent walking.[8] It usually is impossible to elicit newborn stepping past the first month of life, until stepping movements emerge again after 8 or 9 months of age. One hypothesis used to explain this seeming disappearance of newborn stepping is that the spinal circuitry involved in newborn stepping comes under control from higher centers within the central nervous system.[9] During this process, the spinal pattern may not be elicited. Thus, a seemingly regressive period (the disappearance of stepping) may herald the developmental period during which later walking abilities are organized. If stepping behavior was recorded during the first year of life, the graphed record may resemble a U-shaped function. The change in function has been attributed to neurologic maturation.

Thelen has an alternative hypothesis for the evolution of newborn stepping.[10] Although this response clearly cannot be elicited in the upright position in infants after approximately the first month of age, Thelen suggests that kicking in supine is isomorphic to the newborn stepping pattern. Thus, the reason for the disappearing behavior is the increased biomechanical demands put on the infant in the upright position. Thelen argues that the rapid increase in mass of the legs during the first months of life is primarily made up of fat, not muscle. When the infant attempts to lift this heavy mass in the upright position, the task is too difficult for a time, and stepping movements cease. Stepping ability is regained as the infant matures both neurologically and in terms of muscle mass and strength. Growth during the first few years of life is rapid; however, the effects of rapid physical growth on motor development have not been fully considered or evaluated.[11]

The apparent U-shaped function that characterizes newborn stepping may be explained with both neurologic and biomechanical factors. Neurologic approaches to intervention often invoke purely neurologic explanations for early developmental change, ignoring biomechanical explanations that could augment understanding of developmental processes. Another example is the rationale for the successful use of inhibitive casting to decrease spasticity. The increased range of motion following the use of casting is often explained by the inhibition of muscle tone. An alternative explanation is the documented increase in length of muscle following prolonged stretch in a lengthened position.[12,13] Sarcomeres are added and lost in response to maintained elongation or shortening of the muscle, respectively.

Models of development shape strategies for therapeutic intervention. Our expectations concerning development are translated into clinical practice through our recommendations. Our concept of the environmental influences on motor development also shapes therapy. Ecologic psychology is one approach to an understanding of the relationship between the developing organism and the environment. This approach is described in the next section.

AFFORDANCE

The term *affordance*, created by the psychologist J. J. Gibson,[14] names a concept that links humans to their environment. It may seem an obvious link, that of person and place, but in psychology it has been a unique way of conceptualizing human action. The behaviorist notion of a passive human organism being stimulated by the environment has given way to the concept that human action is a function of environmental affordances. Instead of the dichotomy of the actor and the environment for action, the concept of affordance suggests that the two are linked. Separation of the two is artificial just as the dichotomy of sensory and motor systems may be artificial.[15] Gibson[16] defines affordance as follows:

> The affordances of the environment are what it offers the animal, what it provides or furnishes, either for good or ill. The verb to afford is found in the dictionary, but the noun affordance is not. I have made it up. I mean by it something that refers to both the environment and the animal in a way that no existing term does. It implies the complementarity of the animal and the environment.

The concept of affordance fits into the larger approach to psychology referred to as the *ecological approach*.[16,17] Although these may be new terms, clinicians already acknowledge and utilize these concepts therapeutically.

The original work in ecological psychology and the concept of affordance have been applied to development by Eleanor Gibson, a developmental psychologist.[17] She suggests that infants spend the first year of life exploring and defining the affordances in their world; that is, infants reveal the properties of objects and the environment and the relationship between themselves and the physical world. They discover how they can act on the world and the consequences of those actions. These may sound like ideas similar to those of Piaget, Bruner, or other developmentalists, but there is uniqueness in the ecological approach.[18,19] The uniqueness is in the view that the environment elicits action from the infant. The infant is constrained to act in ways that are precipitated by the environment. The Greenough et al. concept of an experience-expectant process is similar in that the organism has a genetic endowment that is then further elaborated through environmental interaction. The infant is organized *for* specific affordances in the world. For example, there is evidence that the newborn has depth perception, suggesting that the visual system is organized at birth to perceive a three-dimensional (3-D) world, and will take advantage of the 3-D world it is exposed to after birth. This 3-D world is not constructed with experience.[20–22] In this way, the infant and environment are attuned to each other from the start.

A classic example of an affordance in the animal world is that of the pecking behavior of the herring gull. Gulls are born organized to peck at a red spot. This may seem like a splinter skill, except that adult gulls have a red spot on their bills. A peck from "Junior" is a signal for the adult gull to open its bill and offer the food content of the bill to the offspring. The affordance in the gull world is the organization between the baby gull's inborn ability to peck at red spots and the adult's coloring and feeding behavior—a useful fit.

Infants spend the first year in what Gibson refers to as *exploration*, a common and useful term. She describes the infant as an active participant in the world, not as a passive creature who is acted on.[17]

> We don't simply see, we look. The visual system is a motor system as well as a sensory one. When we seek information in the optic array, the head turns, the eyes turn to fixate, the lens accommodates to focus. . . .[17]

The sensory and motor systems converge around the united function of providing the infant with knowledge about the world. Why is this important for physical therapy? Or, perhaps more importantly, haven't we understood this all along? In any case, the concept is important in that an entire approach to psychology acknowledges the environment as critical in eliciting the type of action (e.g., movement) that is adaptive. The environment constrains the action. We exploit this principle each time we put a toy on a chair to encourage a child to kneel or to increase hip extension. As developmental therapists, we have figured out that in order to work with children (who, of course, do not always follow oral instructions), we need to create environments that elicit opportunities for normal, or at least preferred, movement patterns. We know how differently a child may move in the clinic versus the home environment and, as a consequence, we often observe or treat children in their homes. Finnie was instrumental in developing the therapeutic ideas of the Bobaths for use in home and school environments, thus increasing the ecologic validity of the neurodevelopmental treatment approach.[23-25] We construct affordances in the environments of children with disabilities to elicit the type of movement that is functional for exploration. Children often will not continue activities unless these activities allow for exploration and knowledge gathering, two key aspects of the ecological approach.

Knowledge of ecological psychology is important for at least two reasons. First, it provides a theoretic foundation for developmental therapy that has been lacking. Second, it reminds us that movement is always linked to sensation and exploration. If we work toward movement for its own sake, forgetting the context in which it must and will take place, we are not likely to help children become more functional.

The ecological approach to psychology and the concept of affordance complement the previous ideas within a transactional system of development. Both concepts provide a dynamic perspective of the child–environment interaction, with the child viewed as an active participant in a world for which the human organism is uniquely organized.

When disorganization occurs within the child or the environment, both are affected. Thus, the child with sensorimotor problems develops unique and perhaps atypical relationships with the environment. These relationships may still serve the exploratory needs of the child; however, children may use patterns of movement that are atypical or potentially harmful in the long term. Therapists can assist children and families in providing an ecology for movement that supports functional movement while diminishing atypical movement that may hamper function in the long term.

Children will persist in exploring their environment regardless of the type of movement used. An example of this is the use of "W" sitting; that is, sitting with the legs folded back so that the heels touch the buttocks (Fig. 2-1). Therapists who have tried to discourage this type of sitting soon realize what they are up against. The child with poor sitting balance still wants to explore objects and the world. This exploratory behavior is primary, and whatever stable posture is available will be used. W sitting often affords the most stable posture and will be constantly used during exploration. The posture is not the focus for the child, only a means to an end—exploratory ability. For therapists, the sitting position may be the focus. We may want to discourage the hamstring tightness that may be facilitated in this position, but we need to remember the utility of the position for the child. Unless exploratory behavior can continue, any new sitting posture will quickly be abandoned. In Fig. 2-2, for example, the long sitting posture was achieved, but required use of the arms and hands for support. Exploratory behavior with the hands is impossible in this position. Substitution of a new sitting posture must facilitate exploration. Creating a game that requires "ring" sitting may provide the necessary incentive. Knocking over containers of water with the knees from a ring-sitting position may create the necessary enthusiasm to sustain the posture. A remote sensor can be attached to a computer and the sensor hit with the knees to activate a game. These methods may seem elaborate and contrived, but if change is to occur,

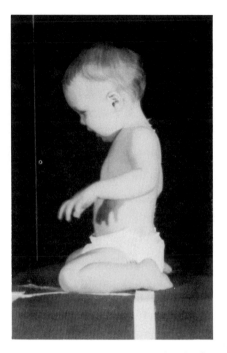

Fig. 2-1.   The W sitting position allows a stable base for the free use of hands and head for exploration. (Courtesy of Suzann K. Campbell.)

the new patterns must incorporate the behaviors that will drive movement, exploration, and knowledge gathering.

A decrease in exploratory behavior has been documented in premature infants, infants with Down syndrome, and children with cerebral palsy.[26–28] Infants in these three diagnostic groups used visual exploration to a greater extent than manipulation. The decreased frequency of exploratory action may suggest an a priori lack of exploratory interest or motivation. The decreased frequency might also be due to difficulty exploring because of atypical sensorimotor abilities. The infant discovers fewer affordances in the environment, perhaps due to the lack of "fit" between infant and the environment. This decrease in discovery behavior may lead to continued lack of motivation and fewer experiences during which the complexities of the world can be sorted out.

The goals of the therapist and family might include increasing the exploratory experiences of the child (something we already do); in addition, we might encourage and practice modeling exploration for children with sensorimotor problems.[28] If a child has difficulty exploring cause and effect relationships because of lack of exploratory interest or an inability to carry out the necessary motor acts to explore, then a cause and effect demonstration might be useful. Dropping a cup of water off the tray for an infant might seem like promoting anarchy, but if the infant cannot perform the act, or never thought to try, why

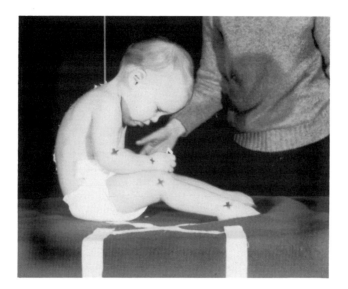

Fig. 2-2.　The same child, now in the long sitting position, does not have free use of the hands and head. (Courtesy of Suzann K. Campbell.)

not spill some water to elicit the effect? Watching family members, particularly siblings, explore materials and relationships between their actions and the world provides much needed exploratory material to infants with sensorimotor impairment. The movement itself and the consequences of the movement are of equal importance—in part for perceptual and cognitive development and also to provide further motivation for movement and exploration of the world.

This concept of fit in the world is important. The human organism comes to the world organized to experience certain of its aspects. If the infant is deficient in some areas of the typical organization, poor motor coordination, for instance, the environment will provide very different affordances to this infant.

I am making the assumption that all humans have what I refer to as *species-specific movement*. That is, movement that is shared by all other humans. For instance, the drive to stand and walk could be described as a species-specific movement. If a child is born with this species-specific movement drive but does not have the coordination of muscles to perform the action normally, what results is movement toward the species-specific goal (i.e., standing), but with atypical movement patterns. The affordances within the environment may elicit the motivation to stand, but the movement result is not accomplishing the goal. In this situation, therapists can rearrange the environment, thus creating affordances that will yield the desired movement. Prior to this or, rather, in conjunction with this, we may need to work with the child on components of movement. We can put a toy on a chair so that the child will pull to stand up, but if the child is too weak, or has decreased range of hip motion, the action may not be possible. What then? We need to work on the component skills and then elicit these components in a functional movement sequence. The component skills, however, will best be elicited by exploiting the characteristics of the environment that encourage movement. For instance, the child with decreased hip extension and poor strength in the hip extensor muscles might work on kicking while prone in the bathtub. It would be fun (it makes a sufficient mess) and stirs up the bubble bath. Encouraging a child to lie prone on a mat and extending the hip might in principle bring about the same goal, but there would be little in that environment to elicit the action naturally. The bath is an ecologically valid stimulus for the desired action, while mat activities are not.

The use of therapeutic balls in treatment offers another example. We often move the ball under the child or with the child to stimulate balance and righting reactions. This is a somewhat artificial mechanism for eliciting these responses. The resulting movement is also a response to an external stimulus, not a pre-planned postural strategy used in a voluntarily generated movement. We might design a more ecologically valid intervention by eliciting these reactions through the child's self-initiated movement rather than by moving the child on the ball. Creating games in which the child must move may cause balance and righting reactions to occur without conscious effort in the context of normally occurring action.

Although we often may need to work on the components of functional movement, we should always exploit the affordances within the environment that will naturally or automatically elicit movement. Parents are the natural resources to develop ecologically valid treatment: they frequently offer creative, practical suggestions, and they can implement these suggestions on a daily basis. Effective treatment must not only include parents; the family–child environment *should* be the vehicle for change.

THE NEED TO RE-EVALUATE REFLEXES

The Case for Reflexes as Adaptive Movements

Development is characterized by change. Understanding the causes of sensorimotor change and the models used to conceptualize change will assist us in planning the most effective therapeutic intervention. The development of primary reflexes is fundamental to the human organism. These reflexes (e.g., automatic stepping, placing, and asymmetric tonic neck reflex [ATNR]) are often viewed as interfering with normal sensorimotor abilities and have become an integral aspect of developmental assessment.

Reflexes have been described as final vestiges of our animal heritage.[29,30] The phrase "ontogeny recapitulating phylogeny" suggests that during normal human development we move through the developmental stages that have characterized animals in our ancestral tree. We finally arrive at that period of time (adulthood) during which our true human characteristics are supposedly manifest. This brief window in our lifespan then gives way to the gradual decline in function from this optimal adult state.

There exists a somewhat different perspective on development, one that suggests that each period in development is unique, important unto itself, has its own unique movement (and many other) patterns, and is not measured in importance by its distance from the optimal state of adulthood. This is an approach described and shaped by many developmentalists. Oppenheim has been one of the most eloquent among them.[15]

> Although there are undoubtedly many important continuities, interactions and antecedent relationships between the behavioral characteristics expressed at different periods of the life cycle beyond infancy, it seems unlikely that the early stages merely represent important preparations for some ultimate adaptations later in life. Rather, I propose as a working hypothesis that even the changes that occur in adulthood, including aging, may represent adaptations for specific periods of life.[15]

The term *adaptation* fits with the notion of affordance in that the organism is fitting into or adapting to the environment at each point in development.

What does this hypothesis have to do with primary reflexes? Viewed in this context, attempts can be made to describe the adaptations necessary during infancy, the period during which primary reflexes are the most necessary. Having described the necessary adaptations, the patterns that occur during this period can be fit to particular adaptations.

One of the important tasks for the human organism is birth. Viewed as one of life's necessary adaptations, birthing requires skills from both mother and baby. The positive support reaction and automatic stepping can be viewed as excellent adaptive movement patterns to complement the maternal birth process.[15] The flexed, cramped baby can "walk" to the head-down position using automatic stepping and then push out through the birth canal with the positive support reaction. Having completed this miraculous life adaptation, the reflexive nature of this movement (if not the behavior altogether) may dissipate.

Another example is the ATNR. This biasing of the limbs based on head position probably never disappears, but limb position certainly becomes less yoked to the position of the head as the infant matures. What is occurring during the months when the ATNR is the most evident (1 to 4 months of age)? The infant's visual system is maturing, while longer periods of time are spent awake. The infant can now spend more time in visual processing, and the hand is now in a position to be seen. That is, when the ATNR is elicited, the viewed arm is extended. This affords the opportunity for the infant not just to see the hand, but to *look* at the hand, to use Gibson's term.[17] Coryell and Michel suggest that this looking·behavior is biased toward the right side and may consequently bias the human toward the right handedness that is characteristic of the older child and adult.[31] The timing of this reflexive ability then coincides (although perhaps not merely coincidentally) with other infant adaptations to afford the infant visual experience with the hand. Once the head and hand can be independently positioned and controlled with finesse, the postural adaptation linking the eyes to the hands is no longer functional or needed.

Primitive Reflexes in Treatment

Reflexes are often assessed in relation to what they indicate about the integrity of the nervous system.[9,29,30] In addition, those that persist past the time of their natural demise are assumed to be interfering in some way with the expression of more mature movement patterns. Viewing primary reflexes as adaptive responses, however, leaves at least two alternative possibilities to the view that these persistent reflexes are necessarily harmful. First, perhaps the adaptive response (primitive reflex) is still useful to the infant. Primary stepping may be too difficult because the legs are too heavy, but the movement pattern may subserve other reciprocal movement patterns, such as kicking and crawling. The ATNR might continue to be useful to achieve arm extension in the presence of flexor hypertonus. Before reflexes are viewed as culprits, we may need to ask what adaptations they may allow.

Second, the lack of expression of more mature movement patterns is most probably due to many difficulties, but not to the presence of primary responses. Causing the inhibition of primary reflexes will not, in all likelihood, facilitate the appearance of mature responses unless concomitant motor learning of more functional behaviors occurs. The assessment of primary reflexive status is most useful in sorting out the question of adaptations. The assessment of patterns of movement both in quantity and quality is the most important task of the developmental therapist. To the end that primary reflexes are adaptive responses, we should evaluate and, perhaps, under some conditions, promote their use. When more mature patterns of movement are absent, we need to create affordances within the environment that precipitate the movement that enables the greatest functional movement.

CONCLUSION

Human development is complex and fascinating. Understanding developmental models and principles will assist us in the task of promoting optimal function for children with atypical development. The human infant–family complex has a natural tendency to self-right—to accomplish the abilities that are common to all humans, including motor abilities. Therapists can work with and facilitate this self-righting ability by promoting movement that is ecologically valid (natural to the human infant) in an appropriate context. This means working with families in their home, school, and community environments. It means moving away from more isolated clinical treatment and moving into the world of the family. Creating and exploiting natural environments for movement provides a challenge for developmental therapists to promote ecologically valid assessment, treatment, and outcome.

REFERENCES

1. Sameroff AJ: Early influences on development: fact or fancy? Merrill Palmer Q 21:267, 1975
2. Sameroff AJ, Chandler MJ: Reproductive risk and the continuum of caretaking

casualty. p. 187. In Horowitz FD, Hetherington M, Scarr-Salapatek S et al (eds): Review of Child Development Research. Vol. 4. University of Chicago Press, Chicago, 1975

3. Greenough WT, Black JE, Wallace CS: Experience and brain development. Child Dev 58:539, 1987
4. Bever TG: Regressions in Mental Development: Basic Phenomena and Theories. Lawrence Erlbaum Associates, Hillsdale, NJ, 1982
5. Bower TGR: Development in Infancy. WH Freeman, San Francisco, 1974
6. von Hofsten C: Eye-hand coordination in newborns. Dev Psychol 18:450, 1982
7. Bergmeier S: Reaching in newborns. Unpublished dissertation, Program in Therapeutic Studies, Sargent College of Allied Health Professions, Boston University, 1989
8. Zelazo PR: The development of walking: new findings and old assumptions. J Motor Behav 15:99, 1983
9. Peiper A: Cerebral Function in Infancy and Childhood. Consultants Bureau, New York, 1963
10. Thelen E: Learning to walk: ecological demands and phylogenetic constraints. p. 213. In Lipsitt LP, Rovee-Collier C (eds): Advances in Infancy Research, Vol. 3. Ablex, Norwood, NJ, 1984
11. Campbell SK, Wilhelm IJ, Slaton DS: Anthropometric characteristics of young children with cerebral palsy. Pediatric Phys Ther 1:105, 1989
12. Rose SJ, Rothstein JM: Muscle mutability. Part 1. General concepts and adaptations to altered patterns of use. Phys Ther 62:1773, 1982
13. Gossman MR, Sahrmann SA, Rose SJ: Review of length-associated changes in muscle. Phys Ther 62:1799, 1982
14. Gibson JJ: The Ecological Approach to Visual Perception. Houghton Mifflin, Boston, 1979
15. Oppenheim RW: Ontogenetic adaptations and retrogressive processes in the development of the nervous system and behavior: a neuroembryological perspective. p. 73. In Connolly K, Prechtl HFR (eds): Maturation and Development: Biological and Psychological Perspectives. JB Lippincott, Philadelphia, 1981
16. Gibson JJ: The Senses Considered as Perceptual Systems. Houghton Mifflin, Boston, 1966
17. Gibson EJ: Exploratory behavior in the development of perceiving, acting, and the acquiring of knowledge. Annu Rev Psychol 39:1, 1988
18. Piaget J: The Origins of Intelligence. International University Press, New York, 1952
19. Bruner J: Organization of early skilled action. Child Dev 44:1, 1973
20. Bower TGR: Object perception in infants. Perception 1:15, 1972
21. Bower TGR, Broughton J, Moore MK: Infant responses to approaching objects: an indicator of response to distal variables. Percept Psychophys 9:193, 1971
22. Dodwell PC, Muire D, DiFranco D: Infant perception of visually presented objects. Science 203:1138, 1979
23. Finnie N: Handling the Young Cerebral Palsied Child at Home. EP Dutton, New York, 1970
24. Bobath K: A neurophysiological Basis for the Treatment of Cerebral Palsy. JB Lippincott, Philadelphia, 1980
25. Bobath K, Bobath B: Cerebral palsy. p. 162. In Pearson P, Williams C (eds): Physical Therapy Services in the Developmental Disabilities. Charles C Thomas, Springfield, IL, 1972

26. Ruff HA, McCarton C, Kurtzberg D et al: Preterm infants' manipulative exploration of objects. Child Dev 55:1166, 1984
27. MacTurk RH, Vietze PM, McCarthy ME et al: The organization of exploratory behavior in Down syndrome and nondelayed infants. Child Dev 56:573, 1985
28. Fetters L: Object permanence development in children with cerebral palsy. Phys Ther 61:327, 1981
29. McGraw MB: The Neuromuscular Maturation of the Human Infant. Hafner, New York, 1960
30. Easton TA: On the normal use of reflexes. Am Scientist 60:591, 1972
31. Coryell J, Michel G: How supine postural preferences can contribute toward the development of handedness. Infant Behav Dev 1:245, 1978

3 | Assessing Motor Development in Children

Thomas J. Stengel

The evaluation of a child with a neurologic disorder is a multidimensional process involving assessment of various aspects of development. Physical, communication, cognitive, and psychosocial development and self-help skills may be assessed individually and in relationship to each other, in an attempt to obtain a comprehensive and yet understandable profile of a child's strengths and weaknesses.

Subareas of the aspects of development mentioned above may vary in organization and content according to the experience, interest, and educational background of an individual tester or the orientation of an individual service agency. Subareas of physical development may include gross and fine motor performance, reflexes, range of motion (ROM), muscle tone, quality of movement, muscle strength, posture, and the processing and organization of sensory information. Subareas of communication include expressive language, receptive language, and nonverbal communication. Psychosocial subareas may include behavior, temperament, caregiver–child interaction and attachment, and peer interactions. Cognitive subareas are attention, problem solving, and responses to eliciting situations similar to those described initially by Piaget[1] involving assessment of concepts such as imitation, operational causality, object permanence, and object relations. Self-help skills may include feeding, dressing, and bathing.

It is essential to mention other areas that require assessment for comprehensive program planning for the child with neurologic dysfunction, for example, cardiopulmonary status, medical and developmental history, family structure, home environment, and adaptive equipment.

33

Because of space limitations, however, this chapter is limited primarily to a discussion of motor evaluation of children, although one test is considered a functional assessment measure. Included in the discussion are evaluation and assessment principles, including the role of parents, test selection, specific testing instruments, and clinical applicability.

PRINCIPLES OF EVALUATION AND ASSESSMENT

In the regulations for Public Law 99-457 (PL99-457),[2] the terms *evaluation* and *assessment* are differentiated. Evaluation is defined as the "procedures used by appropriate qualified personnel to determine a child's initial and continuing eligibility" under Part H (p. 26320). Assessment is defined as "the ongoing procedures used by appropriate personnel throughout the period of a child's eligibility under this part to identify—

(i) The child's unique needs;
(ii) The family's strengths and needs related to development of the child; and
(iii) The nature and extent of early intervention services that are needed by the child and the child's family" to meet the needs in (i) and (ii) (p. 26320).

For the purpose of discussion in this chapter, the terms *evaluation* and *assessment* will be used interchangeably.

Meisels and colleagues[3] discuss three principal types of assessment activities. The first is developmental screening, which identifies those children who have a high probability of exhibiting delayed or abnormal development. Second, developmental assessment instruments are used to determine whether a child has special needs, to ascertain the nature and character of a child's problems, and to propose possible remediation strategies. These instruments should be used in the context of a multidisciplinary team effort. The assessment team should involve parents as a source of assessment data and as a potential focus of intervention. Third, assessment for individual program planning occurs after the assessment team, including the parents, decides that a child needs early intervention. Program planning assessments are generally criterion referenced and focus on how well a child masters specific skills or tasks. The latter instruments are useful for program evaluation and planning. In summary, screening sorts out those children who, as a next step, require diagnostic assessment, while assessment determines if the decision to go to a next step is correct. Table 3-1 further clarifies the three types of assessment activities.

The characteristics of the screening and assessment process are parental participation, clinical interviewing, and formal and informal observation. Meisels and colleagues[3] suggest that the screening and assessment process should be done in both formal and informal settings.

The family-focused emphasis of PL 99-457 mandates that parental participation be central to the screening and assessment process. This law challenges

Table 3-1. Varieties of Assessment Activities

	Purpose	Personnel	Activities
Screening	To identify children who may need further diagnostic assessment	Professionals, parents, and lay professionals	Administration of screening instruments, medical examinations, hearing and vision testing, parent questionnaires, and review of records
Diagnostic assessment	To determine existence of delay or disability, to identify child and family strengths and needs, and to propose possible strategies for intervention	Multidisciplinary team of educators, psychologists, parents, clinicians, physicians, social workers, therapists, and nurses	Formal testing, parent interview, home observation, and team meetings
Individual program planning	To determine individual educational plan, program placement, and instructional activities	Parents, teachers, assessment team personnel, and other professionals	Home and/or program observation, informal assessment, and development of instructional objectives

professionals to examine the manner in which assessments are conducted so that parental collaboration is facilitated. The technical assistance team suggests that clinicians need to address the questions outlined in Table 3-2.

Meisels and colleagues[3] also address the subject of parental reporting. Reports should focus on functional abilities of the child and not test scores. According to this task force,[3] the information provided to parents should include "the conditions under which the child was assessed, the child's responsiveness, the family's judgement about whether the child's performance was optimal, measures that are used (including scores if appropriate), examiner's interpretation of what the scores mean, and the rationale for that inter-

Table 3-2. Questions Concerning Parent Involvement in Assessments

What is the purpose of the assessment and what outcomes are to be achieved?

Will the assessment address the questions and concerns of the parents?

Are the parents involved in determining the nature of the assessment process and the extent of their participation?

Will the assessment consider the child's developmental and adaptive functioning within the context of the family unit and parent–child interaction?

Does the climate of the assessment process encourage optimal comfort and sharing by family members and by professionals?

Are assessment findings presented in a jargon-free, integrated manner that promotes understanding and that emphasizes the child's strengths as well as vulnerabilities?

Are the parents involved in developing the IFSP/IEP and in determining the future course of action?

Abbreviations: IFSP, Individual family service plan; IEP, Individual educational plan.
(From Meisels et al,[3] with permission.)

Table 3-3. Guidelines for Screening and Assessment

Screening and assessment should be viewed as services—as part of the intervention process—and not only as means of identification and measurement.

Processes, procedures, and instruments intended for screening and assessment should only be used for their specified purposes.

Multiple sources of information should be included in screening and assessment.

Developmental screening should take place on a recurrent or periodic basis. It is inappropriate to screen young children only once during their early years. Similarly, provisions should be made for reevaluation or reassessment after services have been initiated.

Developmental screening should be viewed as only one path to more in-depth assessment. Failure to qualify for services based on a single source of screening information should not become a barrier to further evaluation for intervention services if other risk factors (e.g., environmental, medical, familial) are present.

Screening and assessment procedures should be reliable and valid.

Family members should be an integral part of the screening and assessment process. Information provided by family members is critically important for determining whether to initiate more in-depth assessment and for designing appropriate intervention strategies. Parents must be accorded complete informed consent at all stages of the screening and assessment process.

When screening or assessing developmental problems, the more relevant and familiar the tasks and setting are to the child and the child's family, the more likely it is that the results will be valid.

All tests, procedures, and processes intended for screening or assessment must be culturally sensitive.

Extensive and comprehensive training is needed by those who screen and assess very young children.

(From Meisels et al,[3] with permission.)

pretation.'' The use of professional jargon, identification of assessment participants, dissemination of reports and confidentiality, and the right of parental access also need to be considered.

The guidelines[3] for the process of screening and assessment are outlined in Table 3-3. Even though screening and assessment are different processes, the guidelines apply to both.

Meisels and colleagues[3] arrived at three conclusions. First, to identify children in need of early intervention as early as possible, data need to be obtained on a periodic basis from multiple sources, including the child's family. Second, caregiving and environmental variables should be considered along with a child's biologic status during the screening and assessment process. Finally, quantitative measurements of child development should always be used in combination with other sources of data from the caregiving and environmental domains.

Regarding future direction, the technical assistance team recommends 10 tasks that need to be addressed and explored by clinicians, researchers, and policy makers. These tasks are presented in Table 3-4.

TEST SELECTION AND REVIEW

The purposes of this section are to provide the reader with a format for evaluating developmental tests, to review the structure and uses of various testing instruments, to critically review selected instruments, and to propose

Table 3-4. Future Policy Directions for Screening and Assessment

Expand the concept of screening and assessment to include prevention efforts rather than primarily remediation programs.
Create decision-making models that assist in determining the eligibility of children and families for service.
Refine existing infancy and early childhood developmental screening measures and develop new measures that are valid and reliable.
Systematically incorporate clinical interviewing skills into the screening and assessment process.
Analyze the meaning and implications of parent–child interaction measures.
Develop additional measures of family functioning.
Focus on measures for screening the environment that are multicultural and that are appropriate for various social and economic groups.
Restandardize assessment to include disabled children in the normative sample.
Develop more systematic and effective training programs.
Collect longitudinal data that will help to devise more accurate risk indices that can be used for prevention and intervention.

(From Meisels et al,[3] with permission.)

a clinical application for some of the tests. The tests reviewed measure motor development; however, some, such as the Bayley Scales of Infant Development, also measure other areas of development. Some tests, such as the Neonatal Behavioral Assessment Scale, can be used only during the newborn period while others can be used for a considerably larger age span (e.g., the Gesell Developmental Schedules [1 month to 72 months of age]).

Specific developmental tests were chosen for discussion for several reasons. I have used some of the tests for clinical and research purposes and consider them to be useful and reliable measurement tools. Some of the tests are potentially useful for clinicians as intervention tools. The more popular tests are discussed, excluding tests that have a similar conceptual and structural framework. Finally, some tests were included because they seem appropriate for a specific clinical setting. Primary sources of information other than the specific test manuals are *The Eighth Mental Measurements Yearbook,*[4] *Psychological Abstracts*, periodicals such as *Physical and Occupational Therapy in Pediatrics*, and books such as *Screening Growth and Development: A Guide for Test Selection,*[5] *Handbook of Infant Development,*[6] and *Linking Developmental Assessment and Curricula: Prescriptions for Early Intervention.*[7]

Test Criteria

The need for clinicians to become more informed about developmental testing was highlighted by Lewko[8] in a survey assessing current practices in evaluating motor behavior in a sample of 207 facilities providing services to children in the United States and Canada. The 207 respondents, of whom 59 were physical therapists, identified 256 different motor evaluations being used[8]; 91 of these tests were published and 165 were not published. Furthermore, the data indicated that the motor functioning of a great number of children was not being evaluated, particularly in larger facilities. Only four of the 91 published tests were used with any consistency: the Denver Developmental Screening Test,[9] Gesell Developmental Schedules,[10] the Lincoln-Oseretsky Motor Development Scale,[11] and the Purdue Perceptual-Motor Survey.[12] The respondents generally indicated they misused the tests in some fashion. Based on these findings, Lewko[8] recommended that a single reference source including a large number of published tests of motor development should be made available to guide practitioners in the selection of appropriate tests.

Stangler and colleagues[5] partially fulfilled Lewko's recommendation in a book on selection of screening tools. These authors proposed six criteria for evaluating a screening tool: acceptability, simplicity, cost, appropriateness, reliability, and validity.

Acceptability is defined as acceptance by all who will be affected by screening, including the children and families screened, the professionals who receive resulting referrals, and the community as a whole.[5] Screening test simplicity is determined by the ease of teaching, learning, and administering the tool.[5] The cost of a screening test includes the cost of equipment, training and paying personnel, and inaccurate test results. Also included are the costs to the individual being screened (for example, charges and transportation) and the total screening test cost in relation to the benefits of early detection.[5] Test appropriateness is based on the prevalence of developmental delay in the population to be screened and on the application of the test to the population under consideration.[5]

Reliability is the ability of a test to yield consistent results when the same test is given to the same individual more than once.[13] The two types of reliability are stability over time (test–retest reliability) and observer consistency (interobserver reliability).[14] Acceptable reliability is usually indicated by a correlation coefficient above 0.80 or a percentage of agreement above 90 percent.[15]

Test–retest reliability is measured when the same test is given to the same child twice with some interval of time between the two administrations.[5] When this measure, expressed as a correlation coefficient or as percent agreement, is high, it is likely that a test is reflecting the actual abilities of a child. Distractions in the environment that may cause children to perform differently at each test administration are inconsistent methods of test administration, the child's state of health, and the time of day when the tests are administered.

Observer consistency or interobserver reliability is defined as the amount of agreement between two persons interpreting the same test performance.[14] This reliability coefficient is obtained by having two people independently observe and score the behavior of the same individual or by having two people reading and interpreting the same set of test results.[5] When interobserver reliability is high, the behavior under consideration is relatively easily observed and scored in the same way by more than one person.

The final criterion, the validity of a developmental test, is defined as its ability to separate persons with a developmental problem from those without a problem.[13] Validity is concerned with what a test measures and how well it measures it.[15] Validity is determined by comparing performance on one instrument with other independent observations of the same characteristic.[14]

Important validity aspects for screening tests are percent of agreement with a diagnostic measure; sensitivity, specificity, and overreferral and underreferral rates; and predictive validity of positive and negative findings.[5] These aspects of test validity pertain to how well a screening test in question relates to a diagnostic measure. Screening test validity may be expressed as a correlation coefficient between screening test results and the results of corresponding diagnostic tests. The higher the validity, the more efficient the screening test. Instrument *sensitivity* is defined as how well the instrument identifies abnormal cases as being abnormal.[16] Instrument *specificity* is defined as how well an instrument identifies normal cases.

In nonscreening tests, four types of validity should be considered.[16] These are predictive validity, concurrent validity, content validity, and construct validity. Predictive validity, expressed as a validity coefficient, indicates the extent to which an individual's future level of functioning or performance on a criterion variable, for example, intellect at age 15, can be predicted from knowledge of a developmental test administered to a preschool child. Concurrent validity, also expressed as a validity coefficient, represents the relationship between a test (e.g., the Neurological Examination of the Full Term Newborn Infant[17,18]) and a concurrent criterion variable (e.g., a clinical diagnosis of brain damage). Content validity is applicable when it is necessary to measure the extent to which a test, for example, a school test, covers some field of study.[16] It is not expressed as a validity coefficient. "The test items can be regarded as a sample from a population representing the content of the aims of the course. Content validity is determined by the extent to which the sample of items in a test is representative of the total population."[16] When examining a developmental test of "motor" function, one might assess how well the items cover both gross and fine motor performance, as well as motor planning or other constructs.

The construct validity concept is useful when tests measure traits for which external criteria are not readily available.[16] It is not a single measure of correlation between test scores and criterion scores; rather construct validity is determined by showing that consequences are predicted by a theory developed on the basis of test results. These consequences can be confirmed by a series of testings or experiments.

Newborn Tests

In this section, several newborn tests will be reviewed, including the Neurological Examination of the Full Term Newborn Infant by Prechtl and Beintema,[17,18] the Neonatal Behavioral Assessment Scale by Brazelton,[19] and the Neurological Assessment of the Preterm and Full-Term Newborn Infant by Dubowitz and Dubowitz.[20] These tests represent three types of newborn assessments: neurologic, behavioral, and behavioral–neurologic.

Parmelee and Michaelis[21] proposed that a newborn neurologic examination has three purposes:

1. The immediate diagnosis of an evident neurologic problem, such as extreme hypotonia, convulsions, coma, or localized paralysis, to determine what therapy to institute.
2. The evaluation of the day to day changes of a known neurologic problem to determine the evolution of a pathologic process, such as a hypoxic episode, or to follow the evolution of the neurologic signs of a systematic disease, such as respiratory distress.
3. The long-term prognosis of a newborn who is recovering from some neonatal neurologic problem or is considered at risk due to abnormalities of the pregnancy or delivery.

The neurologic examination should contain a properly balanced selection of items to represent the important subsystems of the neural repertory.[22] It is essential to consider that the occurrence and/or intensity of many newborn responses are determined by the behavioral state in which they are examined. The Prechtl and Beintema scale[17,18] is an example of a neurologic examination and is discussed in detail later in this section.

The purpose of a behavioral test is to determine the behavioral makeup of an individual newborn.[22] Behavioral tests should cover a wide selection of behavior patterns that are important in the infant's daily life. The process of selecting test items should be based empirically on an extensive ethogram of the mother–infant dyad and not on preconceptions about what newborns should do. Finally, the obtained behavioral test results should correspond with the actual behavior of the individual baby in the natural mother–infant interaction. The Brazelton scale[19] is an example of a behavioral test.

The third test discussed in this section, the Dubowitz and Dubowitz scale,[20] is an example of a behavioral–neurologic newborn examination, combining elements of both the neurologic and the behavioral asessments.

Neurological Examination of the Full Term Newborn Infant

Prechtl and Beintema[17] published a standardized neurologic test for the full-term newborn infant, which was revised slightly in 1977.[18] The manual states that the test is valid for full-term infants between the gestational ages of 38 and 42 weeks and for preterm infants once they have reached the same postconceptional age. The test was developed to diagnose neurologic abnormalities and to predict future neurologic problems. In addition, a screening test is available to determine the need for low-risk neonates to undergo more detailed testing.[18]

The test[17] was standardized on a large sample of infants whose mothers had a history of obstetric complications. The aspects of the test that were standardized are the external conditions (e.g., the testing environment), the behavioral state of the infant, and the handling of the infant (e.g., position and stimulation). Prechtl[23] reported that interobserver reliability on the test was high (0.80 to 0.96). Beintema[24] tested 49 infants with the neurologic examination starting at 1 day of age and ending at 9 days of age. He found that the infants changed considerably over that time. Beintema concluded that neurologic examinations administered to infants during the first 3 days of postnatal life were less valid than those administered later in the neonatal period. He also pointed out that an infant's behavioral state during testing significantly influenced test results.

The items of the test are scored on variable scales.[17] No total score is obtained, but Prechtl and Beintema have noted that abnormal neurologic findings in full-term newborn infants frequently appear in particular combinations. They have identified four syndromes: (1) the apathy syndrome, characterized by generally depressed responses; (2) the hyperexcitability syndrome, characterized by a low-frequency, high-amplitude tremor and easily elicited Moro reflex; (3) the hemisyndrome, consisting of at least three asymmetries of motility, posture, or response; and (4) the comatose syndrome, characterized by depressed respiration and absent or weak arousal to various stimuli. In a study of 150 newborns with one of more of the abnormal syndromes, Prechtl[25] found that 73 had neurologic abnormalities at 2 to 4 years of age. Certain patterns of movement identified in the neonatal testing were also found to be predictive of later central nervous system (CNS) dysfunction.[26] These were (1) consistent lateral asymmetry of reflex responses, (2) hypertonic or hypotonic muscular responses, (3) athetoid movements, (4) obligatory tonic neck responses, (5) constant strabismus and poor suck, and (6) Moro reflexes.

Some major strengths of the Prechtl and Beintema assessment are that it has well-standardized instructions for administration of each item, that reflexes and responses are quantified as to intensity, that reflex or response asymmetries are noted, and that the state of the infant is recorded before each major section of the assessment. A disadvantage is that it is a long and complex test to administer; however, the authors caution against abbreviating it because, in the course of the examination sequence, findings are consistently verified by repeating certain items. The authors believe this adds to test validity.

Brazelton Neonatal Behavioral Assessment Scale

The Brazelton Neonatal Behavioral Assessment Scale (BNBAS)[19] is an infant behavior analysis instrument developed to distinguish individual differences among normal infants, especially with respect to social interactive behaviors.[27] The test is appropriate for infants from birth to the approximate postterm age of 1 month. The BNBAS was developed on the view that full-term healthy newborns are essentially social beings structured in such a way that they reliably elicit from the caretaker the organization that they themselves still lack.[28] The test includes 26 behavioral items that assess the neonate's capacity (1) to organize states of consciousness, (2) to habituate reactions to disturbing events, (3) to attend to and process simple and complex environmental events, (4) to control motor activity and postural tone while attending to these events, and (5) to perform integrated motor acts.[19,29] The test also includes 20 reflex items[19] purported to assess the neonate's neurologic intact-ness.[27] Contrary to this viewpoint, Prechtl[22] maintains that the BNBAS reflex items are inadequate to assess neural intactness or impairment. Prechtl points out that even though the BNBAS reflex items are based on the descriptions of neurologic assessment he and Beintema outlined in 1964,[17] they are not tested in the same way as was originally described.[22] In addition, the BNBAS reflex scale does not include the most sensitive items for detection of neurologic deviancy.

The reflex items and the biobehavioral items of the BNBAS are scored individually, reflecting the infant's best performance. No total score is ob-tained; however, the items can be clustered into four categories: interactive processes, motoric processes, state control, and physiologic response to stress.[28] Each of these clusters are then graded as exceptional, average, or worrisome. Als[28] recommends that specific clusters should be developed for the population of infants being tested, and to fit the purposes for testing in any given setting.

No formal standardization sample has been used in the development of the BNBAS nor have norms been derived for any large sample. Instead, re-searchers using the scale have provided their own normative data with the population they were testing.[28] In addition, Brazelton reported that the mean score for each item is based on the expected behavior of an infant who is an averge 7 pound, full-term, normal, white infant; whose mother did not have more than 100 mg of barbiturates for pain or 50 mg of other sedative drugs as premedication in the 4 hours prior to delivery; and whose Apgar ratings were no lower than 7/8/8 at 1, 5, and 15 minutes after delivery.[19] Tester–observer reliability and test–retest reliability are reported to be high (≥ 0.85 and ≥ 0.80, respectively).

The predictive validity of the BNBAS was investigated by Tronick and Brazelton[29] in a study involving 53 children examined during the neonatal pe-riod and at 7 years of age. They found that a standard but crude neurologic examination and the BNBAS were similar in their capacity for detecting ab-normal infants, but that the BNBAS was far superior to the neurologic ex-amination in detecting suspect abnormal infants. The latter conclusion is re-jected by Prechtl[22] because of the small number of subjects and because neurologic conditions during early life may be transient. The low number of BNBAS false-positive cases, therefore, may indicate an insensitivity on the part of the BNBAS to detect the presence of abnormal neurologic conditions.

Divitto and Goldberg[30,31] found that sick and healthy premature infants had significantly more worrisome scores on the interactive and motoric clusters of the BNBAS than did the full-term infants they tested. When the infants were retested, the same pattern was found, but the differences were not significant. Divitto and Goldberg[30] also tested the same infants on the Bayley Scales of Infant Development during the first year and found that the premature infants lagged behind the full-term infants and were less responsive to testing materials and tasks, more difficult to test, and less attentive. Finally, Bakow and colleagues[32] reported that the BNBAS items of alertness, motor maturity, tremulousness, habituation, and self-quieting were correlated with infant temperament at 4 months.

The following clinical uses of the BNBAS have been proposed[33]: (1) screen infants for behavioral or motor problems, (2) educate parents about their infant's development and behavior, (3) assess, in part, what impact an infant's behavior will have on the process of parent–infant bonding, (4) help plan a behavioral and/or motor intervention program, (5) provide a developmental and behavioral baseline on infants who will receive future developmental assessments, and (6) help objectively monitor the medical status of an insulted infant, (e.g., one with a central nervous system bleed).

Horowitz and Dunn[34] and Lancioni and colleagues[35] revised the Brazelton Neonatal Behavioral Assessment Scale with Kansas Supplements (BNBAS-K). The BNBAS-K provides for scoring both best and most typical behavior on several items to better reflect the range and variability of infant behavior observed during an assessment.

Field and associates[36] also modified the BNBAS so it could be used by mothers. The instrument was named The Mother's Assessment of the Behavior of Her Infant (MABI). To determine the validity of this instrument, Field and associates trained testers to administer the BNBAS to 32 normal infants and to 32 postterm postmature infants; the mothers in this group administered the MABI to the same infant groups. No differences were found between mothers' and testers' assessments, except that the testers assigned more optimal interactive process scores. Normal-term infants received more optimal scores than postmature infants from both mothers and testers. The mothers' motoric process scores and the testers' motoric process scores correlated with 8-month Bayley[37] motor scores at the 0.34 to 0.42 level. Widmayer and Field[37] found that teenage mothers who observed the BNBAS administered to their preterm infants and who also administered the MABI to their infants during the first month and another group of mothers who only administered the MABI to their infants demonstrated more optimal interactions during feeding and play with their babies than the mothers who did not administer the MABI or observe the BNBAS.

The BNBAS is not intended for use with infants of a gestational age of less than 37 weeks; its use is inappropriate for premature or stressed newborns whose normative performance is not known.[38] For premature infants, the Assessment of Preterm Infants' Behavior (APIB)[39] is used.

Als and Duffy[40] postulate that there exists a consistency in the manner in which newborns interact with their environment and how they behave as children later in life. The difficulties that exist in defining this consistency are related to the difficulties inherent in finding analogs of behavioral functioning at different age points. Developmental competence is defined by the degree of smoothness and modulation, regulation, and differentiation of five behaviorally observable subsystems of functioning: the autonomic system, the motor system, the state regulatory system, the attention–interactive system, and the self-regulatory system. Another aspect of this developmental model is the degree of external facilitation necessary to assist in the regulation of the subsystems when they become disorganized.

Several principles of development are inherent in this developmental model. First is the principle of species adaptedness, in which the organism is described "in any stage of development as having evolved to competency at that stage, rather than as an imperfect precursor model of later stages."[40] Second is "the principle of continuous organism–environment interaction, from the unicellular stage of development throughout the lifespan and implicated in such domains of human functioning as neuroembryologic, motor, cognitive, and language development."[40] The third principle is that "of orthogenesis and syncresis, which postulates that wherever development occurs it proceeds from a state of native globality to a state of increasing differentiation, articulation, and integration."[40] Fourth is "the principle of dual antagonist integration, which postulates that the organism always strives for smoothness of integration, and that underlying this striving is a tension between two basically antagonistic physiologic types of responses, the explorator or reaching out response, and the avoiding or withdrawing response."[40] These principles are synthesized into a principle called *synaction*, which postulates "that development proceeds through the continuous intraorganism subsystem interaction and differentiation and organism–environment interaction aimed at bringing about the realization of hierarchically ordered species-unique developmental agenda."[40]

The assessment of a newborn infant within the above model of development requires the identification of the current standing of a child on the matrix of subsystem development and focuses on the way in which individual infants adapt to their environment rather than on skills. At each developmental stage within this model, various subsystems of functioning exist side by side. They are costly to each other when development is disorganized, and are mutually supportive when development is smooth. During assessment of the infant, smoothness, modulation, and differentiation are evaluated as the child is systematically manipulated within a "paradigm designed to express the newly emerging developmental agenda of a given age point."[40] The manipulation impacts on all the major systems of infant functioning (autonomic, motor, state regulation, attention/interaction, and self-regulation) simultaneously.

The APIB[39] has been developed within the theoretic framework described above as an extension of the BNBAS for premature infants. The maneuvers of the BNBAS are presented to the premature infant as a graded sequence of increasingly demanding environmental inputs or packages, moving from distal stimulation presented during sleep to mild tactile stimulation, to medium tactile stimulation paired with vestibular stimulation, to more massive tactile stimulation paired with vestibular stimulation.[41] The social interactive items of the BNBAS are presented during the course of the examination whenever the infant's behavioral organization indicates an availability for these items. The reactions and behaviors of the infant are monitored along five systems of functioning: physiologic system, motor organizational system, attentional–interactive system, state regulatory system, and self-regulatory system. The kind of graded examiner facilitation is also monitored. The systems are scored from

9 (disorganized performance) to 1 (well-organized performance) and can be graphed on a summary grid.

Test administration takes at least 30 minutes and the scoring takes less than 1 hour. It is better for the APIB to be administered to premature infants closer to a "next feeding." With full-term infants, it is better for the BNBAS to be administered about midway between feedings. The APIB is appropriate for the premature infant who is in an open isolette or crib, in room temperature and room air. The behavioral manipulations necessary for the APIB are often inappropriate and too stressful when the infant is maintained in oxygen or with other life support lines.[41]

The APIB can be used clinically to measure behavioral changes over time, to document behavioral strengths and problems, to document specific sensory input and handling procedures that are appropriate and that positively foster organization, and to help parents become attuned to their infant's actions and reactions.[41] A group of premature infants who received carefully designed caregiving modifications by the primary nursing team based on the results of the APIB had a significantly decreased number of days on the respirator, on supplemental oxygen, and on gavage tube feeding than did another group of premature infants who did not receive caregiving modifications.[42] At 36 months of age, the intervention infants were better modulated in terms of motor system and self-regulation ability.

The APIB appears to be very sensitive to gestational age.[43] Earlier-born babies showed much greater sensitivity and reactivity and a lower threshold to disorganization. Additionally, behavioral group membership in the newborn period as determined by the APIB is predictive of neuropsychologic functioning at later ages.[44] Low-threshold reactive newborns tended to show much greater difficulty in motor and spatial planning, social interactive modulation capacity, and attentional regulation at 5 years of age.

Neurological Assessment of the Preterm and Full-Term Newborn Infant

The Neurological Assessment of the Preterm and Full-Term Newborn Infant by Dubowitz and Dubowitz[20] was devised in response to the authors' need for a single instrument that would meet a number of basic requirements: (1) to be suitable for use by staff without expertise in neonatal neurology, (2) to be usable with preterm and full-term neonates, (3) to be reliable very soon after birth, (4) to require no more than 10 to 15 minutes to administer and score to encourage routine clinical use, and (5) to be suitable for sequential assessment of infants after birth.[20] The opportunity to test sequentially permits the clinician (1) to compare preterm infants after birth with newborn infants of corresponding postgestational age, (2) to document the normal evolution of neurologic behavior in the preterm infant after birth, and (3) to detect deviations in neurologic signs and their subsequent resolution.

The test incorporates items from the systems of Saint-Anne Dargassies,[45]

Prechtl,[18] Parmelee and Michaelis,[21] and Brazelton,[19] and a recording method similar to the gestational age assessment of Dubowitz and associates.[46] Items are scored on a five-point ordinal scale, and it is not essential that all items be administered.[20] No single total score is recorded; rather, the patterns of responses may reflect variations in neurologic function. Some patterns typical of particular groups of infants have begun to be identified and are described in the manual in a series of case histories.

No reliability information on the final version of the scale is presented in the manual. Concurrent validity was investigated by Dubowitz and associates.[47] The investigation consisted of a comparative study of neurologic assessment and ultrasound examination of 100 infants consecutively admitted to a neonatal unit over a 9-month period. All infants received at least three neurologic assessments consisting of six items from the Dubowitz and Dubowitz scale. These items were selected because they could be elicited in even the most severely ill infants. The infants also received a variable number of ultrasound scans, depending on their gestational age and medical condition. The results revealed that 24 of the 31 infants born at less than 36 weeks' gestation with ultrasound evidence of an intraventricular bleed had three or more abnormal clinical signs, compared with only 2 of 37 infants without intraventricular hemorrhage who were also born at less than 36 weeks' gestation. Of the 37 infants without intraventricular hemorrhage, 21 had no abnormal signs. In comparison, only 1 of 31 infants with an intraventricular bleed had no abnormal signs. The researchers suggested that repeated, careful examination of the infants in the sample and the recognition of abnormal signs provide an objective means of alerting the clinician to the probable presence of an intraventricular hemorrhage, which can be verified by ultrasound. Unfortunately, long-term studies of predictive validity for later outcome are not yet available.

Graziani and Korberly[48] address the issue of predictive limitations of neurologic and behavioral assessments in the newborn period. They suggest that several factors may influence the predictability of these instruments. One of these is the ability of the infant who is severely depressed in the newborn period, because of perinatal hypoxia or trauma, to recover completely, provided that brain structures are not damaged. The severity and acuteness of the insult and the maturation and capacities of the infant's subcortical neuroanatomic structures may influence this ability to recover. Other factors are the effects of the environment, human maturation, and psychosocial influences on developmental outcome.

Another factor influencing the predictability of neonatal measures is test–retest reliability. Despite standardization procedures (for example, testing an infant on the BNBAS midway between feedings), test–retest reliability may be affected by changes in an infant's chronologic age, behavioral state, and internal physiologic state. The standardization procedures themselves may alter test performance. Casaer and Akiyama[49] found that an infant's postural position during assessment may affect the heart rate, respiration, and motor activity. Reliability is also affected by the training, experience, and bias of the examiner.

Prechtl[22] suggests that the prognostic value of a neonatal instrument may be increased by repeated testings; however, he also suggests that there is overconcern when neonatal behavioral tests have low test–retest reliability. This overconcern stems from insufficient appreciation of discontinuities in developmental processes. The ability to detect developmental change during the neonatal period should therefore be considered a positive characteristic for any of the instruments discussed in this section. This characteristic has been demonstrated by the BNBAS in a study involving 10 Zambian and 10 American infants.[50] The Zambian infants demonstrated significant behavioral changes when tested the third time at 10 days of age. The first test was administered on day 1 and the second on day 5.

Graziani and Korberly[48] point out that abnormal neurobehavior in the neonate does not imply abnormal or different brain structure. In addition, an absent or abnormal infant response or reflex is frequently of uncertain significance because local dysfunction within the immature brain is not manifested by a *specific* change in behavior or reflexes.

Although there appears to be no completely satisfactory and valid clinical method for the behavioral or neurologic assessment of the neonate, valuable information may be obtained from any of the instruments discussed in this section. Prechtl[22] has suggested that a standardized neurologic assessment be administered along with the Brazelton scale. The Dubowitz and Dubowitz scale designed to assess premature and term infants and the behavioral and neurologic areas may prove to be the most practical and useful clinical instrument for clinicians.

Non-Newborn Tests

The following tests are discussed in this section: the Bayley Scales of Infant Development (BSID),[51] the Gesell Developmental Scales (GDS),[10,52] the Bruininks-Oseretsky Test of Motor Proficiency (BOTMP),[53] the Miller Assessment for Preschoolers (MAP),[54] the Peabody Developmental Motor Scales (PDMS)[55] and the Pediatric Evaluation of Disability Inventory (PEDI).[56]

Each of these instruments, except the PEDI, is used for diagnostic purposes by clinicians because they are more comprehensive than screening tests. They are also familiar to investigators in a variety of disciplines involved in the management of the child with neurologic dysfunction. Common knowledge of these instruments facilitates communication between disciplines, thereby aiding multidisciplinary management. Finally, these comprehensive developmental tests are statistically designed primarily for diagnostic purposes. The PEDI, on the other hand, is a new *functional* assessment tool. The tests chosen are readily available and fairly easy to learn to administer without the need for extensive special instruction.

Bayley Scales of Infant Development

The California First-Year Mental Scale by Bayley,[57] the California Pre-school Mental Scale by Jaffa,[58] and the California Infant Scale of Motor Development by Bayley[59] contributed heavily to the unpublished 1958 version of the BSID, and most of the specific test items for these early Bayley scales[57,59] were drawn from the Gesell scales. The 1958 version of the BSID was revised and a 1958–1960 version was published for use in assessing children from 1 to 15 months of age. The BSID was again revised, renormed, and expanded to its current form in 1969.

The current BSID[51] edition allows assessment of children from 2 to 30 months of age and consists of three parts: a Mental Scale, a Motor Scale, and an Infant Behavior record. For the purposes of this chapter, discussion will be focused on the Motor Scale. The Motor Scale is designed to provide a measure of the degree of control of the body, of coordination of the large muscles, and of finer manipulatory skills of the hands and fingers.

Each test item of the Motor Scale is scored passed, failed, or not testable.[51] All scoring is based on tester observations. By adding the number of passes, a raw score is obtained for the Motor Scale. This score is then converted to a standard score (PDI). Basal and ceiling levels and a motor age equivalency can also be obtained.

The 1958–1960 version of the BSID was normed on a national sample of 1,400 normal children.[51] The current 1969 version was normed on a national sample of 1,962 normal children ranging in age from 2 to 30 months. The original sample design called for testing 100 children at 14 different ages. The sample was controlled for sex, race, residence (urban–rural), and education of the head of the household. This sample reflected the proportions of children from 2 months through 30 months of age in selected strata of the United States population, as described in the 1960 US Census of Population. Using the 1958–1960 version of the scale, Bayley[60] demonstrated that in a nationwide sample of 1,400 children, there were no differences in test scores due to sex, birth order, geographic location, or parents' education; however, a consistent tendency for black children to obtain significantly higher scores on the Motor Scale at all ages from 3 through 14 months was found.

Four different methods were used to measure reliability for the BSID.[51] Split-half reliability coefficients were obtained from each of the 14 age groups of the standardization sample. The reliability coefficients for the Motor Scale ranged from 0.68 to 0.92, with a median value of 0.84. The second statistic calculated was the standard error of measurement (SEM). The SEM for the Motor Scale ranged from 4.6 to 9.0. Finally, high tester–observer reliability (>89 percent agreement) and test–retest reliability (>75 percent agreement) were demonstrated by Werner and Bayley[61] using the 1958–1960 version of the Mental and Motor Scales.

The validity of the BSID was investigated by Ramey and associates,[62] who suggested that, in situations in which natural environmental variation is reduced, there is a high correlation between the scores of the Bayley Mental and

Motor Scales and Stanford-Binet scores. Their sample consisted of 24 subjects who attended day-care facilities and were tested on the Bayley Scales at 6 to 8 months, at 9 to 12 months, and at 13 to 16 months of age, and on the Stanford-Binet at 36 months of age. Mental Scale–Stanford-Binet correlations were 0.49, 0.71, and 0.90, respectively, while Motor Scale–Stanford-Binet correlations were 0.77, 0.56, and 0.43, respectively.

The next topic of discussion is the usefulness of the BSID in diagnosing handicapping conditions. Honzik and associates[63] compared the 8-month Bayley Mental Test scores of a group of infants suspected of having neurologic handicaps with the scores of a matched normal control group from the same hospital. The total number of infants tested was 197. The testers were blind to the grouping of the infants they tested. The Bayley Mental Test scores differentiated the suspect from the control group at a probability of less than 0.05.

Berk[64] conducted a study to determine the discriminative efficiency of the BSID for identifying infants with possible neurologic impairments. The sample consisted of 194 subjects, including 105 randomly selected normal subjects and 89 neurologically suspicious subjects selected incidentally. The Bayley Mental and Motor Scales were administered at 8 months of age. Neurologic examinations were administered to all subjects at ages 1 and 7 years for classification of the children as neurologically normal or suspicious. Berk concluded that the Bayley Motor Scale provides modest discriminating power and that the information contributed by the Mental Scale in linear combination with the Motor Scale is not substantial and meaningful enough to warrant its administration when attempting to discriminate infants with neurologic impairment; however, the findings should be considered tentative until cross-validation studies are completed.

Coryell and colleagues[65] investigated whether the Bayley Motor Scale Psychomotor Index (PDI) scores are stable in high- and low-risk infants during the first year of life. The study sample consisted of 15 low-risk infants (full-term) and 28 high-risk infants (full-term and preterm). The Bayley Motor Scale was administered to these infants at least four times during the first year of life. The infant PDI scores were found to be unstable. It was suggested that the instability was related to the test itself, to the nature of the subjects (recovery from perinatal insult), or to the nature of infant development (inconsistent rate). A similar, very high identification of non-normal subjects was found by Harris[66] when 4-month Bayley Motor Scores were compared with outcomes at 3 years of age.

Clinically, the BSID provides the clinician with a comprehensive evaluation of an infant's level of development.[51] The standard scores (MDI, PDI) provide the basis for establishing a child's current status, in comparison to children in the normative sample, and the extent of any deviation from normal expectancy. The mean standard score for each age range of the standardization sample is 100. A standard deviation (SD) is 16 standard score points; 68 percent of the children in the standardization sample for age range scored between 1 SD below the mean of 100 and 1 SD above the mean of 100. Based on my experience with the BSID, a standard score above the 16th percentile indicates normal development; a score between 1 and 2 SD below the mean of 100 indicates a possible developmental problem or environmental deprivation and a score 2 or more SD below the mean indicates retarded development relative to age peers.

Clinicians using the BSID should be aware, however, that the test norms are out of date and that the test is currently being renormed. Coryell and colleagues, for example, found that 4-month Motor Scale scores appeared especially inflated relative to later outcomes and may lead to the unfounded assumption of early normality.[65] Similarly, Campbell and colleagues showed that 12-month Motor Scale scores in a population-based sample of 305 children averaged 10 points above the normative mean.[67]

With regard to program planning, the instrument's (BSID) developmental sequencing of skills provides a useful starting point for goal planning.[7] The value of the instrument for program planning, however, is diminished for several reasons. The number of developmental items contained in the BSID is insufficient to allow the program planner to pinpoint targets precisely for interaction in any particular developmental domain. The time increments between sequenced developmental items are too broad for precision programming with handicapped children. However, an infant's performance on selected BSID items within the developmental sequences can provide the planner with an idea of the upper and lower intervention limits. The clustering of BSID items may be useful when planning intervention programs.[68]

Gesell Developmental Schedules

The GDS[10,52] is the patriarch of traditional developmental measures on which all other scales have been directly or indirectly modeled. It is a functional and clinical assessment of the infant's and preschooler's (1 to 72 months of age) broad range of developmental skills not contained in many developmental tests.[7] The scales are not an intellectual measure but a vivid sampling of interrelated behaviors across maturity-age levels and developmental areas. Scoring does not provide a global index. Instead, five areas, including language, fine motor, gross motor, adaptive (problem-solving), and personal–social skills, are assessed.[52] In addition, the test includes a developmental history and a neurologic survey.[10] Information is obtained from observation and parental reports.

The original standardization procedure involved three normative samples. The first normative sample was composed of 90 normal and abnormal infants who were tested from the time they were less than 3 months of age until they were more than 48 months of age.[69] The second was composed of 107 normal children of the middle socioeconomic class.[70] The third was composed of 107 normal children of the middle socioeconomic class who were examined at 15 months, at 18 months, and at 2, 3, 4, 5, and 6 years of age.[71]

The normative basis and organizational format of the GDS for age levels 2.5 to 6 years was minimally revised in 1974.[10] The sample for this revision was composed of 640 normal children who were socioeconomically stratified according to the US census figures for 1960. All the children lived in Connecticut and were mostly white. The revision included dividing the original motor behavior category into separate gross and fine motor behavior categories.

The most recent revision of the Gesell schedules was published in 1980.[52] It involved the birth to 36 months age range and included alterations in item placement and sequence. The revision was based on tests conducted on 927 children in the Albany, New York, area. Twenty-four children were tested at 4 weeks of age, 28 at 8 weeks and at 12 weeks, 52 at 28 weeks, 47 at 36 months, and 50 at 15 other age levels. Race distribution for this sample reflected the US distribution. The mean education in years for white mothers was similar to that of the US population; for the black mothers, it was slightly higher than the US average. Revisions in the gross motor area included alteration of the sequencing of items, and gross motor tasks were achieved 17 percent earlier. In the fine motor area, the tasks were achieved 5 percent earlier only in the children in the age range of 56 weeks to 36 months.[52]

Performance is assessed by deriving separate developmental ages, instead of a global score, for each of the five developmental domains.[7] Thus, individual developmental differences are revealed. A flexible scoring system, although somewhat confusing, allows the rating of emerging capabilities and qualitative performance features. Developmental skills are rated as absent, fully acquired, advanced for age, or emerging. Developmental performance in a specific developmental area is described as an age range. A rating of 21 months in the language area represents a skill range of 18 to 24 months. This means that the child typically performs at the 21-month level, but shows scattered and emerging skills spanning the 18- to 24-month range. This scoring system is flexible, thereby facilitating the assessment of individual developmental variations, a useful asset when assessing handicapped children. A handicapped child may perform relatively well in the gross motor area but poorly in the fine motor and language areas. Such a developmental profile could be documented by the GDS scoring system. One drawback is that a specific age level cannot be derived if there is a wide scatter of items passed and failed in a particular area. A developmental quotient (DQ) can be derived for each developmental area by using the formula[52]

$$DQ = \frac{\text{maturity age}}{\text{chronologic age}} \times 100$$

Gesell never investigated the problem of examiner–observer reliability; however, Knobloch and Pasamanick[10] reported the reliability of DQ assignment to be 0.98 among 18 pediatric residents. Test–retest reliability was investigated by Gesell in 1928:[69] the sample for this investigation was composed of 90 infants tested 492 times. Reliability was found to be high. An 80 percent agreement was obtained when the scores were within the normal range; a 96 percent agreement was obtained when the scores were subnormal. In 1974, Knobloch and Pasamanick[10] reported test–retest reliability for 65 infants over a 2- to 3-day time span to be 0.82. An interobserver reliability study was also done using the 1980 version of the scale and a sample of 48 children ranging in age from 16 weeks to 21 months.[52] The overall percentage of agreement for 305 behavior patterns was 93.7 percent; however, agreement varied from 88 percent in fine motor behavior to 97 percent in language. Interrater reliability was also found to be high. In the area of predictive validity, the GDS performances of 26 normal male children at 7, 9, and 15 months correlated significantly and consistently with performance on the visual motor channel of the Illinois Test of Psycho-linguistic Abilities[72] at 5 years.[73]

With regard to program planning, the five domains tested by the GDS are congruent with the skills focused on in many early intervention curricula.[7] The results of research in programs for both disabled and nondisabled preschoolers indicate that the GDS is highly correlated with developmental curricula. The schedules also have utility as a diagnostic device for educational programming.

Bruininks-Oseretsky Test of Motor Proficiency

BOTMP[53] assesses the gross and fine motor functioning of children from 4.5 to 14.5 years of age. The specific motor areas evaluated by subtests are running speed and agility, balance, bilateral coordination, strength, upper limb coordination, response speed, visual motor control, and upper limb speed and dexterity. The test was developed to provide educators, clinicians, and researchers useful information to assist them in assessing the motor skills of individual students, in developing and evaluating motor training programs, and in assessing serious motor dysfunctions and developmental handicaps in children. A shortened version of the BOTMP has also been developed.

The BOTMP provides global and differentiated information about a child.[53] The test yields a Gross Motor Composite Score, a Fine Motor Composite Score, and a Battery Composite Score; these are standard scores. Age equivalencies and standard scores are also obtained for each subtest.

The BOTMP[53] consists of 30 items previously contained in the Oseretsky Tests of Motor Proficiency.[74] The BOTMP was standardized on 765 subjects representative of the 1970 US census according to sex, race, community size, and geographic distribution.[53]

The validity of the BOTMP is based on how well it assesses the construct of motor development or proficiency.[53] Several researchers proposed that motor development consists of a number of constructs.[75–80] The BOTMP measures (1) 6 of 7 constructs identified by Guilford,[75] (2) 4 of 6 constructs postulated by Cratty,[76,77] (3) 12 of 20 constructs described by Fleishman[78] (4) 10 constructs identified by Harrow,[79] and (5) 6 of 8 constructs identified by Rarick and Dobbins.[80]

Construct validity of the BOTMP is also demonstrated by the statistical characteristics of the test.[53] One study revealed that the scores of each subtest correlated significantly with the chronologic age of the children in the standardization sample. For the total sample, the correlations ranged from 0.57 to

0.86, with a median of 0.78. For each subtest, the mean point scores showed the expected increase from one age group to the next.

The final method whereby validity is measured is by comparing contrast groups.[53] The manual reports that normal subjects perform significantly better than mildly retarded subjects, moderately to severely retarded subjects, and learning disabled subjects of the same chronologic age. Part of the difference may be due to difficulty encountered when testing retarded or learning disabled children, specifically giving instructions that are often complex. Reliability for the BOTMP was measured by three methods.[53] A test–retest reliability study was conducted with a sample of 63 second graders and 63 sixth graders. The BOTMP was administered to each group twice within a 7- to 12-day period. The test–retest reliability coefficients for the Gross and Fine Motor Composites were 0.77 and 0.88, respectively, for the sixth graders. The reliability coefficient for the Battery Composite was 0.89 for the second graders and 0.86 for the sixth graders. Test–retest coefficients for the separate subtests ranged from 0.58 to 0.89 for the second graders and from 0.29 to 0.89 for the sixth graders. The second method to measure reliability was the determination of the SEM for the composites and the subtests. Generally, the SEM for the subtests was found to be 2 or 3 standard score points while the SEM for the composites was found to be 4 or 5 standard score points. The final method was the determination of interrater reliability on the eight items of the visual motor control subtest, chosen because scoring the items in this subtest requires more tester judgment than the items of the other subtests. The interrater reliability coefficient for one group of raters was 0.98; it was 0.90 for a second group.

Sabatino[81] describes the BOTMP as well developed, well standardized, and useful to professionals from several disciplines. It is also reported that the test items are administered easily with no special training required.

Miller Assessment for Preschoolers

The MAP[54] is a screening test for identifying children (2 years 9 months to 5 years 8 months) who exhibit moderate "preacademic problems" that may affect one or more areas of development, but who do not have obvious or severe problems.[82] It was not originally developed to predict or diagnose disability. It can be used effectively to identify children who are at risk of experiencing later school-related problems and who merit further professional evaluation and follow-up.[83]

Miller has prepared and tested five editions of the MAP since 1972. During this process, over 800 items were administered to several independent samples totaling over 4,000 preschool children. The most recent normative sample of 1,200 preschool children was randomly selected, stratified, and national in scope; however, there was a disproportionate share of children of well-educated, professionally employed parents in the sample.[82]

The test consists of 27 "core" items that include variations on items that have been widely used for decades (e.g., the draw a person) and many neurologically based items. The responses can be grouped into five subscores for more detailed interpretation.[84] Supplemental Observations have also been developed. These are highly structured clinical observations that may be helpful in describing in qualitative terms a child's weaknesses and strengths and in suggesting possible remediation approaches.[84] The 27 core items were designed to be administered by examiners with minimal test-specific training. The Supplemental Observations require administration by examiners with test-specific training.

The theoretic framework underlying the 27 core items includes a threefold classification of abilities and a performance index within each of the three classifications.[84] Only the Sensory and Motor Abilities classification will be discussed here. Within this classification is the Foundation Index, which examines major or basic motor tasks and sensations, such as finger localization, essential to activities of higher complexity. A second index is the Coordination Index, which reflects increasingly complex motor tasks that join basic sensory and motor factors, such as motor accuracy. A third index is the Combined Foundations and Coordination Indexes, which includes items, such as rapid alternating movements, that integrate factors from the previous two indexes.

For sets of items included in the performance indices, interrater reliability varied between 0.84 and 0.99. The total MAP score interrater reliability was 0.98. Percentages of examiners who did not switch a final scoring category on retest ranged from 72 to 94 on the indices and was 81 for the total MAP score. In terms of validity, the MAP correctly identified as "at risk" 80 percent of a sample of 80 children identified by teachers, doctors, or parents as having preacademic problems.[54] Results of predictive validity studies were not included in the manual; Miller, however, reported that the MAP's classificational accuracy for prediction to achievement and intelligence 4 years later was comparable to that of other tests after shorter intervals.[85]

A strong feature of the MAP is the detailed information presented in the manual for administration and scoring of the items. Another helpful feature is the interpretive information provided.[84] The scoring process is another strong feature.[82]

Peabody Developmental Motor Scales

The PDMS[55] is a standardized, norm-referenced test for assessing the fine and gross motor development of children from birth to 83 months of age.[86] The test consists of 170 gross motor items that are classified into five categories including reflexes, balance, nonlocomotor, locomotor, and receipt and propulsion of objects. The 112 fine motor items are classified into four categories including grasping, hand use, eye–hand coordination, and manual dexterity.

Normative data for the PDMS were collected in 1981 and 1982 on 617 children. The percentage (25 percent) of 5- to 7-year-old children in the normative sample is smaller than the percentage (42 percent) of children from birth to 2 years of age.[86] The children in the sample were not randomly selected and were primarily from middle income families.

With regard to reliability, gross and fine motor scores were found to be stable over time and between raters.[86] However, several areas of concern regarding the reliability methodology were identified by Hinderer and colleagues, including the method of subject and examiner selection, the training and experience of the testers, and the method used to calculate the SEM.[86]

The PDMS manual reports data that suggest concurrent validity of the PDMS with the Bayley Motor Scale and the West Haverstraw Motor Development Test.[86,87] In another study, Palisano[88] reported moderate to high correlations between the Bayley Motor Scale and the PDMS, suggesting good concurrent validity for both measures. Provost and colleagues[87] reported weak to moderate correlations between the PDMS and the MAP, suggesting that each test measures different aspects of sensorimotor functioning.

Regarding construct validity, the PDMS discriminates between children at different age levels except those within the 48 to 59 month age range.[86] Provost and colleagues reported that the PDMS Fine Motor Scale identified the most children as delayed, followed in descending order of frequency by the PDMS Gross Motor Scale and the MAP.[89] Additionally, 38 and 15 percent of the cases who scored as delayed on the MAP Total Score are not identified as delayed on the PDMS Gross and Fine Motor Scales, respectively.[89] In the area of predictive validity, Palisano[88] reported that age equivalent scores of the PDMS at 12 months of age were not predictive of 18-month scores.

Hinderer and colleagues[86] and Palisano[90] identified areas of concern for the PDMS, including vague scoring criteria for partial credit, inefficient presentation of test materials, inappropriate item placement within various age ranges, and missing data and errors on certain percentile rank tables. Despite these shortcomings, Hinderer and colleagues describe the PDMS as a clinically useful test.[86]

Pediatric Evaluation Of Disability Inventory

The Developmental Edition of the PEDI is a functional assessment instrument for the evaluation of disabled and chronically ill children ranging in age from 6 months to 7 years. The PEDI measures functional status and functional change in three areas: functional skill level, caregiver assistance, and modifications of adaptive equipment used.[56] Defined as instruments that measure the actual ability of a child to perform necessary daily activities,[91] the focus of functional assessments is to determine the extent of independence and the maximization of function achieved within the limits of existing physical and cognitive deficits.[92]

The PEDI includes items related to self-care, bowel and bladder control, mobility and transfers, communication, and social function. It can be used as a global evaluation tool in various settings and provides a uniform mechanism for reporting functional disability for data registries.[56] Administration is done by parent report and interview.

Feldman and colleagues[56] conducted a study that assessed the concurrent and construct validity of the PEDI. The study sample included 20 children between the ages of 2 and 8 years with arthritic conditions or spina bifida and

20 nondisabled children. The disabled and nondisabled children were matched for age and sex. The PEDI and the Battelle Developmental Inventory Screening Test (BDIST)[93] were administered to all children and results were compared.

The BDIST was developed from the Battelle Developmental Inventory (BDI).[93] The BDI consists of 341 test items from five domains including motor and adaptive. It has been reported that the BDI discriminates well between disabled and nondisabled children.[94–96] Limitations of the BDIST are a large item pool and the 2 hours needed to complete the test.[96]

The BDIST consists of 96 items and can be administered in approximately 20 to 35 minutes. The BDIST is a strong predictor of performance on the BDI.[56] The BDIST can be used to identify children who are developmentally delayed, to identify strengths and weaknesses of children who are developing normally, and to measure the progress of groups of children with developmental delays.[56]

Concurrent validity of the PEDI was supported by moderately high Pearson product–moment correlations between the summary scores of the PEDI and the BDIST ($r = .70$ to .80). Construct validity was established by results that indicated significant differences between the PEDI scores of the disabled and nondisabled children. Using discriminant analysis, the PEDI scores were determined to be better group discriminators than the BDIST scores.[56]

Intervention Tools

In this section, two selected instruments will be reviewed: the Vulpe Assessment Battery (VAB)[97] and the Carolina Curriculum for Handicapped Infants and Infants At Risk (CCHI.)[98] The primary usefulness of these instruments is in the formulation of developmental intervention programs because they have not been statistically designed for diagnostic purposes.

Vulpe Assessment Battery

The VAB[97] is comprised of assessment items that attempt to cover comprehensively essential areas of child development from birth through 6 years of age. The battery provides a method for obtaining and organizing the information necessary to plan an individualized learning program for an atypical child. The battery utilizes the child's strengths and compensates for areas of weakness using a teaching method approach with which the child learns most effectively. The VAB assesses a number of areas including basic senses and functions, gross motor behaviors, fine motor behaviors, and activities of daily living. Also included in the VAB are tests of reflexes, motor planning, muscle strength, and balance.

Conceptually, the VAB views the child to be actively constructing an understanding of the world on the basis of perceptual organization and adaptation.[97] "The child interacts with the world in a manner which adds new content to learning and which progressively alters the structure of thinking so that the child can interact with the world in a developmentally more mature fashion."[97]

The VAB is not standardized in a formal sense; however, it is not designed to compare children with their age peers.[97] The battery is a product of Vulpe's 15 years of experience working with children with a wide range of developmental disabilities. No reliability or validity information is provided in the manual.

The advantages of the VAB are numerous. First, it is applicable to normal as well as to disabled children. Second, it is comprehensive in nature. Third, the battery can be individualized to each child's learning and developmental pattern. Fourth, it is competency oriented so that the child can succeed. Fifth, scoring of the child's performance considers the teaching technique utilized and the child's learning style; therefore, the VAB can be used simultaneously for assessment and programming. Sixth, an accountability schema is built into the assessment process, which facilitates reporting of assessments and the evaluation of developmental programs. Seventh, references for the original inclusion of each item in the test are provided.[97]

Carolina Curriculum for Handicapped Infants and Infants At Risk

The CCHI was developed to provide appropriate intervention strategies for children with developmental delays functioning in the birth to 24-month developmental age range.[98] The goal of the CCHI is to help teachers and others to optimize the positive interactions of a child with the world and the people in it.[99]

The CCHI is divided into 24 areas of development, including feeding, grooming, dressing, reaching and grasping, object manipulation, bilateral hand activity, gross motor activities—stomach, gross motor activities—back, and gross motor activities—upright.[98] Items from the 24 areas of development (sequences) are incorporated into an assessment log. For assessment purposes, the child needs to demonstrate a skill only one time. Items are credited based on observation or parent reporting. When the assessment is finished, a developmental progress chart is completed. A teaching activity exists for each item as depicted in the developmental progress chart.

As the result of field testing of the 0- to 12-month curriculum, interventionists found the CCHI to be useful for assessing infants with developmental delays and developing programs for them. The interventionists reported that the major reservation was the limitation of the curriculum when used with profoundly handicapped children. The data collected suggest that the use of the CCHI is effective in promoting developmental progress in children with mild to moderate handicaps in a relatively short time period (3 to 6 months).[98]

The Carolina Curriculum for Preschoolers With Special Needs (CCPSN) was developed as an upward extension of the CCHI.[100] The extension follows the basic philosophy and format of the CCHI, but includes a greater emphasis on the integration of intervention activities into the daily life of children in group care settings.

TESTS UNDER DEVELOPMENT

Therapists have long been aware that tests developed by members of other professions have shortcomings for use in physical therapy. A major weakness is that tests developed by nontherapists are concerned primarily with achievement of motor milestones and lack information for discerning problems with posture and coordination. Clinicians should be aware of several new tests under development by physical and occupational therapists that show promise for assessing the more qualitative aspects of motor development. These tests will be reviewed briefly in this section.

Campbell, Kolobe, and Girolami are developing a test for newborns called the Test of Infant Motor Performance (unpublished manuscript, 1989). The Test of Infant Motor Performance has 26 tested items and 22 spontaneously observed motor behaviors that assess functional movements used by young infants, such as changing position and attending to environmental events. The test covers the age range from 32 weeks postconception to 3 months postterm. The Alberta Infant Motor Scale is a 58-item observational instrument for assessing motor maturation from birth to 18 months of age.[101] Unlike most motor milestone tests, the focus of the Alberta Infant Motor Scale is on the sequential development of postural control. The test has shown good reliability and validity and is currently being normed on a Canadian population.

The Chandler Movement Assessment of Infants (unpublished manuscript, 1983) is a revision of the Movement Assessment of Infants[102] that promises to take less time and to have improved item and interrater reliability as well as norms for motor development. Like the original, the test covers approximately the first year of life and assesses motor milestones and postural reactions.

The Gross Motor Function Measure was developed specifically to document change in children with cerebral palsy that might be expected to result from physical therapy.[103] The Gross Motor Function Measure has 88 items that can be scored for several levels of ability; many of the items reflect ability to make transitions from one position to another. The manual should be available by the time of publication of this book. Twenty items on the Gross Motor Function Measure can also be scored for qualitative aspects of movement, such as postural alignment and ability to dissociate body parts during movement. These items are known as the Gross Motor Performance Measure, which is still under development.

The Miller Infant and Toddler Test is intended for use in early intervention programs.[104] The Miller Infant and Toddler Test has items in each of the five required assessment areas under PL 99-457: motor, language, cognitive, behavior, and self-help. The motor assessment is unique in its documentation of sequences of spontaneous movements typically performed by infants and toddlers.

SUMMARY

In this chapter, I have discussed principles of evaluation and assessment, parent involvement in the assessment process, and test selection criteria, and have reviewed a number of motor assessments or the motor components of the assessments and one functional assessment. The assessments were classified into newborn instruments, nonnewborn instruments, and intervention tools.

A clinician should be extensively familiar with the testing instruments he or she is administering and should keep abreast of the literature pertaining to a specific instrument or similar instruments. It is my opinion that a clinician involved in the formal testing of children with neurologic dysfunction should periodically test normal children and should periodically have his or her reliability with other testers evaluated.

For a specific child or clinical setting, each test chosen for evaluation will possess certain strengths and weaknesses, for example, cost, reliability, validity, popularity, time of administration, and purpose. These factors require thorough consideration when deciding which test to use. Physicians and other health professionals should not only be provided with test results, but also the interpretation of these results (e.g., information regarding long-term prognosis) when appropriate. Finally, the results of formalized testing should be used in combination with other information obtained (e.g., posture, range of motion, reflexes, and the quality of movement) to produce a comprehensive evaluation of a child with a neurologic disability.

In light of current fiscal considerations that public and private service providers are facing, it is imperative that clinicians involved in the assessment of children with developmental delays continue to use instruments that are well standardized, valid, reliable, and clinically useful, and not sacrifice quality assessment approaches for the purpose of cost containment. On the other hand, clinicians need to better coordinate the assessment process so that personnel are utilized efficiently. For example, a multidisciplinary assessment may be administered in an arena format that is less time intensive for families, less intrusive to a child, and less costly for providers.

Another example is when a 4-month-old child with a questionable developmental delay is initially assessed by a developmental pediatrician, an occupational therapist, a physical therapist, and a psychologist. The above disciplines do contribute a distinct piece to an assessment, but also duplicate roles to a certain degree. In this specific example, does the utilization of all the disciplines warrant the cost associated with it? If the answer is no, the implications are enormous for traditional methods of service delivery and personnel preparation. If the answer is yes, the cost will be high.

Clinicians need to better coordinate service delivery systems so that evaluations done at a community-based program are not duplicated at a tertiary hospital center where a child attends specialty clinics. In Baltimore, I have observed that it is not uncommon for a child with a developmental delay to be assessed at two or three agencies. This is costly not only to service providers but also to families in terms of time and effort.

In light of the family emphasis of PL 99-457, clinicians need to assess how they are involving parents in the assessment process. In addition, to test validity, standardization, reliability, and other factors, a clinician needs to consider how well a specific testing instrument promotes the parents' participation during the testing process and the parents' understanding of the developmental strengths and weaknesses of their child.

REFERENCES

1. Piaget J: The Origins of Intelligence in Children. Cook M, Trans. International Universities Press, New York, 1936
2. Department of Education: Early Intervention Program for Infants and Toddlers With Handicaps (Public Law 99-457—Final Regulations). 34 CFR Part 303, RIN 1820-AA49. Washington, DC, June 22, 1989
3. Meisels SJ, and the Expert Team on Screening and Assessment (National Center for Clinical Infant Programs, National Early Childhood Technical Assistance System): Guidelines for the Identification and Assessment of Young Disabled and Developmentally Vulnerable Children and Their Families (Draft). Washington, DC, December 20, 1988
4. Buros OK (ed): The Eighth Mental Measurements Yearbook. Gryphon Press, Highland Park, NJ, 1978
5. Stangler S, Huber C, Routh D: Screening Growth and Development: A Guide for Test Selection. McGraw-Hill, New York, 1980
6. Osofsky JD (ed): Handbook of Infant Development. John Wiley & Sons, New York, 1979
7. Bagnato SJ, Neissworth JT: Linking Developmental Assessment and Curricula: Prescriptions for Early Intervention. Aspen Systems Corporation, Rockville, MD, 1981
8. Lewko JH: Current practices in evaluating motor behavior of disabled children. Am J Occup Ther 30:413, 1976
9. Frankenberg WK, Dodds JB, Fandal AW et al: Denver Developmental Screening Test Reference Manual. LADOCA Project and Publishing Foundation, Denver, 1975
10. Knobloch H, Pasamanick B: Gesell and Amatruda's Developmental Diagnosis: The Evaluation and Management of Normal and Abnormal Neuropsychologic Development in Infancy and Early Childhood. Harper & Row, Hagerstown, MD, 1974
11. Sloan W: The Lincoln-Oseretsky Motor Development Scale. Genet Psychol Monogr 51:183, 1955
12. Roach E, Kephart N: Purdue Perceptual-Motor Survey. Charles E Merrill, Columbus, OH, 1966
13. Thorner R, Reimein QR: Principles and procedures in the evaluation of screening for disease. Public Health Monogr 67 (846), 1961
14. Frankenberg WK: Criteria in screening test selection. In Frankenberg WK, Camp BW (eds): Pediatric Screening Tests. Charles C Thomas, Springfield, IL, 1975
15. Anastasi A: Psychological Testing. 5th Ed. Macmillan, New York, 1982

16. Magnusson D: Test Theory. Addison-Wesley Publishing, Reading, MA, 1967
17. Prechtl HFR, Beintema D: The Neurological Examination of the Full Term Newborn Infant. Clinics in Developmental Medicine, No. 12. JB Lippincott, Philadelphia, 1964
18. Prechtl HFR: The Neurological Examination of the Full Term Newborn Infant. Clinics in Developmental Medicine, No. 63. JB Lippincott, Philadelphia, 1977
19. Brazelton TB: Neonatal Behavioral Assessment Scale. Clinics in Developmental Medicine, No. 50. JB Lippincott, Philadelphia, 1973
20. Dubowitz L, Dubowitz V: The Neurological Assessment of the Preterm and Full-Term Newborn Infant. Clinics in Developmental Medicine, No. 79. JB Lippincott, Philadelphia, 1981
21. Parmelee AH, Michaelis R: Neurological examination of the newborn. p. 7. In Hellmuth J (ed): Exceptional Infant. Vol. 2: Studies in Abnormalities. Butterworth, London, 1971
22. Prechtl HFR: Assessment methods for the newborn infant, a critical evaluation. p. 78. In Stratton P, Chichester J (eds): Psychobiology of the Human Newborn. John Wiley & Sons, New York, 1982
23. Prechtl HFR: The mother-child interaction in babies with minimal brain damage. In Foss BM (ed): Determinants of Infant Behavior II. John Wiley & Sons, New York, 1963
24. Beintema DJ: A Neurological Study of a Newborn Infant. Clinics in Developmental Medicine, No. 28. Heinemann, London, 1968
25. Prechtl HFR: Prognostic value of neurological signs in the newborn period. Proc R Soc Med 58:3, 1965
26. Prechtl HFR, Dijkstra J: Neurological diagnosis of cerebral palsy in the newborn. In tenBerge BS (ed): Prenatal Care. Noordhoff, Groningen, 1960
27. Als H, Tronick E, Lester BM et al: Specific neonatal measures: the Brazelton Neonatal Behavioral Assessment Scale. p. 185. In Osofsky JD (ed): Handbook of Infant Development. John Wiley & Sons, New York, 1979
28. Als H: Assessing an assessment: conceptual considerations, methodological issues and a perspective on the future of the NBAS. Monogr Soc Res Child Dev, ser 177 43(5–6):14, 1978
29. Tronick E, Brazelton TB: Clinical uses of the Brazelton Neonatal Behavior Assessment. p. 137. In Friedlander BZ, Sterritt GM, Kirk GE (eds): Exceptional Infant: Assessment and Intervention. Vol. 3. Brunner/Mazel, New York, 1975
30. DiVitto B, Goldberg S: The effects of newborn medical status on early parent-infant interaction. p. 311. In Field TM (ed): Infants Born at Risk. SP Medical and Scientific Books, New York, 1979
31. Goldberg S, Bachfield S, Divitto S: Feeding, fussing and play: parent-infant interaction in the first year as a function of prematurity and perinatal medical problems. In Field TM. High-risk Infants and Children. Academic, San Diego, 1980
32. Bakow H, Samaroff A, Kelly P et al: Relation between newborn and mother-child interactions at four months. Paper presented at the biennial meeting of the Society for Research in Child Development, Philadelphia, 1973
33. Stengel TJ: The Neonatal Behavioral Assessment Scale: description, clinical uses, and research implications. Phys Occup Ther Pediatr 1:39, 1980
34. Horowitz FD, Dunn M: Infant intelligence testing. p. 21. In Minifie FD, Lloyd LL (eds): Communicative and Cognitive Abilities: Early Behavorial Assessment. University Park Press, Baltimore, 1977
35. Lancioni GE, Horowitz FD, Sullivan JW: The NBAS-K. 1. A study of its stability and structure over the first month of life. Infant Behav Dev 3:341, 1980

36. Field TM, Dempsey JR, Hallock NH et al: The mother's assessment of the behavior of her infant. Infant Behav Dev 1:156, 1978
37. Widmayer SM, Field TM: Effects of Brazelton demonstrations on early interactions of preterm infants and their teenage mothers. Infant Behav Dev 3:79, 1980
38. St Clair KL: Neonatal assessment procedures: a historical review. Child Dev 49:280, 1978
39. Als H, Lester BM, Tronick EC, Brazelton TB: Manual for the Assessment of Preterm Infants' Behavior (APIB). In Fitzgerald HE, Lester BM, Yogman MW (eds): Theory and Research in Behavioral Pediatrics. Plenum, New York, 1982
40. Als H, Duffy FH: Neurobehavioral assessment in the newborn period: opportunity for early detection of later learning disabilities and for early intervention. In Paul NW, Golia SR (eds): Birth Defects Original Article Series (25:6). March of Dimes Birth Defects Foundation, White Plaines, NY, 1989
41. Als H, Lester BM, Tronick EC, Brazelton TB: Toward a research instrument for the Assessment of Preterm Infants' Behavior (APIB). In Fitzgerald HE, Lester BM, Yogman MW (eds): Theory and Research in Behavioral Pediatrics. Plenum, New York, 1982
42. Als H, Lawhon G, Brown E, et al: Individualized behavioral and environmental care for the very low birth weight preterm infant at high risk for bronchopulmonary dysplasia: neonatal intensive care unit and developmental outcome. Pediatrics 78:1123, 1986
43. Als H, Duffy FH, McAnulty GB: Behavioral differences between preterm and fullterm newborns as measured with the APIB system scores: I. Infant Behav Dev 11:305, 1988
44. Als H, Duffy FH, McAnulty GB: Preterm and fullterm behavior as assessed with the APIB: prediction to 3 years. (In preparation.)
45. Saint-Anne Dargassies S: Neurodevelopmental symptoms during the first year of life. I: Essential landmarks for each key-age. Dev Med Child Neurol 14:235, 1972
46. Dubowitz LMS, Dubowitz V, Goldberg C: Clinical assessment of gestational age in the newborn infant. J Pediatr 77:1, 1970
47. Dubowitz LMS, Levene MI, Morante A et al: Neurologic signs in neonatal intraventricular hemorrhage: a correlation with real-time ultrasound. J Pediatr 99:127, 1981
48. Graziani LJ, Korberly B: Limitations of neurological and behavioral assessments in the newborn infant. In Gluck L (ed): Intrauterine Asphyxia and the Developing Fetal Brain. Year Book Medical Publishers, Chicago, 1977
49. Casaer P, Akiyama Y: Is body posture relevant for neonatal studies? Acta Paediatr Belg 27:418, 1973
50. Brazelton TB, Koslowski B, Tronick E: Neonatal behavior among urban Zambians and Americans. J Acad Child Psychiatry 15:97, 1976
51. Bayley N: Bayley Scales of Infant Development. Psychological Corporation, New York, 1969
52. Knobloch H, Stevens F, Malone AF: Manual of Developmental Diagnosis. Rev Ed. Harper & Row, New York, 1980
53. Bruininks RH: Bruininks-Oseretsky Test of Motor Proficiency: Examiner's Manual. American Guidance Service, Circle Pines, MN, 1978
54. Miller LJ: Miller Assessment for Preschoolers. The Foundation for Knowledge in Development, Littleton, CO, 1982
55. Folio M, Fewell R: Peabody Developmental Motor Scales and Activity Cards. DLM Teaching Resources, Hingham, MA, 1983

56. Feldman AB, Haley SM, Coryell J: Concurrent and construct validity of the Pediatric Evaluation of Disability Inventory. Phys Ther 70:602, 1990

57. Bayley N: The California First-Year Mental Scale. University of California Press, Berkeley, 1933

58. Jaffa AS: The California Preschool Mental Scale. University of California Press, Berkley, 1934

59. Bayley N: The California Infant Scale of Motor Development. University of California Press, Berkeley, 1936

60. Bayley N: Consistency and variability in the growth of intelligence from birth to eighteen years. J Genet Psychol 75:165, 1949

61. Werner EE, Bayley N: The reliability of Bayley's revised scale of mental and motor development during the first year of life. Child Dev 37:39, 1966

62. Ramey CT, Campbell FA, Nicholson JE: The predictive power of the Bayley Scales of Infant Development and the Stanford-Binet Intelligence Test in a relatively constant environment. Child Dev 44:790, 1973

63. Honzik MP, Hutchings JJ, Burnip SR: Birth record assessments and test performance at eight months. Am J Dis Child 109:416, 1965

64. Berk RA: The discriminative efficiency of the Bayley Scales of Infant Development. J Abnorm Child Psychol 7:113, 1979

65. Coryell J, Provost B, Wilhelm IJ, Campbell SK: Stability of Bayley Motor Scale scores in the first year of life. Phys Ther 69:834, 1989

66. Harris SR: Early detection of cerebral palsy: sensitivity and specificity of two major assessment tools. Perinatology 7:11, 1987

67. Campbell SK, Siegel E, Parr CA et al: Evidence for the need to renorm the Bayley Scales of Infant Development based on the performance of a population-based sample of 12-month-old infants. Top Early Child Special Edu 6:83, 1986

68. Yarrow LF, Pederson FA: The interplay between cognition and motivation in infancy. p. 379. In Lewis M (ed): Origins of Intelligence: Infancy and Early Childhood. Plenum, New York, 1976

69. Gesell A: Infancy and Human Growth. Macmillan, New York, 1928

70. Gesell A, Thompson H, Amatruda CS: Infant Behavior: Its Genesis and Growth. McGraw-Hill, New York, 1934

71. Gesell A, Halverson HM, Ilg FL et al: The First Five Years of Life. Harper & Row, New York, 1940

72. Kirks A, McCarthy JJ, Kirk WD: Illinois Test of Psycholinguistic Abilities. Rev Ed. University of Illinois Press, Urbana, 1968

73. Roe KV: Correlations between Gesell scores in infancy and performance on verbal and non-verbal tests in early childhood. Percept Mot Skills 45(3, pt 2):1131, 1977

74. Doll EA (ed): The Oseretsky Tests of Motor Proficiency. Translation from the Portuguese (adaptation). American Guidance Service, Circle Pines, MN, 1946

75. Guilford JP: A system of psychomotor abilities. Am J Psychol 71:164, 1958

76. Cratty FJ: Movement Behavior and Motor Learning. Lea & Febiger, Philadelphia, 1967

77. Cratty BJ: Perceptual and Motor Development in Infants and Young Children. Macmillan, New York, 1970

78. Fleishman EA: The Structure and Measurement of Physical Fitness. Prentice Hall, Englewood Cliffs, NJ, 1964

79. Harrow AJ: Taxonomy of the Psychomotor Domain: A Guide for Developing Behavioral Objectives. David McKay, New York, 1972

80. Rarick GL, Dobbins DA: Basic Components in the Motor Performance of Ed-

ucable Mentally Retarded Children: Implications for Curriculum Development (Grant No. OEG-0-70-2568-610). US Office of Education, Washington DC, 1972

81. Sabatino DA: Test #174. In Mitchell JV (ed): The Ninth Mental Measurements Yearbook. University of Nebraska Press, Lincoln, 1985

82. Deloria DJ: Test #706. In Mitchell JV (ed): The Ninth Mental Measurements Yearbook. University of Nebraska Press, Lincoln, 1985

83. Slaton DA: The Miller Assessment for Preschoolers: A clinician's perspective. Phys Occup Ther Pediatr 5:65, 1985

84. Michael WB: Test #706. In Mitchell JV (ed): The Ninth Mental Measurements Yearbook. University of Nebraska Press, Lincoln, 1985

85. Miller LJ: An overview of the predictive validity of the Miller Assessment for Preschoolers. Dissertation abstract. Phys Occup Ther Pediatr 10:101, 1990

86. Hinderer KA, Richardson PK, Atwater SW: Clinical implications of the Peabody Developmental Motor Scales: a constructive review. Phys Occup Ther Pediatr 9:81, 1989

87. West Haverstraw Motor Development Test. New York State Rehabilitation Hospital, West Haverstraw, NY, 1964

88. Palisano R: Concurrent and predictive validities of the Bayley Motor Scale and the Peabody Developmental Motor Scales. Phys Ther 66:1714, 1986

89. Provost B, Harris MB, Ross K, Michnal D: A comparison of scores on two preschool assessment tools: implications for theory and practice. Phys Occup Ther Pediatr 8:35, 1989

90. Palisano RJ: Commentary. Phys Occup Ther Pediatr 10:1, 1990

91. Haley SM, Hallenborg SC, Gans BM: Functional assessment in young children with neurological impairments. Top Early Child Special Educ 9:106, 1989

92. Allen D: Measuring Rehabilitation Outcomes for Infants and Young Children: A Family Approach. Paul H Brooks Publishing, Baltimore, 1987

93. Newborg J, Strock J, Wnek L: Battelle Developmental Inventory. DLM Teaching Resources, Allen, TX, 1984

94. Mott S: Concurrent validity of the Battelle Developmental Inventory for speech- and language-disordered children. Psychol Schools 24:215, 1987

95. Guidubaldi J, Perry J: Concurrent and predictive validity of the Battelle Developmental Inventory at the first grade level. Educ Psychol Measure 44:977, 1984

96. Cole KN, Harris SR, Eland SF, Mills PE: Comparison of two service delivery models: in-class and out-of-class therapy approaches. Pediatr Phys Ther 1:49, 1989

97. Vulpe SG: Vulpe Assessment Battery: Developmental Assessment. Performance Analysis, Individualized Programming for the Atypical Child. National Institute on Mental Retardation, Toronto, 1977

98. Johnson-Martin N, Jens KG, Attermeier SM: The Carolina Curriculum for Handicapped Infants and Infants at Risk. Paul H Brookes Publishing, Baltimore, 1986

99. O'Donnell K, Ogle P: Teaching suggestions. p. 7. In Johnson-Martin N, Jens KG, Attermeier SM (eds): The Carolina Curriculum for Handicapped Infants and Infants At Risk. Paul H Brookes Publishing, Baltimore, 1986

100. Johnson-Martin NM, Attermeir SM, Hacker B: The Carolina Curriculum for Preschoolers with Special Needs. Paul H Brookes Publishing, Baltimore, 1990

101. Piper MC, Darrah J, Pinnell L et al: Alberta Infant Motor Scale (Preliminary Manual). University of Alberta Faculty of Rehabilitation Medicine, Edmonton, 1989

102. Chandler L, Andrews M, Swanson M: Movement Assessment of Infants. Infant Movement Research, Rolling Bay, WA, 1980

103. Russell D, Rosenbaum P, Cadman D et al: The Gross Motor Function Measure: a means to evaluate the effects of physical therapy. Dev Med Child Neurol 31:341, 1989
104. Miller LJ: Test development on the installment plan or "How I Developed a Test in 27,000 Easy Steps." p. 185. In Miller LJ (ed): Developing Norm-Referenced Standardized Tests. The Haworth Press, New York, 1989.

4 | The Neurologically Suspect Neonate

Irma J. Wilhelm

The role of the physical therapist in the care of high-risk neonates has been described by a number of therapists who are experienced in the special care nursery setting.[1] Neonatal practice requires preparation beyond that included in the basic physical therapy curriculum.[2] The Section on Pediatrics of the American Physical Therapy Association has published a set of guidelines/competencies for physical therapists planning to enter neonatal practice.[3]

One aim of this chapter is to provide the reader with background information about high-risk infants, their care and the settings in which care is delivered, and their neurodevelopmental outcome. A second purpose is to review some recent research on assessment and intervention with high-risk infants with the aim of gleaning from it general principles and rationales for use in physical therapy programs for these infants. Finally, some suggestions will be presented for physical therapists to consider in preparing for, developing, and evaluating therapeutic programs for high-risk neonates.

EVENTS CONTRIBUTING TO RISK FOR CENTRAL NERVOUS SYSTEM DYSFUNCTION

Clusters of antenatal and perinatal problems rather than single events, in combination with suboptimal socioeconomic and environmental conditions in infancy, contribute most to poor long-term developmental outcome.[4] In addition, even the most sensitive neonatal screening program will not identify all infants who will develop neuromotor dysfunction, as most cases of cerebral palsy (CP) do not come from recognizable high-risk groups.[5]

Low Birth Weight

Many infants born at extremely low birth weight (ELBW; <1,000 g) are now surviving. A decade ago, only approximately 25 percent of ELBW infants survived; today, over 50 percent survive.[6] The current theory is that technology probably cannot lower the biologic threshold for survival (now considered to be 23 weeks), but that improved technology will further increase the survival of ELBW infants more than 23 weeks of age.[6] These infants represent less than 1 percent of live births in the United States, but account for 60 percent of neonatal deaths and have a rate of severe handicap of approximately 30 percent.[6,7] The rate of handicap in these infants has not changed in the last 20 years, but the actual numbers of both handicapped and nonhandicapped survivors has increased because of the lowered neonatal mortality rate.[6] The actual fact of low birth weight is not the major contributor to later handicap; rather, low birth weight is a marker for factors operating before delivery that may contribute to premature labor and delivery and compromise the fetus before birth.[8]

Infants of ELBW are at high risk neonatally for multiple system disorders, including bronchopulmonary dysplasia (BPD), patent ductus arteriosis (PDA), sepsis, necrotizing enterocolitis (NEC), intraventricular hemorrhage (IVH), and retinopathy of prematurity (ROP).[6] Some of these conditions contribute to the increased risk in these infants for developing CP, seizure disorders, neurosensory disorders, and developmental delay. In addition, ELBW infants are subject to frequent rehospitalization for recurrent respiratory disorders and surgery; growth retardation (44 percent remain below the 10th percentile for weight and height); behavioral problems such as sleep disturbance, colic, temper tantrums, overactivity, and distractibility; and learning disabilities.[8–13] In one study, 36 percent of preterm infants required special educational services in preschool and school settings.[13] The two primary lesions contributing to neuropathology in premature infants, however, are periventricular leukomalacia (PVL) and periventricular hemorrhagic infarction (PVHI).[14] With the increasing use of cranial ultrasonography, these lesions are now better understood.

Periventricular Leukomalacia

Periventricular leukomalacia is necrosis of the cerebral white matter dorsal and lateral to the external angle of the lateral ventricles. Its incidence is 25 to 40 percent in very low birth weight (VLBW; <1,500 g) infants. The necrosis occurs in arterial border and end zone areas; very premature infants may also have secondary hemorrhage within the necrotic area.[14] Bilateral echodensities (flares) in the predilection sites or diffusely distributed in the periventricular white matter are the first signs of PVL on ultrasound scans. The flares either resolve or evolve into multiple small cysts 2 to 3 weeks after their appearance. After 1 to 3 months the cysts disappear, leaving enlarged ventricles expanded into the space left by the cysts, and decreased cerebral myelin.[14]

The periventricular region is particularly vulnerable to ischemia because arterial border and end zones are vulnerable to decreased perfusion pressure and decreased cerebral blood flow. Premature infants, especially ill ones, have pressure-passive cerebral circulation (lack of autoregulation of cerebral blood flow when systolic blood pressure falls). Hypotension occurs frequently in fragile premature infants as a result of perinatal asphyxia, myocardial failure, respiratory disease, sepsis, PDA, apnea and bradycardia, and handling during caretaking.[14]

Periventricular Hemorrhagic Infarction

Periventricular hemorrhagic infarction is most common in the very smallest premature infants and is, therefore, still new to the medical literature. It is characterized by a large region of hemorrhagic necrosis in the periventricular white matter that is usually either unilateral or bilaterally asymmetric. Eighty percent of PVHI lesions are associated with large IVHs and are sometimes incorrectly described as extensions of the IVH. The lesion is probably a venous infarction, as it follows the fan-shaped distribution of the medullary veins. It can be distinguished pathologically from secondary hemorrhage into PVL, but this difference cannot be detected clinically. On ultrasound, PVHI lesions appear as fan-shaped echodensities radiating from the external angle of the lateral ventricle. The echodensities evolve into single, large porencephalic cysts that rarely disappear over time. The pathogenesis of PVHI is not completely known. It may evolve from periventricular venous obstruction caused by IVH or germinal matrix hemorrhage, resulting in ischemia and infarction.[14]

Intraventricular Hemorrhage

Periventricular/intraventricular hemorrhage (PVH/IVH) is the most common neonatal intracranial hemorrhage (ICH) and is characteristic of the premature infant. With improved neonatal intensive care its incidence is decreasing in some neonatal centers, but it will remain a problem with increased survival of ELBW infants.[15,16] The overall incidence of IVH in premature infants is approximately 30 percent, but it can be over 70 percent in ELBW infants weighing less than 750 g at birth.[16]

The site of origin of PVH/IVH is the subependymal germinal matrix, ventrolateral to the lateral ventricles. In approximately 80 percent of cases, the hemorrhage spreads into the lateral ventricles and throughout the ventricular system. The neuropathology includes destruction of the germinal matrix and the glial precursor cells being formed there and posthemorrhagic hydrocephalus secondary to impaired cerebrospinal fluid absorption or ventricular outflow obstruction caused by the blood clot. Fifteen percent of infants with PVH/IVH also have PVHI, 75 percent may also have PVL, and 45 percent have pontine necrosis.[16]

The pathogenesis of PVH/IVH is both multifactorial and interactive and includes fluctuations of cerebral blood flow (CBF) reflective of fluctuating arterial blood pressure, and increased CBF reflecting abrupt increases in arterial blood pressure resulting from the pressure-passive state of the central circulation. Decreases in CBF are also dangerous, as fragile germinal matrix blood vessels can easily rupture on reperfusion.[16]

Since PVL and PVHI cannot be distinguished from each other clinically, outcome studies often do not provide specific results for each. Some characteristic outcomes, however, may serve to differentiate the two. The clinical correlate of severe PVL is usually spastic diplegia, sometimes with intellectual deficit. The lesion is located specifically in the area of motor tracts to motoneurons of lower extremity muscles and, when severe, may also damage posterior white matter subserving visual, auditory, and somesthetic association fibers.[14] The clinical correlate of PVHI is primarily spastic hemiparesis (or asymmetric quadriparesis) with intellectual deficit, because the larger lesion often involves motor tracts to arms as well as legs. In general, extensive ischemic lesions are associated with over 80 percent mortality and over 90 percent morbidity in the form of CP and intellectual deficit in survivors.[14] Transient echodensities (flares) are considered to be the mild end of the PVL/PVHI spectrum, but are still associated (especially if they persist more than 10 days) with signs of transient dystonia and neurologic sequelae. These children may also be at increased risk for later attentional and learning problems.[17]

Grades III and IV IVH are frequently associated with major neurologic sequelae (although grade IV IVH may actually be either PVHI or secondary hemorrhage into a PVL lesion).[18] The neurologic prognosis for infants with various combinations of ischemic and hemorrhagic brain lesions depends primarily on the amount of parenchymal damage and, to a lesser extent, on the occurrence of posthemorrhagic hydrocephalus and the extent of IVH. Intraventricular hemorrhage, however, frequently occurs in conjunction with parenchymal lesions and, therefore, may be a marker for cerebral insults of various kinds.[19,20]

These three primary lesions of the premature/ELBW infant may be preventable. Management of premature infants in which emphasis is placed on monitoring circulatory status and prompt correction of events that contribute to systemic hypotension and intraventricular hemorrhage could have a significant effect on reducing PVL and PVHI.[14,20]

Sepsis Neonatorum

Sepsis in the newborn infant is relatively rare (one to five per 1,000 live births), but is still a major cause of morbidity and mortality. Mortality is 30 to 50 percent and has not declined in the past two decades. The most common neonatal pathogens are *Escherichia coli*, group B streptococcus, *Staphylococcus epidermidis*, *Listeria monocytogenes*, and *Staphylococcus aureus*.[21] Most infants are infected near the time of delivery by swallowing amniotic fluid contaminated from maternal genital tract colonization. Viral infections are transmitted from mother to infant in the blood via the placenta. Nosocomial infections occur in 25 percent of infants who have lengthy hospital stays. Neurologic handicap occurs in approximately 35 percent, especially in those with meningitis.[21]

Neonatal Seizures

Neonatal seizures are the clinical manifestation of serious underlying neurologic disease and may cause additional brain injury.[22,23] Seizures are difficult to diagnose in the neonate, and new information from continuous electroencephalographic (EEG) monitoring with simultaneous observation provides some evidence for why this is so. Some observable motor and behavioral phenomena previously classified as seizures have no EEG correlates; conversely, some seizures identified electrographically have no observable behavioral alteration.[22,23] Clinically, nonepileptic motor activity usually increases with sensory stimulation (e.g., shows properties of temporal and spatial summation and irradiation), can be suppressed easily by gentle passive restraint, and has no accompanying autonomic phenomena.[22,23]

The prognosis of infants having neonatal seizures depends on the etiology and duration of the convulsions. Overall, about 45 percent have mild to severe disabilities (25 percent neuromotor, 20 percent sensory). Recurrent seizures occur in approximately 20 percent. The worst prognoses are for infants with tonic seizures (73 percent with major disabilities), seizures resulting from IVH (72 percent) or hypoxic-ischemic encephalopathy (HIE) (57 percent), and seizures lasting more than 3 days (66 percent).[24]

Respiratory Distress Syndrome and Chronic Lung Disease

The long-term sequelae of the common respiratory problems of ELBW infants are just beginning to be understood as greater numbers of ELBW survivors are observed developmentally through childhood. Most premature infants of ELBW develop some degree of respiratory distress syndrome (RDS) that results from a deficiency of pulmonary surfactant. The unopposed surface tension forces lead to alveolar collapse (atelectasis) and greatly increased work of breathing to re-expand collapsed alveoli.[25] Although RDS contributes significantly to neonatal mortality and morbidity, the long-term outcome of infants with mild to moderate RDS does not appear to differ greatly from that of healthy premature infants unless chronic lung disease develops.[26]

Chronic lung disease (CLD), the most well-known type being BPD, occurs primarily in premature infants who, as neonates, had severe RDS requiring mechanical ventilation and oxygen therapy.[27] The diagnosis is made when the infant's clinical lung disease persists, oxygen therapy is required longer than

28 days, and chest radiograms reveal cystic areas interspersed with radiodense strands. The incidence of BPD varies with maturity and birthweight, and ranges from about 3 to 65 percent of survivors of mechanical ventilation. The etiology of BPD is thought to be mechanical ventilation and oxygen therapy for RDS, both of which can injure the immature lung via barotrauma and toxic effects, respectively.[27] From 25 to 90 percent of infants with CLD survive at least 6 months, the rate varying with birth weight.

The sequelae of CLD are varied and multifocal. Respiratory sequelae are common and include frequent lower respiratory tract infections, respiratory failure, and continued abnormal chest radiography. Later in childhood, children have symptoms such as frequent upper respiratory infections, otitis media and wheezing, and evidence of airway obstruction and hyperinflation on pulmonary testing.[28,29] On exercise stress tests they demonstrate increased $tcPCO_2$ before exercise and at maximal work load, decreased minute ventilation at maximal O_2 consumption, fall in SaO_2 from pre-exercise to maximum work load, and exercise-induced bronchospasm (an indication of airway hyperreactivity).[29] The oldest survivors of CLD are just entering their second decade. Whether, as adults, they will be at increased risk for chronic obstructive pulmonary disease remains to be seen.[28]

Campbell and colleagues[30] identified two syndromes of neurologic disease in survivors of BPD. Infants with severe BPD developed intractable seizures and demonstrated progressive neurologic deterioration until they died of respiratory failure. Another group demonstrated nonprogressive neurologic disease associated with increased incidence of IVH, PVL, bronchospasm, acidosis, and decreased head growth. The rate of CP in CLD survivors is approximately 5 percent.[26] In addition, Perlman and Volpe[31] have identified a movement disorder syndrome in infants with severe BPD consisting of rapid, random, jerky movements of distal limbs similar to chorea in adults; extensor posturing of the neck; darting, thrusting tongue movements with intermittent wide mouth-opening; and lip puckering and chewing movements similar to oral-buccal-lingual dyskinesia in adults. The movements were increased during respiratory failure episodes, noise, and manipulation of trunk and limbs. Seizure disorders were ruled out. These investigators postulate basal ganglia injury resulting from the prolonged hypoxemia associated with severe BPD as the neurologic explanation for this disorder.[31]

Infants with CLD have increased risk for sudden infant death syndrome. Garg and associates[32] demonstrated that premature infants with BPD and RDS compared with full-term infants had significantly increased periods of severe oxygen desaturation that were not clinically evident (e.g., no apnea, bradycardia, or cyanosis). These desaturation episodes occurred in sleep and awake states; the highest incidence occurred during feeding. Garg et al.[33] reported that infants with clinically silent arterial oxygen desaturation episodes, when challenged with room air at PO_2 of 80 mmHg, demonstrated appropriate arousal responses, but all required vigorous stimulation and supplemental oxygen after the initial response.

Maternal Substance Abuse

Use patterns of alcohol, marijuana, and narcotics have not changed much in the past decade, but the use of cocaine and accompanying polydrug abuse is rapidly increasing.[34] At least 10 percent of women use cocaine at least one time during pregnancy, resulting in around 375,000 exposed neonates per year.[35] Because it is the most prevalent current form of drug abuse and because it seems to have the most potential for producing permanent neuromotor deficits in the offspring of users, this section will concentrate on the effects of maternal cocaine use as opposed to narcotic, alcohol, or nonnarcotic substance abuse.

Cocaine is highly water- and lipid-soluble and readily perfuses from maternal to fetal circulation. The immature fetal liver and kidneys metabolize cocaine slowly, because the fetus has decreased amounts of cholinesterases. The cocaine is metabolized to norcocaine, which is a highly active substance that easily penetrates the central nervous system (CNS). It is also not readily passed back to the maternal system for excretion and, when excreted by the fetus, can be reingested from the amniotic fluid. Cocaine prevents norepinephrine re-uptake at nerve terminals. The increased norepinephrine concentration in the blood produces peripheral and placental vasoconstriction, tachycardia, abrupt increase in blood pressure, probably in both mother and fetus, and increased uterine contractility.[35,36]

The immediate complications in cocaine-using pregnant women include increased incidences of abruptio placentae, spontaneous abortion, fetal death, premature delivery, and acute HIE. Neonates born to cocaine-using women frequently have intrauterine growth retardation, CNS irritability (tremors, startles, irritable behavior), tachypnea, and tachycardia. On neurobehavioral testing, infants demonstrate poor motoric and state control and orientation/interaction ability.[35,36] They often demonstrate abrupt state changes (beyond that expected for the level of stimulation being given) or maintain a very deep sleep and are unavailable for interaction. When awake, they are described as being hyperalert or in a "panicked awake" state.[35]

Cerebral infarction and intracranial hemorrhage have been documented by cranial ultrasound in infants exposed to stimulant drugs (cocaine and methamphetamine) in utero. The incidence of these lesions was equal to that expected in high-risk infants, even though the drug-exposed infants were otherwise normal. Thus, stimulant drugs may actually be a major cause of perinatal brain injury. The mechanism for the brain injury could be direct vasoconstriction of fetal cerebral vessels, or systemic circulatory failure or thromboembolism associated with placental vasoconstriction.[37] Longer-term effects include continued poor neurobehavioral regulation at 1 month of age (hyperexcitability, abrupt state changes, poor orientation); increased tremors, extensor tone, and persistent primitive reflexes at 4 months; and delayed motor milestones, slow movement, and increased lower extremity muscle tone at 8 months.[35]

MANAGEMENT

Since the 1960s, high-risk neonates have been cared for in modern perinatal care networks in most developed countries. These regionalized networks involve three levels of care: level I facilities are equipped for normal newborn care, transitional care for high-risk neonates awaiting transfer, and risk assessment; level II nurseries provide care for moderately ill neonates or those treated initially in a higher level facility who are now stable; and level III units provide neonatal intensive care and maternity care of the highest sophistication in life-support systems, specialized perinatal and maternal care personnel, and transport systems with units equipped to transport infants in utero and to treat neonates in transit. The regional center is responsible for ongoing education programs for personnel in the entire network.[38]

Routine Medical Care of High-Risk Neonates

A better understanding of the physiologic needs of high-risk infants has been translated into routines of care that are aimed at controlling many of the perinatal and neonatal risk factors commonly associated with poor immediate and long-term outcome, especially in ELBW, extremely premature infants. Some of these routines are preventive, some are diagnostic, and others are treatment oriented. They include identification of high-risk mothers, fetal monitoring during labor, and performance of cesarean sections when vaginal delivery is judged to be an additional risk factor. Premature labor can sometimes be arrested or, if preterm delivery seems inevitable, glucocorticoids can be given to decrease the risk of RDS in the neonate.[39]

When the high-risk infant is born, his or her physiologic parameters are continuously monitored electronically to enable prompt intervention should they indicate abnormalities. Transcutaneous monitoring and pulse oximetry serve to decrease the need for frequent blood sampling for laboratory analyses of blood gases and the problems associated with umbilical catheterization.[40–42]

Routine care also includes the use of prophylactic antibiotics, prompt initiation of intravenous feeding, respiratory support, and control of metabolic imbalances. As the infant's condition stabilizes, the infant is monitored closely for weight gain, begins oral feedings, and is weaned from ventilatory support, supplementary oxygen, and automatic temperature controls.

Ultrasonography is routinely used to visualize the brain of the neonate in a relatively noninvasive manner. The ultrasonography apparatus is portable and involves no ionizing radiation, so scans can be repeated frequently to monitor progression or resolution of the condition and the response to therapy.[19]

This impressive armamentarium of care is not without risk. In fact, some of the problems developed by high-risk infants are the result of the efforts aimed at ensuring their survival. Respiratory support has inherent risks, largely related to increased pressure to the lungs and blood vessels and to increased concentrations of oxygen. Continuous distending pressure or positive end-expiratory pressure therapy greatly increases the risk of air leaks. Both high airway pressure and prolonged oxygen therapy are associated with the development of BPD. Oxygen is also toxic to the retina if the arterial oxygen tension is allowed to go too high, resulting in ROP. The incidence of both BPD and ROP is increased in extremely premature ELBW infants.[27]

The use of phototherapy for reducing serum bilirubin levels may also have some side effects, such as diarrhea, abdominal distension, hypocalcemia, and increased insensible water loss, which require close monitoring. Phototherapy, therefore, should not be considered a "routine" procedure for minor elevations of bilirubin.[42]

Finally, the environment of the neonatal intensive care unit (NICU) itself may place an infant at increased risk for poor immediate or long-term outcome. The NICU environment is often one of continuous excessive noise (averaging between 50 and 85 dB) from machinery and personnel, and continuous, brilliant illumination (averaging 90 foot-candles) from overhead lighting and natural sunlight, or more (up to 400 foot-candles) when heat or phototherapy lamps are being used.[42,43] The light exposure may contribute to the development of ROP, and the excessive noise may contribute to hearing loss.[43,44] In addition, the sounds of human voices are muffled by isolettes, and the infant may not develop the ability to match sounds with faces.[45] The constant noise, light exposure, and interruptions for caregiving or medical procedures may contribute to sleep disturbance and sleep problems after discharge because little or no diurnal rhythmicity is introduced in the nursery.[42,45,46] High levels of routine handling for medical care are common, and gentle parental handling or social contact is minimal.[47] The most hypoxemia is evident with endotracheal suctioning and chest physical therapy.[45] Finally, learning opportunities are few because tactile/kinesthetic experiences are largely aversive, auditory experiences are disturbing or vague, meaningful visual experiences are minimal, contingent responses to infant-initiated actions are few, and interactions are mainly staff controlled.[45]

New Management Technology and Approaches

A number of new management techniques are currently being examined as the result of the desire to treat more aggressively the severe cardiorespiratory problems often experienced by ELBW infants and to minimize some of the environmental hazards of neonatal intensive care.

Surfactant Replacement Therapy

Exogenous surfactant replacement is currently undergoing controlled clinical trials in a number of medical centers.[25] Several types of preparations are being tested, including human surfactant isolated from amniotic fluid aspirated during cesarean sections of term pregnancies, bovine and porcine surfactants obtained from minced animal lungs or by lung lavage, and artificial surfactants made from synthetic compounds.[25]

In most of the clinical trial reports, the following results have been obtained in the treated groups when compared with comparable groups of untreated infants: improved neonatal survival, reduced severity of RDS as evidenced by need for lower levels of oxygen supplementation and lower ventilator settings, reduced incidence of air leaks, improved oxygenation in the first 72 hours, increased dynamic lung compliance and tidal volume, and radiographic evidence of lung clearance. The studies have produced mixed results relative to reduction of the incidences of CLD, ICH, NEC, ROP, and PDA,[48–51] with the greatest effects in the smallest, most immature infants.[48]

Some longitudinal data on later outcome of infants treated with surfactant replacement therapy are now available. In general, the researchers have concluded that the treatment has no adverse effects, but does not seem related to any improvements in developmental, respiratory nor neurologic outcome, or growth when treated infants are compared with controls at 1 to 2 years of age, but neither is the increased survival rate accompanied by an increased incidence of handicap.[52,53] Morley therefore recommends giving surfactant therapy prophylactically to all high-risk neonates because it has very few side effects and no complications.[48]

High-Frequency Ventilation

High-frequency ventilation (HFV) is a form of mechanical ventilation using rates that are often more than 900 breaths per minute (bpm) and extremely small tidal volumes (less than anatomic dead space). The exact mechanism for the gas transport is not known; it may be a form of augmented diffusion. At high frequencies, diffusion becomes the primary transport method even in upper airways which, in regular ventilation, takes place through convection.[54]

Three types of HFV are currently in clinical use and under study.[54,55] High-frequency, positive-pressure ventilation is produced by a conventional ventilator operating at 60 to 150 bpm with the aim of achieving gas exchange with low proximal airway pressures to decrease barotrauma, air leaks, and the infant's "fighting the ventilator" on expiration. High-frequency jet ventilation (HFJV) is produced by high-velocity pressurized gas delivered into the trachea or endotracheal tube through a small bore injector at frequencies of 150 to 600 bpm. High-frequency oscillatory ventilation (HFOV) is produced by airway vibrators (piston pumps or vibrating diaphragms) that move gas to and from the airways, producing positive and negative airway pressures at frequencies of 400 to 2,400 bpm.

Several reports of HFOV compared with conventional mechanical ventilation (CMV) with premature infants are available. Gerhardt and colleagues[56] reported no improvements in lung function measures or incidence of BPD in the HFOV-treated group. The HiFi Study Group[57] reported no improvements in BPD incidence or survival in the HFOV-treated group. They also reported that air leaks, grades III and IV IVH, PVL, and postextubation atelectasis were all increased in the HFOV-treated group. For these reasons, HFOV is not currently recommended for use with premature infants. The infants in this study were reassessed at 9 months of age.[58] No differences were noted in pulmonary function tests or any other measures of health in the HFOV- and CMV-treated infants. Both HFOV and HFJV are still experimental and cannot be used except in research protocols approved by the National Institutes of Health.[54]

Extracorporeal Membrane Oxygenator Therapy

Extracorporeal membrane oxygenator therapy (ECMO) is a method of oxygenation via a heart-lung bypass system that allows the lungs to rest and heal free from the iatrogenic effects of high oxygen and ventilator therapy. It requires catheter placements in the right jugular vein and right common carotid artery, which are permanently ligated, and anticoagulation therapy. Criteria for using ECMO are a gestational age of more than 34 weeks, severe respiratory failure in spite of maximal conventional ventilatory and medical support, and less than 20 percent chance of survival. The respiratory disease must be reversible within 10 to 14 days; therefore, ECMO is not useful with CLD, severe RDS in very immature infants, or congenital heart disease. It is also not recommended for infants with ICH or any bleeding disorder because of the need for anticoagulation. Its primary use is in infants with persistent pulmonary hypertension of the newborn.[59,60]

Over 80 percent of infants treated with ECMO survive, compared with 20 percent in comparable infants before ECMO was available and with infants treated with CMV.[59,60] Complications of the treatment include thromboemboli that develop in the membrane oxygenator bypass circuit, which is subjected to repeated changes in flow dynamics[61] and hemolysis from mechanical erythrocyte damage after blood-membrane contact or snagging and fragmentation on fibrin strands in clotted areas of the circuit.[62]

Long-term outcome of infants treated with ECMO is currently being closely monitored. Concerns are that ligation of the right common carotid artery and jugular vein might contribute to hemisyndromes, systemic anticoagulation might predispose to increased ICH and hemorrhagic infarction, and increased survival of hypoxic infants might increase the prevalence of handicaps.[60,63] At 1 to 2 years of age, the majority of children are normal in physical growth (86 percent) and neurologic outcome (60 to 75 percent). Developmental delay is evident in 15 to 20 percent (10 percent severe). Hemorrhagic infarcts are more common, especially in infants younger than 37 weeks' gestational age, but no evidence of hemisyndromes unrelated to documented cerebral lesions has been reported.[63-65]

Developmental/Environmental Neonatology and Individualized Care

Concerns about the effect of the NICU environment on the development of premature infant survivors have been fueled by reports of later developmental problems in the form of subtle neuromotor abnormalities, learning disabilities, and behavior problems in infants who appeared to be developmentally normal and without evidence of neurologic damage at the time of discharge from the special care unit.[66] Attempts to prevent these problems are beginning to be made in some NICUs based on the descriptive studies that have contributed information about the NICU environment and its effect on medical and developmental status of sick infants (environmental neonatology) and on studies of behavioral changes and progress of the neonate while in special care units (developmental neonatology).[45] Als[67] describes the need to provide a nurturing extrauterine environment in the NICU to ameliorate the mismatch between the intrauterine and extrauterine environment, with the primary consideration being protecting the immature, rapidly evolving brain and enhancing its development. The environment of the NICU can be manipulated to provide for improved oxygenation, reduced risk of IVH and hypoxemia, better utilization of nutrition, enhanced neurointegrative functioning, and more sensitive caretaking and parenting.[66]

These goals can be attained through such methods as primary nursing to develop and coordinate individualized caretaking plans, reducing noise and light levels and providing diurnal rhythmicity, clustering caregiving procedures to reduce sleep interruptions and unnecessary handling, positioning and motoric containment, titrating stimulation to reduce stress and enhance behavioral organization and learning opportunities, providing contingent responses to infant signals, and recognizing and managing personal stresses and emotional needs of premature parents and nursery staff.[45,46,66,68]

Als and associates[69,70] have begun to evaluate the outcome of infants who have received individualized neonatal developmental care compared with comparable groups receiving routine care while in the NICU. Their results to date with small groups of subjects have been encouraging. The individual care infants had fewer days of mechanical ventilation and supplemental oxygen therapy, fewer days of hospitalization, reduced incidence of IVH and severity of BPD, increased weight gain, required less time to attain complete breast or bottle feeding independence, and were younger at discharge. On later follow-up, individual care infants were more organized on all systems parameters of the Assessment of Premature Infant Behavior (APIB)[71] at 1 month of age, had higher Bayley Scales of Infant Development (BSID) scores at 3, 6, and 9 months, and displayed better functioning in many areas in a play situation paradigm (kangaroo box) at 9 months. These results suggest that an individualized approach to caregiving in the NICU emphasizing stress reduction and enhancing self-regulatory capacity may improve medical, developmental, and behavioral outcome in the first year of life.[69]

PHYSICAL THERAPY ASSESSMENT

The process of assessment includes selecting who to assess, determining when and what to assess, selecting the most appropriate tools, and considering what options are available for action following evaluation of the results.

Selection of Infants in Need of Assessment

Evidence of risk for poor outcome strongly suggests that the neuromuscular functioning of all infants who are of ELBW or have documented maternal substance abuse, periventricular infarction, intraventricular hemorrhage, major infection, neonatal seizures, or chronic lung disease should be assessed. The therapist may also want to document maternal and neonatal risk factors in a semiobjective way.

Several systems are available in which antepartum, intrapartum, and neonatal risk factors are assigned scores. These include the Problem-Oriented Perinatal Risk Assessment System developed by obstetricians following women with complicated pregnancies,[72] the Obstetric and Postnatal Complications Scales developed as part of a cumulative developmental assessment system to predict cognitive and affective performance,[73] the "optimality" concept developed by Prechtl[74] to assess the events of pregnancy and delivery, and the Fetal Biophysical Profile (FBP).[75] The FBP is used in conjunction with real-time ultrasonography to assess a combination of acute and chronic markers of fetal well-being (fetal body and breathing movements, tone, heart rate reactivity, and volume of amniotic fluid).[75]

Determining criteria for assessment can be done through consultation with the medical and nursing staff. A protocol can then be established that includes referral or blanket permission for assessment of infants meeting the predefined criteria.

Timing of Assessment

If the physical therapy assessment is to be of benefit to the high-risk infant, it should not contribute to that infant's risk for mortality or morbidity. In the same view, if the testing is to provide the physical therapist with useful information about the infant, it should not be done at a time when that infant is either too ill or unstable to respond, or at such an early stage of recovery that present status is unreflective of eventual outcome.

To assist in determining when best to initiate testing, some understanding of the developmental course in high-risk (especially premature) infants and the effects of handling is necessary. Als[66] conceptualized a synactive model of newborn neurobehavioral organization and development based on the concept of continuous interaction among subsystems and between organism and environment. Newborn assessment begins by observation of subsystem funtioning. The autonomic system is observable through respiratory rhythms, color changes, and visceral signals. The motor system is visible via posture, tone, and movement. The state organizational system is observed in patterns of state changes, range of available states, and differentiation and lability of states. The attentional/interactive system is reflected in the infant's ability to maintain a quiet, alert state while taking in stimulation from the environment and producing behaviors indicative of approach or exploration. The regulatory system can be observed in the maneuvers the infant uses to maintain or attain a relaxed, balanced condition, or the degree and type of assistance needed from the environment if the infant's regulatory capacity is exceeded. Because these subsystems are continuously interacting, imbalance or disorganization in one can produce imbalance in any of the others. Thus, the infant who is too ill or too immature to have autonomic stability will be unlikely to demonstrate normal motoric capacity on assessment, and the stress of the procedure could further compromise the already fragile autonomic system.

A number of investigators have documented that high-risk neonates may react negatively to relatively benign caretaking procedures and extremely negatively to painful procedures.[76,77] Of particular interest in the context of assessment is the work of Sweeney,[78,79] who studied the physiologic and behavioral effects of handling on neonates during neurobehavioral testing with the Neurological Assessment of the Preterm and Full-term Newborn Infant.[80] Sweeney reported that both low-risk preterm and full-term neonates showed some physiologic destabilization during testing, but that the preterm group had significantly more, as measured by increased heart rate, respiratory rate, and blood pressure, poor skin color, increased behavioral evidence of stress (finger splay, arm salute, hiccups, yawns), and decreased amount of quiet sleep and active alert states. Both groups demonstrated more stress reactions during the neuromuscular portion of the examination than during the neurobehavioral portion.[2,79] Sweeney concluded that the benefit of neuromotor assessment for high-risk, unstable infants is highly questionable because even low-risk, stable premature infants showed some evidence of stress.[79]

One should use a transcutaneous monitor or a pulse oximeter during testing and be thoroughly instructed in their use and in ways to modify procedures to minimize physiologic stress. Even if the neonate demonstrates some degree of physiologic stability, observation of motor function may be misleading. Premature infants are frequently unable to modulate their motor responses, which tend to be tremulous and jerky, spread to involve the entire motor system from a single stimulus, and are repeated over and over until the infant is exhausted. Or, the musculature may be so weak that a response is inadequate or greatly delayed. Any of these responses can occur in a neurologically uncompromised preterm infant.[81] The initial assessment may, therefore, have questionable value for future prediction, but does serve to describe the current status of the infant as a baseline on which to judge recovery.

Scope of Assessment

Ideally, the neonatal assessment should serve three major purposes: to measure the process and extent of the infant's recovery from perinatal stress, to assess the current status of neurobehavioral organization, and to predict future functioning. From these purposes can be derived several principles of neonatal assessment. One is that assessment must be repeated at a number of points in time in order to document the recovery process; another is that assessment instruments must be sensitive enough to allow discrimination of neurobehavioral deviations most likely to result in significant impairment of future functioning.

In the neonatal period, the physical therapist would seem uniquely qualified to assess neuromuscular maturation and motoric functioning, identify musculoskeletal abnormalities, evaluate oral–motor function, and assess the need of the infant for therapeutic intervention or long-term follow-up. As the infant matures, the physical therapist will provide ongoing expertise in assessing the level and quality of neuromuscular development as well as the need for initiation, continuance, or termination of therapeutic intervention.

Neonatal Assessment Methods

The next step in the evaluation process is the selection of the assessment methods and instruments that will contribute most to meeting the goals of assessment. A number of the available neonatal testing instruments and strategies are discussed in Chapter 3.

Neurobehavioral Assessment

Typically, newborn assessment results do not successfully predict the eventual developmental outcome of a child.[82] Als et al.,[81] however, believe that this reflects a measurement problem rather than a true developmental discontinuity. These investigators state that if broad constructs are assessed that reflect developmentally appropriate organizational issues, continuity will be found between newborn and later functioning. The broad constructs measured in neonatal neurobehavioral tests are newborn competence and behavioral organization.

Because serial tests are necessary in newborn assessment, a sequence of tests based on similar constructs is suggested for assessing high-risk neonates at different stages of their neonatal care. In the NICU, while the infant is still on life-support systems, the appropriate assessment is one requiring no handling, such as the naturalistic observation system that is part of the Neonatal Individualized Developmental Care and Assessment Program (NIDCAP).[83] The NIDCAP checklist of behavioral observations is used to assess the infant's responses before, during, and after a caregiving event or procedure. The observation then forms the basis for caregiving suggestions and environmental modifications designed to avoid stress and enhance the development of emerging capabilities.[69,83] When the infant is more stable, the Dubowitz' examination[80] can be used. Its neuromuscular sections are adapted from the work of the French neurologists[84-86] and it also incorporates some neurobehavioral items adapted from the Brazelton Neonatal Behavioral Assessment Scale (BNBAS).[87] The Neonatal Neurobehavioral Examination[88] is a similar test that can be used at this stage. It consists of items from the French method,[84] the Dubowitz examination,[80] the BNBAS,[87] and a number of primitive reflexes rated on a three-point scale.

A more comprehensive examination is recommended on which to base discharge planning. The APIB[71] is the most comprehensive assessment of newborn behavior available. It does, however, require a great deal of training to attain reliability certification and is a lengthy test to score. Once learned, however, its results are valuable for consulting with parents and other health professionals who will be caring for the infant after discharge. The BNBAS can also be used for discharge planning, if the infant has attained a postconceptual age of 37 weeks and is medically stable. It contains some supplementary items which, along with the Kansas supplements,[89] are useful for describing the high-risk infant who has reached term-equivalent age. The BNBAS requires slightly less time to administer than the APIB and much less time to score. Training and certification are also highly recommended for clinical use of the BNBAS.

Oral–Motor Assessment

To assess the adequacy of the high-risk neonate's oral functioning, the therapist must have a thorough understanding of oral–motor development and normal oral functioning in infancy. A discussion of these topics is beyond the scope of this chapter, but a number of excellent resources are available for the interested reader.[90-94]

The oral–motor assessment must include feeding time requirements; tactile responsiveness of the mouth and facial area; oral reflexes; tongue position and mobility; coordination of breathing, sucking, and swallowing; jaw structure and stability; facial musculature balance; feeding behaviors; response to handling and positioning for feeding; amount of nourishment ingested; and an estimate of the energy required to complete a feeding.[90,91]

The Neonatal Oral–Motor Assessment Scale (NOMAS)[95] shows promise as a semiobjective observational method to assess neonatal tongue and jaw movements during nutritive (NS) and non-nutritive sucking (NNS). The NOMAS and its revised version[96,97] have been shown to distinguish infants with normal sucking from those with some disorganization and those with definite dysfunction, to identify infants whose nurses have reported poor feeding abilities, and to distinguish inefficient from efficient feeders on the basis of oral intake.[95,96]

The final stage of evaluation, that of determining what action should occur as the result of the assessments, may lead to a number of options. *Option one* might be to delay extensive assessment if the infant is too ill or physiologically unstable for testing to be both safe and meaningful. *Option two* might be to plan for a series of assessments if the initial assessment was, in some way, inconclusive or unsatisfactory, the infant demonstrated some questionable responses on initial testing, or the infant demonstrated no questionable functioning on initial evaluation, but sustained subsequent events that would again place the infant at increased risk of CNS dysfunction. Finally, *option three* might be to initiate an intervention program. Those infants who are selected for testing and show cumulative medical, neurologic, and neurobehavioral evidence of deviant maturation or function may benefit from therapeutic intervention aimed at enhancing the recovery process and preventing or minimizing some of the sequelae of perinatal or neonatal complications.

THERAPEUTIC INTERVENTION

Support for the need of intervention with high-risk neonates stems from the numerous studies demonstrating that premature and other high-risk neonates are much more likely to have later developmental problems in almost every area of function than are full-term, low-risk neonates, especially if they are raised in environments with nonoptimal stimulation, such as may be the case in low socioeconomic situations or discordant families.[35,98] These developmental problems stem primarily from two sources: reproductive casualties (infants with medical and physiologic problems stemming from their immaturity or illness that affect later development) and caretaking casualties (infants raised in environments, including the NICU, that are not adequate for fostering normal development).[98,99]

The rationales underlying the various intervention programs for high-risk neonates stem from differing views of the premature infant and the NICU environment. If the premature infant is viewed as an extrauterine fetus, intervention is aimed at mimicking the intrauterine environment. If the premature infant is viewed as an inadequately functioning neonate, intervention is focused on stimulation paradigms. Some investigators consider the special care nursery environment to be one of deprivation of normal sensory input requiring sensory enrichment, while others view it as one of sensory overload requiring decreased input to infants. Still others view it as discordant and strive to introduce rhythmicity and contingency.[98–101] Running throughout are the concepts of plasticity and critical or sensitive periods. Inappropriate inputs or sensory deprivation can damage the CNS, so the CNS should be protected and intervention should take place while the CNS is still plastic enough to adapt to appropriate inputs.[66,98]

Few studies of intervention designed specifically to improve motor control of high-risk neonates have been reported in the literature. In intervention studies designed to improve other areas of development, information on the effects of the programs on neurologic, neuromuscular, or motoric functioning is somewhat sparse.[98] The typical intervention program has as its model the relatively healthy, preterm infant who is not typical of the critically ill, neurologically suspect infant being followed by physical therapists in special care nurseries. The studies may be excluding those infants most in need of early intervention.[102] In addition, many evaluative studies of the effects of early intervention have a number of methodologic problems that limit the interpretation, understanding, and generalizability of their results. They also contain a great deal of variability in methods, which makes comparing studies difficult.[98–102] Still, some theoretic background, rationale, and principles for effective intervention and some areas of focus for intervention with high-risk neonates by physical therapists can be construed from these works. Particularly relevant for the field of physical therapy are reports of the effects of intervention on growth, behavioral state and activity levels, and motor development and control.

Effects on Growth

Postconceptional weeks 24 to 44 are characterized by rapid growth in many systems with concomitant increased nutritional requirements. If those weeks are spent ex utero, the problem is confounded by the premature infant's increased caloric needs to combat cardiorespiratory and other problems of prematurity. The most serious problem is suboptimal head growth (microcephaly secondary to inadequate brain growth).[103] Sick premature infants have a typical triphasic pattern of head growth characterized by an initial phase of suboptimal growth, a phase of catch-up growth, and a phase of growth along standard curves.[104] Neonatal illness is characterized by a period of caloric deprivation below the minimum necessary for head growth. Persistent suboptimal head growth is associated with poor developmental outcome.[104]

Interventions introduced after the complications of prematurity are resolved should include programs to enhance growth. Investigators have reported increased weight gain in experimental groups in studies of tactile/kinesthetic stimulation,[98,102,105] NNS,[102] and vestibular/proprioceptive stimulation.[98,100,106,107] Woodson and Hamilton[108] suggest two possibilities to explain increased weight gain: increased numbers of calories extracted from diet or decreased numbers of calories used in nongrowth processes. Some research with NS and NNS supports the first mechanism. Enhanced rates of NS and increased volume of formula ingested were reported in groups of high-risk neonates during feeding conditions in which perioral stimulation was given.[109,110] Non-nutritive sucking opportunities for premature infants during and following tube feedings resulted in earlier attainment of bottle feeding, fewer tube feedings, earlier discharge, and more rapid weight gain in the experimental group compared with a control group that did not suck.[111] In a recent study, however, Ernst and associates[112] reported no effect on weight gain of NNS during gavage feeding in a group of VLBW infants.

Effects on Behavioral State and Activity Level

Premature infants typically use a lot of energy in poorly coordinated, poorly inhibited motor activity. Their sleep states are, in general, more active than those of the full-term infant, and they spend more time in active than in quiet sleep. They have wide-ranging, uncoordinated, and continuous movements, difficulty maintaining motoric control while attending to other events, and inability to inhibit motor activity once it is elicited.[81] This suggests that intervention designed to enhance quiet states and to decrease activity levels may be beneficial to the infant's growth and development.

Woodson and Hamilton[108] suggest that the effect of NNS on state and activity level may partially explain the association with weight gain noted in most studies. They demonstrated that NNS is associated with significantly decreased heart rate (an indirect measure of nongrowth energy expenditure). Non-nutritive sucking has also been shown to have a pacifying effect and to be associated with decreased restlessness.[113,114]

Vestibular input provided by waterbeds, hammocks, and rocking isolettes has consistently been associated with decreased jitteriness and irritability, increased quiet sleep, decreased active sleep and active alert states, decreased movement, and decreased avoidance and increased approach behaviors.[98,100,115,116] Waterbed use has also been associated with decreased severity of neonatal abstinence syndrome, decreased irritability, and decreased activity during sleep in infants exposed prenatally to narcotics.[107]

Positioning also has effects on behavioral state and activity level. A number of studies have demonstrated decreased wakefulness and crying and increased quiet sleep when high-risk infants are positioned in the prone compared with the supine position.[117–119]

Another recent addition to preterm infant care is skin-to-skin contact, often referred to as *kangaroo care*.[120,121] In this method, naked infants are held directly against the parents' bodies, at about a 60-degree angle from upright. Some of the benefits described in the research on this approach are enhanced regular sleep, decreased crying, and maintenance of adequate temperature and oxygenation.[121]

Tactile stimulation may be somewhat more arousing in nature. In a number of studies and reviews, neonatal massage or stroking regimes have been associated with increased time spent awake, alert, and active; muscle tension; range of states exhibited; and heart and respiratory rates.[100,102,122]

Effects on Motor Development and Control

The preterm infant must be assisted to maintain appropriate postures, as the infant is at the mercy of gravity and has great difficulty changing position and maintaining a flexed posture.[123] The preterm infant is at risk for developing "nursery-acquired positional malformations," including elevated and retracted scapulae; abducted shoulders and flexed elbows (W position of upper extremities); flexed, abducted, and externally rotated hips ("frog" position of lower extremities); neck hyperextension with scapular elevation, especially in infants immobilized for long periods of time for mechanical ventilation; and a generally hyperextended posture of the entire body when hypertonia is severe.[124] If uncorrected, these positional problems can persist. Positioning is necessary to counteract these influences and should be directed toward facilitating flexion of trunk and limbs, symmetric postures, and midline orientation. Infants should be placed in the prone or sidelying position whenever possible to decrease the tendency toward extension and abduction of the trunk and extremities. The results of published research suggest that placing high-risk infants in prone or lateral positions carries little, if any, risk and may benefit the infant physiologically as well as behaviorally, as the prone position is also conducive to regular respiration and improved oxygenation.[117,125–128]

Performance on developmental tests is frequently reported as enhanced in infants receiving various forms of neonatal intervention. Tactile/kinesthetic stimulation has been associated with enhanced performance in habituation, orientation, motor functions, and range of state clusters of the BNBAS,[102,105] as well as with higher BSID scores at later ages.[100,102,105] Similar associations with improved developmental test performance have been reported for vestibular/proprioceptive stimulation[98,99] and multimodal forms of intervention,[100] including individualized contingent care programs and programs that included the parents in the intervention.[69,129,130] Vestibular stimulation (rocking isolette) has also been associated with improved movement and tone, reflex, and neurobehavioral performance on the Dubowitz' neurologic examination.[106]

Neonatal hydrotherapy[131] is recommended for infants with muscle tone abnormalities resulting in excessive extension in neck, trunk, or extremities and limitation of joint motion; and for infants with behavioral state abnormalities such as intolerance to handling. Benefits of hydrotherapy are cited as decreased extensor tone, increased spontaneous movement, and improved orientation, interaction, and feeding.

The efficacy of physical therapy based on Neurodevelopmental therapy (NDT) principles for infants at risk for developmental disability was evaluated in a controlled, clinical trial by Piper et al.[132] with 115 VLBW and neurologically suspect infants who were survivors of neonatal intensive care. After 1 year of treatment, the treated and untreated groups did not differ on the outcome assessments, which included tests of gross motor, general development, and reflex integration, neurologic assessment, and growth measures. In addition, no longer-term effects were evident when the infants were re-examined at the age of 24 months.[133] The major determinant of poor outcome was a birth weight of less than 750 g. The ELBW children consistently performed more poorly than the heavier children on all measures. One possible explanation for the lack of treatment effects is that very few children in either the treated or untreated group were actually disabled. Another is that the outcome measures may not have been sensitive enough to pick up effects of treatment. That possibility is supported to some extent by the work of Girolami, who examined the effects of NDT on motor control in infants with suspect motor performance at 34 weeks' postconceptional age.[134] Preterm infants who received NDT 14 to 28 times during a 7- to 17-day period while in the special care nursery demonstrated improved performance on a supplemental test specifically designed to assess motor control, when compared with a preterm comparison group that received handling without the specific NDT component. No differences between the two groups were evident on a general neurobehavioral test, the BNBAS.

In summary, the intervention research suggests that as long as intervention is not overly vigorous with fragile infants, almost all modalities appear to have some beneficial effects, although much work is needed on developing the appropriate tools to measure those effects. A number of motor developmental goals may be attainable through neonatal intervention, including (1) improved growth through interventions for oral–motor control, behavioral state regulation, and reduction of nongrowth-related activity; (2) prevention of postural deformities by positioning and activities to reduce joint immobility; (3) general developmental enhancement through individualized programs designed to reduce stress and enhance emerging developmental tasks; and (4) enhancement of motor control through programs of hydrotherapy and therapeutic handling, as well as control of behavioral state.

In addition to these suggestions, several other points are mentioned in the literature that can serve to guide methods of treatment. Intervention programs appear to enhance development more readily when both infants and caretakers are active participants and when nursery intervention is followed by a home-based program with continued individualized care.[100,102,130] The effects of intervention may go undetected if only short-term measures are used, as the early intervention may set up transactional effects that appear later.[99]

Precautions in Therapeutic Intervention

Although the potential benefits of therapeutic intervention have been cited, the risks must also be considered. Sweeney and Chandler[2] list a number of risks during physical therapy assessment and treatment of high-risk neonates, including fractures, dislocations, and joint effusions during joint mobilization; apnea, bradycardia, and hypothermia during handling for movement therapy; regurgitation or aspiration during oral–motor therapy; and propagation of infection. Others warn of subtle and gross distress during chest physical therapy and close social interaction,[135] apnea and bradycardia during feeding,[136] and increased heart and respiratory rates during tactile/kinesthetic stimulation.[137]

Kelly and associates,[138] for example, reported no changes in oxygen saturation, but increases in heart rate in 14 stable preterm infants at 34 to 38 weeks' postconceptional age during a developmental physical therapy program. The heart rate increase was considered a normal "exercise effect." Several infants, however, had a decrease in SaO_2 during the postexercise recovery period.

These reports are evidence that monitoring the physiologic responses of infants during assessment and treatment is mandatory, and should be extended through the postactivity recovery period to be sure that later destabilization does not go unnoticed.

Follow-up of the High-Risk Infant

Diagnosis of definite CNS dysfunction is rarely possible during the period of critical illness. When the infant is medically stable, early signs of dysfunction may be predictive of eventual prognosis. As the infant matures, subtle signs may appear that were previously masked by the initial perinatal problems or that become evident as more complex behaviors develop.

Just before the infant is discharged, the therapist may wish to repeat a "risk assessment" to select those infants most in need of continued developmental follow-up. A number of researchers suggest that extremely important prognosticators for eventual outcome are the speed and degree to which the infant responds to the management provided in the special care setting,[80] the persistence of deviant signs beyond the neonatal period,[139] and the cumulative effects of perinatal and later nonoptimal events.[73] The therapist, armed with the results of a series of assessments during the infant's nursery stay, should be able to identify infants who consistently demonstrated poor performance, responded poorly to intervention, and suffered a large number of perinatal insults. Arrangements for continued assessment and treatment of these infants must be explored if they are not followed within the same facility. Typically, most tertiary care facilities maintain follow-up clinics to which high-risk neonates are referred for specified lengths of time and which employ developmental therapy personnel. Those infants who reside a great distance from the referral hospital may need specific referral to a developmental facility in their home community.

A number of tools for assessment of the older infant are discussed in Chapter 3 and will not be reiterated here. Several new tools have recently been reported or cited in the literature that may also prove useful to assess the early development of special care nursery graduates. These tools are discussed below.

The Infant Neurological International Battery,[140,141] an instrument for assessing the neurologic integrity of infants from birth through 18 months' postconceptional age, is based on the Milani-Comparetti examination,[142] the French "angles" method,[143] primitive reflex assessment,[144] and the standard pediatric neurologic examination.[145] It was developed particularly for use in follow-up programs for neonatal intensive care.[140]

The Infant Motor Screen[146,147] is a screening tool for assessing the quality of movement patterns and motor milestones in infants aged 4 to 16 months. Its purpose is to identify infants in need of referral for comprehensive neuromotor evaluation to rule out cerebral palsy. It is adapted from the Milani-Comparetti examination[142] and the Movement Assessment of Infants (MAI).[148]

The Posture and Fine Motor Assessment of Infants[149,150] is a test of the quality of motor function in infants at a developmental age between 2 and 6 months. Its fine motor section is based on the observations of Touwen,[151] Kopp,[152] Gesell et al.,[153] and Erhardt.[154] The posture section is based on the MAI[148] and the Test of Motor and Neurological Functions.[155]

The Test of Sensory Functions in Infants[156,157] is designed to quantify sensory processing dysfunction in infants 4 to 18 months of age. The items were generated from domain specifications of tactile and vestibular functions considered important in early sensory experience and relevant for later learning and emotional behavior. These are reactivity to tactile deep-pressure and vestibular stimulation, adaptive motor responses, visual–tactile integration, and ocular–motor control.

A major question is likely to be "How soon can we be sure that physical therapy is indicated"? This question stems from a limited amount of information about the typical course of development in infants who have sustained significant perinatal insults. The studies of their eventual outcome do not usually provide descriptions of the developmental behavior that occurred between the neonatal period and the age of outcome assessment. Do high-risk infants have delayed attainment of developmental milestones, delayed integration of automatic responses, or delayed appearance of postural reactions? In a prospective, longitudinal study, Campbell and Wilhelm[158] reported that unevenness in standardized motor test scores can be expected throughout the first year, but that 1- and 2-year motor outcome in infants at very high risk for poor outcome was correlated with BSID scores at as early as 3 months of age. Harris[159] reported that increased risk scores in all sections of the MAI at 4 months were predictive of CP at 36 months.

The decision as to when to initiate intervention in the older high-risk infant must be judiciously made. The results of assessments may show tremendous variability in the first year or two of life in infants whose outcome will be normal, yet early deviations can also predict later poor motor performance.[133,160,161] In addition, early motor deviations may be predictive of later nonmotoric problems, such as the generalized developmental delay typical of the child with mental retardation. Deviant early motor assessment results, therefore, should not be used to label a child with a diagnosis of motoric dysfunction, but rather as warning signs requiring careful follow-up of the child's total development.

PARENT INVOLVEMENT

In recent years, the special care nursery has been made increasingly more accessible to parents and close relatives of high-risk neonates. They are encouraged to visit early and frequently, to make contact with their infants, and to take part in their care when possible.[99,162] If parents are encouraged to visit and participate in their high-risk neonate's program, special care nursery personnel must be alert to their needs and aware of the family dynamics involved.[66,163] Chapter 12 provides more information on this topic.

Campbell[164] reminds us that high-risk pregnancy and delivery occurs more frequently in families already under stress (economically, socially, health-wise). These families are less prepared than others to handle the added stress of a sick or fragile baby. Parents may need to go through a grieving process for the loss of a healthy baby.[163] Parents also use defense mechanisms as ways to cope with distress. These mechanisms are described by O'Donnell as "crazy things sane people do to stay sane in crazy situations."[165] Thus, parents may be paralyzed with fear that the baby will die, deny or repress knowledge of the seriousness of the infant's condition, be very angry and wanting to place blame somewhere, and feel guilty about having produced an unhealthy child. During these phases, they may be unable to respond to staff explanations or instructions for caretaking, to make decisions, or to interact with their infant.[66,163,165] Staff must be understanding, accepting, and nonjudgmental as parents display these behaviors.

Als[66] suggests that parenting is a gradual letting go process in normal circumstances, but that for parents of high-risk infants the process of letting go is abrupt, complete, and out of the parents' control. These parents need to be helped to "regain" their infant while the infant is in special care. They can be helped to develop confidence in caregiving and understanding of their infant's unique characteristics, behavioral cues, and competencies. This phase should be well under way before the infant is sent home to avoid the common parental practice of overprotection.[66] A particular problem is introduced if staff and parents compete for the care of the infant. Staff may have to become more accepting of less-than-perfect parents; to be too critical of the parents' attempts at interacting with their infant can be devastating to their emerging confidence.[66] A number of possibilities exist for guiding parents. Parent support groups, frequent communications with the baby's nurses, physicians, and therapists, printed materials and videotapes about high-risk babies and caretaking, and regular individualized review and feedback on their performance and the infant's changing capabilities are often used.[164]

Neonatal behavioral tests such as the BNBAS and APIB have been used as interventions to demonstrate to parents of high-risk infants their infant's unique capabilities, to increase their perceptions and awareness of their infant's behaviors, to decrease their anxiety, and to facilitate their interactions with the infant.[100,166–168] Success in these areas has been reported with parents of preterm infants, as well as with parents at risk because of poor socioeconomic conditions.

During the period of posthospitalization follow-up, the physical therapist can contribute a great deal to education of parents and other family members. Because many preterm infants are discharged to their parents before or very close to their expected birth dates, families should be made aware of some of the basic differences in appearance, behavior, and functioning between preterm infants reaching 40 weeks' postconceptional age and infants born at term.[169–171] As the child matures, if a disability is diagnosed, parents must be helped to cope with this new problem and guided to seek appropriate therapeutic help. Such support and follow-up should continue at least through the preschool years, as problems in school readiness, disorders of attention, and learning disability may become evident in infants approaching school age.

STAFF EDUCATION

The contribution of physical therapists to the care of the high-risk neonate is not complete unless it includes a contribution to the ongoing education of their colleagues. Most level II and III special care nurseries are located in facilities in which ongoing postgraduate education is an integral part of the institution's program. The physical therapist must participate in this educational program both as a learner and a teacher.

This implies that the therapist must become an integral member of the nursery team, not just receive referrals for treatment of individual infants. Participation in nursery rounds, inservice education programs, on-the-job training programs, individual consultations, staff conferences, and ongoing research projects provides avenues for staff education to supplement daily presence in the nursery for assessment and intervention. Before a physical therapy program is initiated, the therapist should perform a needs assessment to determine the needs for direct care, environmental modifications, parent involvement and education, consultation, staff education, team participation, and discharge planning. A formal protocol should be developed that outlines the purposes and goals of the service; referral mechanisms and criteria; administrative mechanisms; job descriptions; direct, team, and consultative services to be provided; and methods to ensure accountability.[164]

Therapists tend to assume that special care nurses, because they are in constant attendance in the nursery, are available and eager to carry out daily therapy programs. This assumption should be critically evaluated, not taken for granted. Nurses are subject to an almost impossible set of demands. The full-time routine nursing care of the very sick neonate demands a huge proportion of their time and emotional energy. This is complicated by the constant need to be ready to respond to life-threatening crises, admissions at any time of the day or night, transport system coverage, the needs of visiting parents, and other interruptions.[172] Small wonder that some may offer resistance to the suggestion that they must also be responsible for programs of developmental therapy. Physical therapists must be practical, innovative, realistic, and, most of all, available if they are to gain the support of nursing colleagues. They must carefully evaluate what care can reasonably be given by the nurses and be innovative about incorporating developmental care into the nursery routine.

Last, but definitely not least, to gain acceptance as valued special care nursery team members, physical therapists must be accountable for their programs. The fact that very little evidence exists of the effectiveness of physical therapy with high-risk neonates should be acknowledged and every effort made to remedy this situation. Some ways to establish accountability are to develop protocols for standardized methods of collecting patient data during treatment and long-term follow-up, establish therapeutic goals that can be objectively measured, and contribute to the professional knowledge base through participation in planning and conducting clinical research at whatever level one's education permits. This includes publishing one's results in the professional literature or presenting them at scientific meetings, whether these be well-documented case reports, single-subject experiments, or the results of more formal research. To this end and to ensure the safety of their practice in the intensive care nursery environment, physical therapists must undergo extensive preparation for nursery practice.

PREPARATION FOR SPECIAL CARE NURSERY PRACTICE

Neonatal physical therapy, as a subspeciality of general pediatric physical therapy, requires advanced-level knowledge and clinical skills.[2,3] The minimal requirements to enter neonatal practice are 2 to 3 years in general pediatric practice, specialized training in infant assessment and the management of children in intensive care, and 3 to 6 months of precepted clinical neonatal experience.[2,3,164]

Minimum competencies include risk management, screening and comprehensive assessment of the high-risk neonate in neurobehavioral, neurodevelopmental, and motor developmental areas, and treatment design, implementation, and modification. Highly desirable are competencies in consultation, coordination, communication, research knowledge and participation, education of professional students and colleagues in other disciplines, and administration.[3] Specific areas of study should include normal fetal and early infant development, physiology and energy costs, neonatal medical problems, nursery ecology, and family dynamics.[3,164]

Options for obtaining professional training include master's level graduate programs with a neonatal track, university-affiliated postgraduate fellowships with a neonatal component, and individualized precepted training with clinical specialists. Eased entry into neonatal practice is recommended. This might begin with developmental screening of well babies and inpatient management of older children on life-support systems, progressing to participation in an NICU follow-up clinic and discharge planning and then to precepted practice in the intermediate care nursery before beginning NICU practice.[2]

If therapists do not take responsibility to prepare thoroughly for neonatal practice, the risks are high for the infant (physiologic, musculoskeletal risks), the therapist (medicolegal risk), and the medical center (quality control risk), and clearly outweigh the benefits of the therapy program.[2]

REFERENCES

1. Sweeney JK: The High-risk neonate: developmental therapy perspectives. Phys Occup Ther Pediatr 6(3/4), 1986
2. Sweeney JK, Chandler LS: Neonatal physical therapy: medical risks and professional education. Inf Young Child 2:59, 1990

3. Scull S, Deitz J: Competencies for the physical therapist in the neonatal intensive care unit (NICU). Pediatr Phys Ther 1:11, 1989
4. Pederson DR, Evans B, Chance GW et al: Predictors of one-year developmental status in low birth weight infants. J Dev Behav Pediatr 9:287, 1988
5. Nelson KB: Perspective on the role of perinatal asphyxia in neurologic outcome. p. 3. In: Perinatal Asphyxia: Its Role in Developmental Deficits in Children. American Academy for Cerebral Palsy and Developmental Medicine Proceedings, Toronto, 1988
6. Hack M, Fanaroff AA: How small is too small? Considerations in evaluating the outcome of the tiny infant. Clin Perinatol 15(4):773, 1988
7. Amon E: Limits of fetal viability. Obstet Gynecol Clin North Am 15(2):321, 1988
8. Scott DT, Spiker D: Research on the sequelae of prematurity: early learning, early interventions, and later outcomes. Semin Perinatol 13(6):495, 1989
9. Bowman E, Yu VYH: Continuing morbidity in extremely low birth weight infants. Early Hum Dev 18:165, 1989
10. Klein NK, Hack M, Breslau N: Children who were very low birth weight: development and academic achievement at nine years of age. J Dev Behav Pediatr 10:32, 1989
11. Robertson CMT, Etches PC, Kyle JM: Eight-year school performance and growth of preterm, small for gestational age infants: a comparative study with subjects matched for birth weight or for gestational age. J Pediatr 116:19, 1990
12. Astbury J, Orgill AA, Bajuk B, Yu VYH: Neurodevelopmental outcome, growth and health of extremely low-birthweight survivors: how soon can we tell? Dev Med Child Neurol 32:582, 1990
13. Vohr BR, Garcia-Coll C, Oh W: Language and neuro-developmental outcome of low-birthweight infants at three years. Dev Med Child Neurol 31:582, 1989
14. Volpe JJ: Brain injury in the premature infant: is it preventable? Pediatr Res, Suppl. 27:S28, 1990
15. Philip AGS, Allan WC, Tito AM, Wheeler LR: Intraventricular hemorrhage in preterm infants: declining incidence in the 1980s. Pediatrics 84:797, 1989
16. Volpe JJ: Intraventricular hemorrhage and brain injury in the premature infant: neuropathology and pathogenesis. Clin Perinatol 16(2):361, 1989
17. DeVries LS, Regev R, Pennock JM et al: Ultrasound evolution and later outcome of infants with periventricular densities. Early Hum Dev 16:225, 1988
18. Bennett FC, Silver G, Leung EJ, Mack LA: Periventricular echodensities detected by cranial ultrasonography: usefulness in predicting neurodevelopmental outcome in low-birth-weight, preterm infants. Pediatrics, Suppl. 85:400, 1990
19. Volpe JJ: Intraventricular hemorrhage and brain injury in the premature infant: diagnosis, prognosis, and prevention. Clin Perinatol 16(2):387, 1989
20. Ment LR, Ehrenkranz RA, Duncan CC: Intraventricular hemorrhage of the preterm neonate: prevention studies. Semin Perinatol 12(4):359, 1988
21. St. Geme JW III, Polin RA: Neonatal sepsis: progress in diagnosis and management. Drugs 36:784, 1988
22. Volpe JJ: Neonatal seizures: current concepts and revised classification. Pediatrics 84:422, 1989
23. Mizrahi EM: Consensus and controversy in the clinical management of neonatal seizures. Clin Perinatol 16(2):485, 1989
24. Tudehope DI, Harris A, Hawes D, Hayes M: Clinical spectrum and outcome of neonatal convulsions. Aust Paediatr J 24:249, 1988
25. Kendig JW, Shapiro DL: Surfactant therapy in the newborn. Pediatr Ann 17:504, 1988

26. Skidmore MD, Rivers A, Hack M: Increased risk of cerebral palsy among very low-birthweight infants with chronic lung disease. Dev Med Child Neurol 32:325, 1990

27. Goldson E: Bronchopulmonary dysplasia. Pediatr Ann 19:13, 1990

28. Samuels MP, Warner JO: Bronchopulmonary dysplasia: the outcome. Arch Dis Child 62:1099, 1987

29. Bader D, Rames A, Lew CD et al: Childhood sequelae of infant lung disease: exercise and pulmonary function abnormalities after bronchopulmonary dysplasia. J Pediatr 110:693, 1987

30. Campbell LR, McAlister W, Volpe JJ: Neurologic aspects of bronchopulmonary dysplasia. Clin Pediatr 27:7, 1988

31. Perlman JM, Volpe JJ: Movement disorder of premature infants with severe bronchopulmonary dysplasia: a new syndrome. Pediatrics 84:215, 1989

32. Garg M, Kurzner SI, Bautista DB, Keens TG: Clinically unsuspected hypoxia during sleep and feeding in infants with bronchopulmonary dysplasia. Pediatrics 81:635, 1988

33. Garg M, Kurzner SI, Bautista D, Keens TG: Hypoxic arousal responses in infants with bronchopulmonary dysplasia. Pediatrics 82:59, 1988

34. Chasnoff IJ: Drug use in pregnancy: parameters of risk. Pediatr Clin North Am 35(6):1403, 1988

35. Schneider JW, Griffith DR, Chasnoff IJ: Infants exposed to cocaine in utero: implications for developmental assessment and intervention. Inf Young Child 2(1):25, 1989

36. Hadeed AJ, Siegel SR: Maternal cocaine use during pregnancy: effect on the newborn infant. Pediatrics 84:205, 1989

37. Dixon SD, Bejar R: Echoencephalographic findings in neonates associated with maternal cocaine and methamphetamine use: incidence and clinical correlates. J Pediatr 115:770, 1989

38. Korones SB: Physical structure and functional organization of neonatal intensive care units. p. 7. In Gottfried AW, Gaiter JL (eds): Infant Stress Under Intensive Care. University Park Press, Baltimore, 1985

39. Papageorgiou AN, Doray J-L, Ardila R, Kunos I: Reduction of mortality, morbidity, and respiratory distress syndrome in infants weighing less than 1,000 grams by treatment with betamethasone and ritodrine. Pediatrics 83:493, 1989

40. Bowes WA III, Corke BC, Hulka J: Pulse oximetry: a review of the theory, accuracy, and clinical applications. Obstet Gynecol 74:541, 1989

41. Huch A, Huch R: Transcutaneous noninvasive monitoring of pO_2. Hosp Pract 11:43, 1976

42. Peabody JL, Lewis K: Consequences of newborn intensive care. p. 199. In Gottfried AW, Gaiter JL (eds): Infant Stress Under Intensive Care. University Park Press, Baltimore, 1985

43. Glass P, Avery GB, Subramanian KNS: Effect of bright light in the hospital nursery on the incidence of retinopathy of prematurity. N Engl J Med 313:401, 1985

44. Salamy A, Eldredge L, Tooley WH: Neonatal status and hearing loss in high-risk infants. J Pediatr 114:847, 1989

45. Wolke D: Environmental and developmental neonatology. J Reprod Inf Psychol 5:17, 1987

46. Mann NP, Haddow R, Stokes L et al: Effect of night and day on preterm infants in a newborn nursery: randomised trial. Br Med J 293:1265, 1986

47. Blackburn ST, Bernard KE: Analysis of caregiving events relating to preterm

infants in the special care unit. p. 113. In Gottfried AW, Gaiter JL (eds): Infant Stress Under Intensive Care. University Park Press, Baltimore, 1985

48. Morley CJ: Surfactant therapy for very premature babies. Br Med Bull 44:919, 1988

49. Polak MJ, Polak JD, Bucciarelli RL: Perspectives on respiratory distress syndrome of the newborn. Compr Ther 15:28, 1989

50. Couser RJ, Ferrara TB, Ebert J et al: Effects of exogenous surfactant therapy on dynamic compliance during mechanical breathing in preterm infants with hyaline membrane disease. J Pediatr 116:119, 1990

51. Lang MJ, Hall RT, Reddy NS et al: A controlled trial of human surfactant replacement therapy for severe respiratory distress syndrome in very low birth weight infants. J Pediatr 116:295, 1990

52. Vaucher YE, Merritt TA, Hallman M et al: Neuro-developmental and respiratory outcome in early childhood after human surfactant treatment. Am J Dis Child 142:927, 1988

53. Ware J, Taeusch HW, Soll RF, McCormick MC: Health and developmental outcomes of a surfactant controlled trial: follow-up at 2 years. Pediatrics 85:1103, 1990

54. Boros SJ, Mammel MC: A practical guide to high-frequency ventilation. Pediatr Ann 17:508, 1988

55. Milner AD, Hoskyns EW: High frequency positive pressure ventilation in neonates. Arch Dis Child 64:1, 1989

56. Gerhardt T, Reifenberg L, Goldberg RN, Bancalari E: Pulmonary function in preterm infants whose lungs were ventilated conventionally or by high-frequency oscillation. J Pediatr 115:121, 1989

57. HiFi Study Group: High-frequency oscillatory ventilation compared with conventional mechanical ventilation in the treatment of respiratory failure in preterm infants. N Engl J Med 320:88, 1989

58. HiFi Study Group: High-frequency oscillatory ventilation compared with conventional mechanical ventilation in the treatment of respiratory failure in preterm infants: assessment of pulmonary function at 9 months of corrected age. J Pediatr 116:933, 1990

59. Short BL, Lotze A: Extracorporeal membrane oxygenator therapy. Pediatr Ann 17:516, 1988

60. Arensman RM: Developmental outcome of neonates treated with extracorporeal membrane oxygenation. p. 262. In: Developmental Interventions in Neonatal Care. Contemporary Forums Proceedings, New Orleans, 1989

61. Fink SM, Bockman DE, Howell CG et al: Bypass circuits as the source of thromboemboli during extracorporeal membrane oxygenation. J Pediatr 115:621, 1989

62. Steinhorn RH, Isham-Schopf B, Smith C, Green TP: Hemolysis during long-term extracorporeal membrane oxygenation. J Pediatr 115:625, 1989

63. Glass P, Miller M, Short B: Morbidity for survivors of extracorporeal membrane oxygenation: neurodevelopmental outcome at 1 year of age. Pediatrics 83:72, 1989

64. Towne BH, Lott IT, Hicks DA, Healey T: Long-term follow-up of infants and children treated with extracorporeal membrane oxygenation (ECMO): a preliminary report. J Pediatr Surg 20:410, 1985

65. Taylor GA, Short BL, Fitz CR: Imaging of cerebrovascular injury in infants treated with extracorporeal membrane oxygenation. J Pediatr 114:635, 1988

66. Als H: A synactive model of neonatal behavioral organization: framework for the assessment of neurobehavioral development in the premature infant and for sup-

port of infants and parents in the neonatal intensive care environment. Phys Occup Ther Pediatr 6(3/4):3, 1986

67. Als H: Self-regulation and motor development in preterm infants. p. 65. In Lockman J, Hazen N (eds): Action in Social Context: Perspectives on Early Development. Plenum, New York, 1989

68. Lawhon G, Melzar A: Developmental care of the very low birth weight infant. p. 189. In: Developmental Interventions in Neonatal Care. Contemporary Forums Proceedings, New Orleans, 1989

69. Als H, Lawhon G, Brown E et al: Individualized behavioral and environmental care for the VLBW preterm infant at high risk for bronchopulmonary dysplasia: NICU and developmental outcome. Pediatrics 78:1123, 1986

70. Als H: The behavior of the preterm infant: basis for prediction of later functioning and for preventive care. p. 25. In: Developmental Interventions in Neonatal Care. Contemporary Forums Proceedings, New Orleans, 1989

71. Als H, Lester BM, Tronick EZ, Brazelton TB: Manual for the Assessment of Preterm Infants' Behavior (APIB). p. 65. In Fitzgerald HE, Lester BM, Yogman MW (eds): Theory and Research in Behavioral Pediatrics. Vol. 1. Plenum, New York, 1982

72. Hobel CJ: Identification of the patient at risk. p. 3. In Bolognese RJ, Schwarz RH, Schneider J (eds): Perinatal Medicine: Management of the High Risk Fetus and Neonate. Williams & Wilkins, Baltimore, 1982

73. Parmelee A, Kopp C, Sigmon M: Selection of developmental assessment techniques for infants at risk. Merrill-Palmer Q 22:177, 1976

74. Prechtl HFR: Neurological findings in newborn infants after pre- and paranatal complications. p. 303. In Jonxis JHP, Visser HKA, Troelska JA (eds): Nutricia Symposium: Aspects of Prematurity and Dysmaturity. Stenfert Kroese, Leiden, 1968

75. Vintzileos AM, Campbell WA, Rodis JF: Fetal biophysical profile scoring: current status. Clin Perinatol 16(3):661, 1989

76. Anand KJS, Hickey PR: Pain and its effects in the human neonate and fetus. N Engl J Med 317:1321, 1987

77. Murdoch DR, Darlow BA: Handling during neonatal intensive care. Arch Dis Child 59:957, 1984

78. Sweeney JK: Physiologic adaptation of neonates to neurological assessment. Phys Occup Ther Pediatr 6(3/4):155, 1986

79. Sweeney JK: Physiological and behavioral effects of neurological assessment in preterm and full-term neonates, abstracted. Phys Occup Ther Pediatr 9(3):144, 1989

80. Dubowitz L, Dubowitz V: The Neurological Assessment of the Preterm and Full-Term Newborn Infant. Clinics in Developmental Medicine, No. 79. JB Lippincott, Philadelphia, 1981

81. Als H, Lester BM, Tronick EZ, Brazelton TB: Toward a research instrument for the assessment of preterm infants' behavior (APIB). p. 35. In Fitzgerald H, Lester BM, Yogman MW (eds): Theory and Research in Behavioral Pediatrics. Vol. 1. Plenum, New York, 1982

82. Marx JA: Predictive value of early neuromotor assessment instruments. Phys Occup Ther Pediatr 9(4):69, 1989

83. Als H: Manual for the Naturalistic Observation of Newborn Behavior (Preterm and Fullterm Infants). The Children's Hospital, Boston, 1984

84. Andre-Thomas, Chesni Y, Ste-Anne Dargassies S: The Neurological Examination

of the Infant. Little Club Clinics in Developmental Medicine, No. 1. National Spastics Society, London, 1960

85. Ste-Anne Dargassies S: Neurological Development in the Full-term and Premature Neonate. Excerpta Medica, New York, 1977

86. Amiel-Tison C: Neurological evaluation of the maturity of newborn infants. Arch Dis Child 43:89, 1968

87. Brazelton TB: Neonatal Behavioral Assessment Scale. 2nd Ed. Clinics in Developmental Medicine, No. 88. JB Lippincott, Philadelphia, 1984

88. Morgan AM, Koch V, Lee V, Aldag J: Neonatal neurobehavioral examination: a new instrument for quantitative analysis of neonatal neurological status. Phys Ther 68:1352, 1988

89. Horowitz FD, Sullivan JW, Linn P: Stability and instability in the newborn infant: the quest for elusive threads. In Sameroff JA (ed): Organization and Stability of Newborn Behavior: A Commentary on the Brazelton Neonatal Behavioral Assessment Scale. Monogr Soc Res Child Dev 43:1978

90. Harris MB: Oral-motor management of the high-risk neonate. Phys Occup Ther Pediatr 6(3/4):231, 1986

91. Medoff-Cooper B, Weininger S, Zukowsky K: Neonatal sucking as a clinical assessment tool: preliminary findings. Nurs Res 38:162, 1989

92. Anderson GC, McBride MR, Dahm J et al: Development of sucking in term infants from birth to four hours postbirth. Res Nurs Health 5:21, 1982

93. Bosma JF, Hepburn LG, Josell SD, Baker K: Ultrasound demonstration of tongue motions during suckle feeding. Dev Med Child Neurol 32:223, 1990

94. Bu'Lock F, Woolridge MW, Baum JD: Development of coordination of sucking, swallowing and breathing: ultrasound study of term and preterm infants. Dev Med Child Neurol 32:669, 1990

95. Braun MA, Palmer MM: A pilot study of oral-motor dysfunction in "at-risk" infants. Phys Occup Ther Pediatr 5(4):13, 1985

96. Case-Smith J: An efficacy study of occupational therapy with high-risk neonates. Am J Occup Ther 42:499, 1988

97. Case-Smith J, Cooper P, Scala V: Feeding efficiency of premature neonates. Am J Occup Ther 43:245, 1989

98. Harris MB: Stimulation of premature infants: the boundary between believing and knowing. Inf Ment Health J 7:171, 1986

99. Korner AF: Preventive intervention with high-risk newborns: theoretical, conceptual, and methodological perspectives. p. 1006. In Osofsky J (ed): Handbook of Infant Development. 2nd Ed. John Wiley & Sons, New York, 1987

100. Heriza CB, Sweeney JK: Effects of NICU intervention on preterm infants: part 1—implications for neonatal practice. Inf Young Child 2(3):31, 1990

101. Heriza CB, Sweeney JK: Effects of NICU intervention on preterm infants: part 2—implications for movement research. Inf Young Child 2(4):29, 1990

102. Field T: Stimulation of preterm infants. Pediatr Rev 10:149, 1988

103. Georgieff MK, Sasanow SR: Nutritional assessment of the neonate. Clin Perinatol 13(1):73, 1986

104. Georgieff MK, Hoffman JS, Pereira GR et al: Effect of neonatal caloric deprivation on head growth and 1-year developmental status in preterm infants. J Pediatr 107:581, 1985

105. Field T, Scafidi F, Schanberg S: Massage of preterm newborns to improve growth and development. Pediatr Nurs 13:385, 1987

106. Clark DL, Cordero L, Goss KC, Manos D: Effects of rocking on neuromuscular development in the premature. Biol Neonate 56:306, 1989

107. Oro AS, Dixon SD: Waterbed care of narcotic-exposed neonates. Am J Dis Child 142:186, 1988
108. Woodson R, Hamilton C: The effect of nonnutritive sucking on heart rate in preterm infants. Dev Psychobiol 21:207, 1988
109. Leonard EL, Trykowski LE, Kirkpatrick BV: Nutritive sucking in high-risk neonates after perioral stimulation. Phys Ther 60:299, 1980
110. Trykowski LE, Kirkpatrick BV, Leonard EL: Enhancement of nutritive sucking in premature infants. Phys Occup Ther Pediatr 1(4):27, 1981
111. Measel CP, Anderson GC: Nonnutritive sucking during tube feedings: effect on clinical course in premature infants. JOGN Nurs 8:265, 1979
112. Ernst JA, Rickard KA, Neal PR et al: Lack of improved growth outcome related to nonnutritive sucking in very low birth weight premature infants fed a controlled nutrient intake: a randomized prospective study. Pediatrics 83:706, 1989
113. Field T, Goldson E: Pacifying effects of nonnutritive sucking on term and preterm neonates during heelstick procedures. Pediatrics 74:1012, 1984
114. Woodson R, Drinkwin J, Hamilton C: Effects of nonnutritive sucking on state and activity: term-preterm comparisons. Inf Behav Dev 8:435, 1985
115. Cordero L, Clark DL, Schott L: Effects of vestibular stimulation on sleep states in premature infants. Am J Perinatol 3:319, 1986
116. Pelletier JM, Short MA, Nelson DL: Immediate effects of waterbed flotation on approach and avoidance behaviors of premature infants. Phys Occup Ther Pediatr 5(2/3):81, 1985
117. Martin RJ, Herrell N, Rubin D, Fanaroff A: Effect of supine and prone positions on arterial oxygen tension in the preterm infant. Pediatrics 63:528, 1979
118. Bottos M, Stefani D: Postural and motor care of the premature baby. Dev Med Child Neurol 24:706, 1982
119. Masterson J, Zucker C, Schulze K: Prone and supine positioning effects on energy expenditure and behavior of low birth weight neonates. Pediatrics 80:689, 1987
120. Anderson GC: Skin to skin: kangaroo care in western Europe. Am J Nurs 89:622, 1989
121. Acolet D, Sleath K, Whitelaw A: Oxygenation, heart rate and temperature in very low birthweight infants during skin-to-skin contact with their mothers. Acta Paediatr Scand 78:189, 1989
122. White Traut RC, Pate CMH: Modulating infant state in premature infants. J Pediatr Nurs 2:96, 1987
123. Carter RE, Campbell SK: Early neuromuscular development of the premature infant. Phys Ther 55:1332, 1975
124. Updike C, Schmidt RE, Macke C et al: Positional support for premature infants. Am J Occup Ther 40:712, 1986
125. Lioy J, Manginello FP: A comparison of prone and supine positioning in the immediate postextubation period of neonates. J Pediatr 112:982, 1988
126. Kishan J, Bhargava SK, Rehman F: Effect of posture on arterial oxygen tension in preterm infants. Indian Pediatr 18:701, 1981
127. Hutchison AA, Ross KR, Russell G: The effect of posture on ventilation and lung mechanics in preterm and light-for-date infants. Pediatrics 64:429, 1979
128. Wagaman MJ, Shutack JG, Moomjian S et al: Improved oxygenation and lung compliance with prone positioning of neonates. J Pediatr 94:787, 1979
129. Resnick MB, Eyler FD, Nelson RM et al: Developmental intervention for low birth weight infants: improved early developmental outcome. Pediatrics 80:68, 1987

130. Resnick MB, Armstrong S, Carter RL: Developmental intervention program for high-risk premature infants: effects on development and parent-infant interactions. J Dev Behav Pediatr 9:73, 1988

131. Sweeney JK: Neonatal hydrotherapy: an adjunct to developmental intervention in an intensive care nursery setting. Phys Occup Ther Pediatr 3(1):39, 1983

132. Piper MC, Kunos VI, Willis DM et al: Early physical therapy effects on the high-risk infant: a randomized controlled trial. Pediatrics 78:216, 1986

133. Piper MC, Maxer B, Silver KM, Ramsay M: Resolution of neurological symptoms in high-risk infants during the first two years of life. Dev Med Child Neurol 30:26, 1988

134. Girolami GL: Evaluating the effectiveness of a neurodevelopmental treatment physical therapy program to improve the motor control of high-risk preterm infants, abstracted. Phys Occup Ther Pediatr 8(2/3):112, 1988

135. Gorski PA, Hole WT, Leonard CH, Martin JA: Direct computer recording of premature infants and nursery care: distress following two interventions. Pediatrics 72:198, 1983

136. Mathew OP: Respiratory control during nipple feeding in preterm infants. Pediatr Pulmonol 5:220, 1988

137. White-Traut RC, Goldman MBC: Premature infant massage: is it safe? Pediatr Nurs 14:285, 1988

138. Kelly MK, Palisano RJ, Wolfson MR: Effects of a developmental physical therapy program on oxygen saturation and heart rate in preterm infants. Phys Ther 69:467, 1989

139. Prechtl HFR: Assessment methods for newborn infants, a critical evaluation. p. 21. In Stratton P (ed): Psychobiology of the Human Newborn. John Wiley & Sons, New York, 1982

140. Ellison PH, Horn JL, Browning CA: Construction of an Infant Neurological International Battery (INFANIB) for the assessment of neurological integrity in infancy. Phys Ther 65:1326, 1985

141. Ellison PH: Scoring sheet for the Infant Neurological International Battery (INFANIB). Phys Ther 66:548, 1986

142. Milani-Comparetti A, Gidoni EA: Routine developmental examination in normal and retarded children. Dev Med Child Neurol 9:631, 1967

143. Amiel-Tison C, Grenier A: Neurologic Evaluation of the Infant and Newborn. Masson, New York, 1983

144. Capute AJ, Accardo PJ, Vining EPG et al: Primitive Reflex Profile. University Park Press, Baltimore, 1978

145. Paine RS, Oppe TE: Neurological Examination of Children. Clinics in Developmental Medicine, Nos. 20/21. Heinemann, London, 1966

146. Nickel RE: The Manual for the Infant Motor Screen. Oregon Health Sciences University, Portland, OR, 1987

147. Nickel RE, Renken CA, Gallenstein JS: The Infant Motor Screen. Dev Med Child Neurol 31:35, 1989

148. Chandler LS, Andrews MS, Swanson MW, Larson AH: Movement Assessment of Infants: A Manual. Rolling Bay, WA, 1980

149. Case-Smith J: Posture and Fine Motor Assessment of Infants. Research Ed. American Occupational Therapy Foundation, Rockville, MD, 1988

150. Case-Smith J: Reliability and validity of the Posture and Fine Motor Assessment of Infants. Occup Ther J Res 9:259, 1989

151. Touwen B: Neurological Development in Infancy. Clinics in Developmental Medicine, No. 58. JB Lippincott, Philadelphia, 1976

152. Kopp CB: Fine motor abilities of infants. Dev Med Child Neurol 16:629, 1974
153. Gesell A, Halverson HM, Thompson H et al: The First Five Years of Life. Harper & Row, New York, 1940
154. Erhardt RP: Developmental Hand Function. RAMSCO, Laurel, MD, 1982
155. DeGangi G, Berk R, Valvano J: Test of motor and neurological functions in high risk infants: preliminary findings. J Dev Behav Pediatr 4:182, 1983
156. DeGangi GA: Test of Sensory Functions in Infants. Western Psychological Services, Los Angeles, 1988
157. DeGangi GA, Berk RA, Greenspan SI: The clinical measurement of sensory functioning in infants: a preliminary study. Phys Occup Ther Pediatr 8(2/3):1, 1988
158. Campbell SK, Wilhelm IJ: Development from birth to 3 years of age of 15 children at high risk for central nervous system dysfunction: interim report. Phys Ther 65:463, 1985
159. Harris SR: Early neuromotor predictors of cerebral palsy in low-birthweight infants. Dev Med Child Neurol 29:508, 1987
160. Nelson K, Ellenberg J: Children who "outgrew" cerebral palsy. Pediatrics 69:529, 1982
161. Coolman RB, Bennett FC, Sells CJ et al: Neuromotor development of graduates of the neonatal intensive care unit: patterns encountered in the first two years of life. J Dev Behav Pediatr 6:327, 1985
162. O'Donnell KJ: The family system in the neonatal setting: theoretical perspectives. p. 105. In Wilhelm IJ (ed): Advances in Neonatal Special Care. University of North Carolina, Chapel Hill, 1986
163. Leander D, Pettett G: Parental response to the birth of a high-risk neonate: dynamics and management. Phys Occup Ther Pediatr 6(3/4):205, 1986
164. Campbell SK: Organizational and educational considerations in creating an environment to promote optimal development of high-risk neonates. Phys Occup Ther Pediatr 6(3/4):191, 1986
165. O'Donnell KJ: Defenses in the nursery. p. 118. In Wilhelm IJ (ed): Advances in Neonatal Special Care. University of North Carolina, Chapel Hill, 1986
166. Worobey J: Review of Brazelton-based interventions to enhance parent-infant interaction. J Reprod Inf Psychol 3:64, 1986
167. Nugent JK, Brazelton TB: Preventive intervention with infants and families: the NBAS model. Inf Ment Health J 10:84, 1989
168. Culp RE, Culp AM, Harmon RJ: A tool for educating parents about their premature infants. Birth 16:23, 1989
169. Howard J, Parmelee AH, Kopp CB, Littman B: A neurologic comparison of preterm and full-term infants at term conceptional age. J Pediatr 88:995, 1976
170. Ferrari F, Grosoli MV, Fontana G, Cavazzuti GB: Neurobehavioral comparison of low-risk preterm and fullterm infants at term conceptional age. Dev Med Child Neurol 25:450, 1983
171. Anderson LT, Coll CG, Vohr BR et al: Behavioral characteristics and early temperament of premature infants with intracranial hemorrhage. Early Hum Dev 18:273, 1989
172. Marshall RE, Kasman C: Burnout in the neonatal intensive care unit. Pediatrics 65:1161, 1980

5 | Brachial Plexus Injury

Roberta B. Shepherd

Although both the occurrence and the severity of brachial plexus injury in the neonate have been reduced by improved obstetric techniques, as Eng[1] has pointed out the current incidence is not negligible, and the resultant handicap can be very severe indeed. The relatively small number of such infants seen by therapists constitutes a problem as there has been little investigation of new and more effective ways of ensuring maximum possible recovery of function. Unfortunately, early treatment for infants with brachial plexus injury is still seen as largely comprising passive movements to prevent soft tissue contractures.[2] A major role of physical therapy, however, is the stimulation of muscle activity and training of effective functional movement.[3]

Recent advances in the broad area of movement science provide the physical therapist with an increased understanding of normal infant reaching and how to elicit it,[4] of the biomechanics and control of reaching and grasping,[5] and of the need for task- and context-specific training of muscles.[6] Furthermore, with modern technology, it is now reasonable to expect physical therapists to test the effectiveness of motor training using, for example, biomechanical data derived from videotape recordings.

Brachial plexus injuries are usually classified under three headings: *Erb or upper plexus type* (involving C5 and C6), *Klumpke or lower plexus type* (involve C7,8 and T1), and *Erb-Klumpke or whole arm type* (involving C5 to T1). Exact localization of the anatomic lesion is often difficult,[7,8] however, and many infants demonstrate a mixed upper and lower type. Considerable variation in the type of lesion occurs, ranging from a mild edema affecting one or two roots to total avulsion of the entire plexus. Involvement is usually unilateral and the results of the lesion are always immediately recognizable.

ETIOLOGY AND INCIDENCE

Injury to the brachial plexus in infants occurs most commonly as a result of a difficult birth.[3,9] The factors implicated include the following: high birth weight, prolonged maternal labor, a sedated, hypotonic, and therefore vulnerable infant, a heavily sedated mother, traction in a breech presentation or rotation of the head in a cephalic presentation, and a difficult cesarean extraction.

During the birth process, the trauma that injures the plexus may also injure the facial nerve, causing a mild facial paralysis.[1] Other complications include fractures of the clavicle or humerus, traction to the cervical cord with signs of upper motoneuron lesion, subluxation of the shoulder, and torticollis. The phrenic nerve (C4) may also be injured, causing an ipsilateral hemiparalysis of the diaphragm. Eng[1] reported an infant with a peripheral radial nerve lesion in addition to bilateral Erb's paralysis.

Trauma to the shoulder region other than birth injury may also result in injury to the brachial plexus, although this is not common. Such trauma may include pressure from a body cast,[10] falls involving traction and hyperabduction of the shoulder, and pressure from the neck seal of a continuous positive airway pressure head box.[11]

The lower plexus may be injured as a result of pressure from congenital abnormalities such as cervical rib, abnormal thoracic vertebrae, or shortened scalenus anticus muscle. An unusual neuritis of the brachial plexus, called *paralytic brachial neuritis*, which is of unknown etiology, has been described by Magee and DeJong.[12]

Although the incidence of severe brachial plexus injury is considered to have declined because of improved obstetric management of difficult labor, some reports indicate that overall incidence has not declined.[9] According to the studies[8,13-15] available, actual incidence seems to vary. Adler and Patterson[8] reported that the incidence had declined from 1.56 to 0.38 per 1,000 live births between the years of 1938 and 1962. However, Specht,[15] in his 1975 review, gave an incidence of 0.57 per 1,000, Davis and associates[16] reported in 1978 that the current incidence was approximately 0.6 per 1,000 live births, and there have been two recent reports[13,14] of incidence between 2.0 and 2.5 per 1,000 births.

PATHOLOGY

To understand the mechanism of injury, it is necessary to study the anatomy of the brachial plexus and its relationship to its surrounding structures. The reader is referred to the many anatomy texts available. Figure 5-1 illustrates diagrammatically the three main trunks of the plexus.

In theory, any force that alters the anatomic relationship between neck, shoulder, and arm may result in injury to the plexus. The plexus is attached

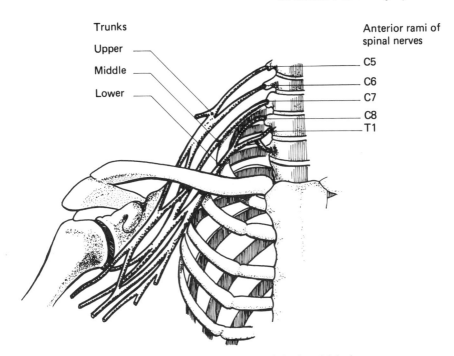

Trunks

Upper

Middle

Lower

Anterior rami of
spinal nerves

C5

C6

C7

C8
T1

Fig. 5-1. The three main trunks of the brachial plexus.

by fascia to the first rib medially and to the coracoid process of the scapula laterally. Lateral movement of the head with depression of the shoulder girdle will stretch the nerves and compress them against the first ribs. Forced abduction (hyperabduction) of the shoulder with traction on the arm will stretch the nerves and compress them under the coracoid process. The former will cause injury to the upper plexus, the latter to the lower plexus. When the trauma is severe and stretch reaches a certain force, complete avulsion of the nerves will result.

Stretching of the nerve roots or trunk of the plexus may result in injuries ranging from swelling of the neural sheath with blocking of nerve impulses, to hemorrhage and scar formation, to axonal rupture with wide separation of fragments.[17] The nerve roots may be completely avulsed from the cord. A combination of these lesions is common and will be reflected in the electromyographic (EMG) findings.[17] If avulsion occurs, there will be some hemorrhage in the subarachnoid space, and the presence of blood in the cerebrospinal fluid will therefore suggest this more serious injury. Some investigators[18,19] recommend the use of somatosensory cerebral-evoked potentials for specific diagnosis of dorsal root avulsion. The presence of Horner syndrome (deficient sweating, recession of eyeball into the orbit, abnormal pupillary contraction, and ptosis) indicates an intraspinal avulsion of the root of T1 with involvement of the sympathetic fibers.

Regeneration of nerves is unlikely following complete axonal rupture. However, most brachial plexus lesions are less severe and, in these cases, recovery occurs due to resolution of edema and hemorrhage or to regrowth of nerve fibers down the sheath. In the latter case, recovery will be slow due to the distance over which regenerating axons must grow. Regrowth, if it occurs, proceeds at approximately 1 mm/d. In the upper arm type, this regeneration is usually complete by 4 to 5 months, in the whole arm type, by 7 to 9 months.[17]

Eng[1] describes serial EMG studies that depict the evolution of the disorder. The lesion is indicated by decreased voluntary motor unit activity and the presence of denervation potentials in the form of fibrillation and sharp wave potentials. Regeneration is signified by the appearance of small polyphasic motor units. As recovery progresses, there is an increase in the number of motor units recorded, a decrease in denervation potentials, and eventually a return of excitability of the nerves to electrical stimuli. Degenerative changes in muscles are indicated by absent motor unit activity and paucity of denervation potentials plus nonconduction.

In adults, denervation of a muscle is followed by changes in the contractile properties of that muscle. A denervated muscle atrophies with shrinkage of individual muscle cells and thickening of endomysium, perimysium, and epimysium. Studies by Stefanova-Uzunova and colleagues[20] suggest that if denervation occurs at birth, there is also impairment of the normal developmental changes in the contractile properties of muscle that should occur postnatally.

DIFFERENTIAL DIAGNOSIS AND PROGNOSIS

The other principal causes of upper limb paralysis in infancy that need to be excluded are upper motoneuron lesions (lesions of the cervical cord or brain) and lower motoneuron lesions (lesions of the anterior horn cell) such as occur in poliomyelitis. Although the clinical appearance of the upper limb in hemiplegia and brachial plexus paralysis may be similar in terms of the arm's posture and absence of movement in either the whole arm or in certain muscle groups, hemiplegia can usually be easily differentiated by careful analysis of lower limb function and by the testing of reflexes. In upper motoneuron lesions, tendon reflexes are present and hyperactive in both limbs on the affected side or in all four limbs. In addition, there may be sustained ankle clonus and a persistent Babinski sign. A spinal cord lesion is also characterized by sensory abnormalities over the trunk and involvement of the bladder.

Poliomyelitis may be confused with the whole arm type of brachial plexus lesion, but can usually be differentiated by the typical clinical picture and by the presence of intact sensation.

Most cases of brachial nerve injury have a favorable prognosis.[3] It is not the extensiveness of the involvement but the severity of the involvement (i.e., the degree of neural damage) that gives the clue to prognosis. Eng[1] reported that EMG findings on the extent of the involvement did not correlate with the rate of recovery. For example, an extensive paralysis that is merely a neura-praxic lesion may recover completely, while a lesion of only C5 and C6, if complete axonal rupture is involved, may not recover at all.

PHYSICAL THERAPY ASSESSMENT

Assessment is necessary as an aid to diagnosis, as a record of progress, and, by providing a detailed analysis of function, as an important stage in the clinical problem-solving process. An important part of the physical therapy assessment is the analysis of motor function, the objective of which is to gain the most complete picture possible of the infant's current status, the reasons for dysfunction, and the problems that may arise in the future. For analysis of motor function to be sufficiently thorough, the therapist must understand the muscle function required for the performance of everyday movements, particularly reaching to grasp. In the case of infants, the therapist must also understand the development of motor control that occurs as the infant's brain matures and it becomes possible to practice increasingly complex motor tasks.

Analysis of motor function is made by observation of muscle contraction and of movement in comparison with normal function at that age, and by passive movement to gauge the length of muscles and to gain a subjective impression of the muscle contraction that occurs in response to these movements. Motor function may be recorded for subsequent analysis on videotape, cine film, or still photograph. Muscle activity may be documented by an EMG recording or on a muscle chart.

Sensory loss may not correspond to the extent of motor loss. Sensory testing is not possible with any degree of accuracy in young infants, and the problem is compounded by the muscle paralysis. Response to pin prick can be tested, using the infant's appearance of discomfort as a guide, and the result can be recorded on a body chart. O'Riain[21] describes a "wrinkle" test that may be helpful. The fingers are immersed in water at 40°C for 30 minutes. Normal skin wrinkles, but denervated skin does not. Wrinkling returns as the skin is reinnervated. In older children, two-point discrimination can be tested using an esthesiometer; however, the functional significance of such testing is not understood.

Analysis of Motor Function

Presence of movement is assessed by *observation* of the following:

1. Spontaneous movement and posture as the infant lies in the supine and prone positions and is moved around, cuddled, and talked to.
2. Motor behavior during testing of reflexes and reactions, particularly the Moro reflex, the placing reaction of the hands, the Galant (trunk incurvation) reflex, the neck-righting reaction, and the parachute reaction.

Observation will give some indication of muscle activity, which can be graded and recorded on a chart as, for example,

    0 = Absent
    1 = Present, but lacking full range of movement
    2 = Present throughout a full range of movement

This chart is upgraded at subsequent visits, the therapist always searching actively for the presence of muscle contraction in different parts of range and different relationships to gravity.

Although it is usual in the literature to see a list of the typically denervated muscles in the various types of lesions, the therapist should take care not to assume weakness and paralysis in certain muscles and normal function in others. Careful analysis of motor function will frequently reveal a mixed lesion. In addition, as time passes, lack of use of the limb will result in disuse weakness of other muscles not involved in the original lesion.

Several authors describe the use of *electromyographic assessment*.[17,22-24] Eng[1] suggests that EMG is useful in topographically delineating the extent and severity of the injury and in giving information about expected recovery. Electromyography would also provide the therapist with the information needed in planning treatment, as EMG signs of return usually precede clinical evidence of function by several weeks. Serial EMGs are commenced within the first 2 weeks after birth and are repeated at 6- to 8-week intervals for as long as is indicated.

The appearance of decreased denervation potentials and the appearance of reinnervation potentials may predate subjective clinical evidence by several weeks. The appearance of these EMG findings should therefore be followed immediately by intensified therapy to stimulate activity in these muscles. Electromyographic information would therefore enable the therapist and parents to concentrate on the eliciting of motor activity in particular muscles and training of functional movements at a time when the therapist may not otherwise be able to recognize the first signs of motor activity. Although excessive fatigue should be avoided, specific motor training at this point in recovery may be crucial to the infant's ability to make the most of neural recovery. It is therefore probable that EMG should be used more extensively than at present in order to guide the motor training program.

Patterns of Muscle Dysfunction

In the *upper arm type*, the dysfunction may involve the following muscles: rhomboids, levator scapulae, serratus anterior, deltoid, supraspinatus, infraspinatus, biceps brachii, brachioradialis, brachialis, supinator and long extensors of the wrist, fingers, and thumb (Fig. 5-2).

In the *lower arm type*, dysfunction involves the intrinsic muscles of the

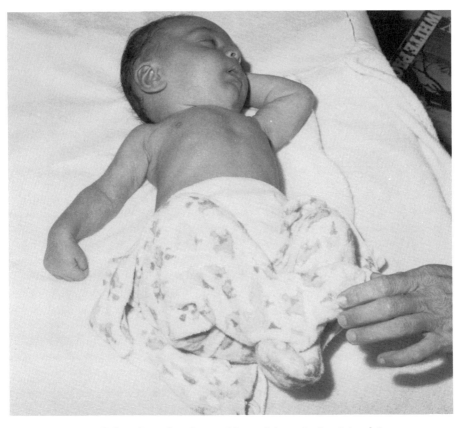

Fig. 5-2. Infant 4 weeks of age with partial paralysis of the right arm.

hand and the extensors and flexors of the wrist and fingers. Many infants demonstrate some mixture of upper and lower type dysfunction.

In the *upper and lower arm types*, problems arise as a result of the paralysis or weakness of certain muscles, the unopposed activity of other muscles, and the resultant muscle imbalance. These problems include persistent and abnormal movement substitutions (Fig. 5-3), abnormal posturing of the arm (Fig. 5-2), soft tissue contracture, glenohumeral subluxation or dislocation (Fig. 5-4), posterior displacement of the humeral epiphysis and posterior radial dislocation, and, eventually, skeletal deformity and poor bone growth.

The resting position of the arm is normally at the side. After brachial plexus injury, this position, plus the paralysis or weakness of the shoulder abductors and flexors and the scapular retractors and protractors, and the overactivity of the unopposed shoulder adductors and medial rotators, eventually result in soft tissue contracture of those muscles held at their shortened length.

Paralysis of the rhomboideus muscle together with the unopposed activity and eventual contracture of the muscles that link the humerus to the scapula

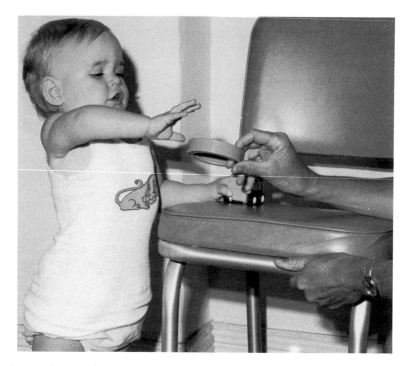

Fig. 5-3. Infant aged 13 months showing abnormal posturing of the arm and trunk, encouraged in this case by the position of the toy and the ease with which it can be grasped with the forearm in pronation.

(muscles subscapularis, teres minor, latissimus dorsi) cause the scapula to adhere to the humerus, and any flexion or abduction movement of the arm will be accomplished in a 1:1 ratio instead of the normal 6:1 humeroscapular relationship in the first 30 degrees of movement.

Abnormal movement of the arm reflects the muscle imbalance and also the substitution of incorrect motor activity. The typical posturing of the neonate with the upper arm type of paralysis (adducted, medially rotated shoulder, extended and pronated forearm, flexed wrist) gives way to an elevated, slightly abducted, medially rotated and pronated arm as some muscle activity returns and as the infant makes compensatory movements in attempts to reach out with the arm.

It is common to see abnormal combinations of movement components, for example, the combination of wrist flexion and forearm pronation with finger extension for grasp. This is similar to the abnormal synergic activity seen as part of the motor dysfunction resulting from central nervous system lesions. It is likely that these abnormal movements are the result of the infant's attempts at reaching in the most biomechanically advantageous way given the state of muscle innervation and muscle length. These substitutions may be reasonably

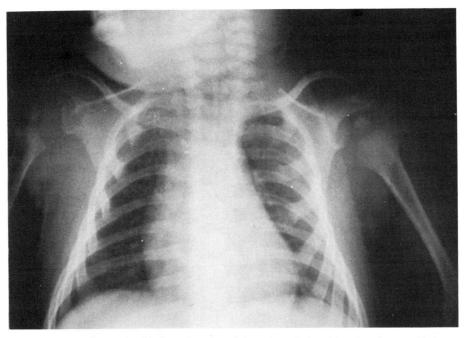

Fig. 5-4. Radiograph of infant showing dislocation of the right glenohumeral joint.

effective in the short term[3] and, hence, will be practiced by the infant and learned.

Some investigators refer to these movements as *synkinetic movements* or *associated movements*. Contractions of the biceps brachii and deltoid muscles have been noted to occur in conjunction with inspiratory movement.[25,26] Esslen[27] found synchronous motor unit potentials in different muscles supplied by the same nerve. De Grandis and colleagues[28] described a 13-year-old girl who was incapable of extending her fingers without flexing the forearm and wrist, and a 15-year-old girl whose strong finger flexion was associated with flexion of the forearm and wrist. These authors concluded that there is simultaneous innervation by the same motoneurons of one or more "motor subunits" in different muscles. They also suggested that inability to perform some movements may be due to simultaneous contraction of antagonistic muscles and not to lack of muscle strength. Tada and associates,[29] in their study of rats, discussed disordered recovery and suggested that functionally different neurons as well as the correct neurons participate in the regeneration of the disrupted nerves.

In the *whole arm type* of muscle dysfunction there may be no apparent muscle activity in the limb. In whole arm paralysis, major problems are caused by the dependent position of the arm with resultant stretch of soft tissues, together with a lack of muscle activity with which to preserve the integrity of the glenohumeral joint. This may result in subluxation and dislocation of the glenohumeral joint.

Other problems that result from muscle paralysis are "learned nonuse," delay in achieving certain motor milestones such as independent sitting, and inability to perform two-handed actions in addition to those actions involving only the affected limb.

Analysis of Respiratory Function

Phrenic nerve paralysis, resulting in decreased movement of the ipsilateral thorax with respiratory distress and cyanosis, may mimic diaphragmatic hernia.[30]

Hemiparalysis of the diaphragm should be suspected whenever there are persistent physical and radiographic findings of atelectasis and unilateral diaphragmatic elevation. However, examination of diaphragmatic function using EMG and fluoroscopy should be carried out for all infants with the upper or whole arm type of paralysis. When EMG is unavailable, assessment will involve observation of thoracic and abdominal movement in order to detect motor asymmetry.

PHYSICAL THERAPY

The infant should rest for the first few days to allow hemorrhage and edema to resolve. Physical treatment then commences, with the major objectives being to ensure the optimal conditions for recovery of motor function, to provide the environmental conditions and the motivation necessary to enable muscles to resume function as soon as sufficient neural regeneration has taken place, and to train motor control by practice of actions such as reaching out.

To ensure the optimal conditions for recovery, the problems of soft tissue contracture, disorganization of movements at the shoulder and shoulder girdle joints, neglect of the limb, and incorrect movement habits (substitution) must be prevented. To ensure that maximal functional recovery will follow neural regeneration, therapy must include specific training of functional movement once the affected muscles are reinnervated and capable of contraction. If recovery does not occur, the objectives of physical therapy will change to provide for the specific training that will be necessary following microsurgery to repair nerves[31] or surgery to transplant muscles or arthrodial joints.

The role of physical therapy must be seen, therefore, to extend beyond the maintenance of soft tissue length and stimulation of movement, and must take into account the need to develop ways of preventing or minimizing disorganized movement in the limb, of training motor control, and of preventing neglect of the arm. In addition, the therapist will train the parents to carry out exercises at home. Treatment follows from a detailed analysis of each problem, both existing and potential, together with an up-to-date understanding of the specificity of muscle training and the biomechanics of, in particular, reaching. The significance of the growing area of movement science to physical therapy in rehabilitation has been pointed out by Carr and Shepherd,[32] and is also relevant when the movement-disabled are infants and children. The effects of each step in therapy should be subject to evaluation to ensure that unproductive methods are discarded and new methods are introduced when necessary.

Motor Training

A program of specific motor training should commence within the first 2 weeks of the infant's life. Although there can be no activity in muscles that are not innervated, this early motor training probably serves several purposes: to stimulate activity in muscles whose nerve supply is only temporarily disconnected; to enable muscles to be activated as soon as nerve regeneration has taken place, and to prevent, or minimize, soft tissue contracture, neglect, and habituation of substitution movements.

Motor training should be specific in that particular actions, such as reaching, are trained. The infant's actions should be carefully monitored, the therapist using manual guidance and verbal feedback to ensure that the infant moves as normally as possible, that is, activates the appropriate muscles for the movement. In selecting the muscles on which to focus attention, it may be helpful to consider that certain of the involved muscles are particularly essential for reaching to grasp an object, for example, the abductors, flexors, and lateral rotators of the shoulder, together with the scapular rotators, retractors and protractors, the supinators of the forearm, the wrist extensors and radial deviators, and the palmar abductor of the thumb. Of course, this is not to suggest that these are the only muscles to be trained, but only to point out that there is an urgent need to train these muscles as early as recovery will allow, before learned substitution of the nonparalyzed muscles and shortening of soft tissues make it difficult for the recovering muscles to demonstrate their optimal activity.

Training should commence under the best possible conditions for each muscle, taking into account leverage, the relationship of the limb to gravity (Figs. 5-5 and 5-6), the fact that an eccentric contraction can often be elicited before a concentric contraction (Fig. 5-7), and the need for optimal alignment to encourage the required muscle action (Fig. 5-8). Hence, the therapist must actively search for the presence of muscle contraction, checking different sectors of the movement range and different relationships of the limb to gravity, and trying to elicit eccentric activity if concentric activity is not present.

Unless the therapist initiates these activities, the earliest manifestations of recovery of motor activity in particular muscles may pass unnoticed. In the earliest stage of recovery, a muscle may not be able to contract under certain conditions of leverage and the task may have to be modified to be achievable. For example, the deltoid may not be strong enough to raise the arm from the side, but may be able to hold the arm and lower it a few degrees from a hor-

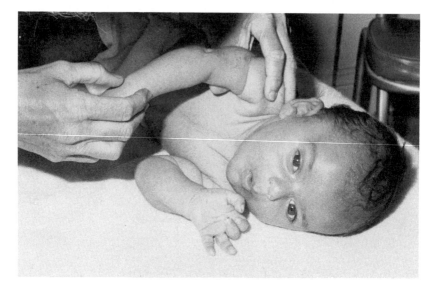

Fig. 5-5. Infant aged 4 weeks. Attempting to elicit activity in the deltoid muscle by encouraging the infant to take his hand to his face. This would require the muscle to work both concentrically and as a fixator.

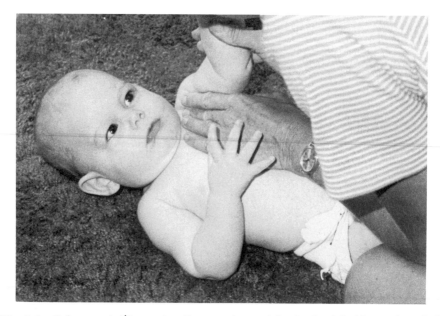

Fig. 5-6. Infant aged 4½ months. Encouraging activity in the deltoid muscle to hold arm in flexion as he reaches up to touch the therapist's face.

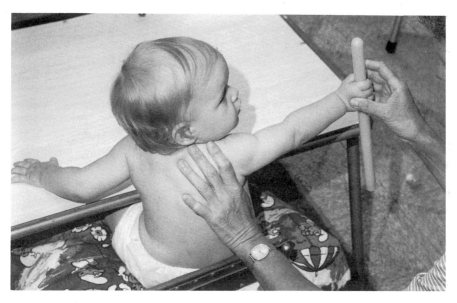

Fig. 5-7. Infant aged 13 months. Attempting to elicit eccentric deltoid activity in the inner range. Therapist guides correct scapula movement with her left hand.

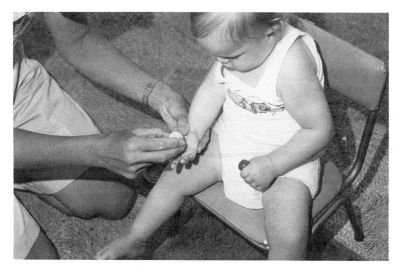

Fig. 5-8. Infant aged 13 months. Encouraging grasp and release with the forearm in supination. She will only spontaneously grasp and release in pronation.

izontal position when sitting (Fig. 5-7) or in a vertical position when lying (Fig. 5-6). Similarly, the wrist extensors may not be able to contract strongly enough to lift the hand from a position of wrist flexion, but they may be able to contract eccentrically from a position in which they are shortened, or the radial extensor may be able to contract to radially deviate or lift the wrist from the table.

Motor training should continue for as long as recovery is still occurring. It may be that nerves have the potential for recovery for a relatively long period of time. Gatcheva[33] reports EMG evidence of reinnervation and the return of nerve conduction for 6 to 8 years after brachial plexus injury and suggests that it is essential to continue rehabilitation for many years. Gatcheva's observation is contrary to the usual opinion that recovery takes place within the first 2 years. However, the therapist should continue with periods of intensive motor training, using EMG to provide guidance as to recovery.

Support through the upper limb when prone and sitting, and reaching to grasp are two actions to concentrate on in training infants and children in upper extremity use because these are the principal functions of the upper limb to be developed for effective everyday life. From recent research by von Hofsten, it is now evident that reaching occurs as a meaningful action considerably earlier than was once thought.[4,34] The clinical implication is that training of reaching can commence in early infancy. From von Hofsten's work, it appears that certain factors would be important for reaching to be elicited in very young infants: the infant may use the arm more effectively sitting in a semireclined and supported posture in a chair, the object used to elicit the action should be irresistible in its form and color and should be graspable (von Hofsten used a fishing lure minus hook), and the object will be more easily detected if it moves across the infant's field of vision, rather than being stationary, at a distance of 5 to 7 inches. As the infant matures and more complex reaching games can be played, the object can be placed to encourage flexion and external rotation of the shoulder during reaching and to discourage internal rotation and abduction.

Practice

Manual and object-mediated guidance is usually essential during practice (Figs. 5-9 and 5-10) in order that the desired muscle activity can be encouraged and incorrect movements prevented. For example, if the therapist attempts to elicit motor activity by encouraging reaching and other movements without appropriate guidance (Fig. 5-3), the infant, who will tend to use the stronger muscles or those that have the greatest advantage, will practice incorrect movements, and these substitution movements will quickly become learned. Manual guidance needs to be used carefully because the movement will be more likely to be learned if the infant is free to make the movement and not restricted or controlled by the therapist. Object-mediated guidance, in which a toy is presented that by its position in space and its shape requires a certain approach, is potentially more effective (see Fig. 5-18).

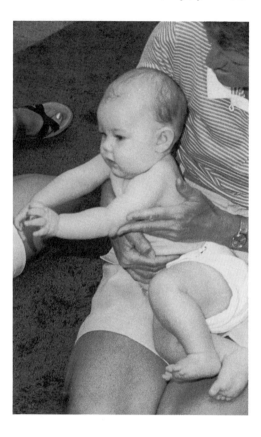

Fig. 5-9. Manual guidance to ensure the infant reaches forward in flexion and external rotation. Without manual guidance he would hold the shoulder in some abduction and internal rotation.

It should be kept in mind even with the young infant that it will be difficult for abnormal substitution movements to be "unlearned" once they have become well established, at least not until the child is old enough to concentrate for longer periods on motor training and practice. In certain cases, muscles with the potential to recover may fail to develop maximal function because of the early establishment of poor movement habits. For this reason, a simple and accurate method of discovering the earliest manifestations of muscle activity by EMG must be developed and utilized so that the therapist and parents can have advance notice of muscle reinnervation and concentrate their attention on organizing practice to ensure the best possible recovery of function. Of course, when there has been severe disruption of nerve supply, there may be no recovery of function, no matter how skilled the therapist.

Fitts[35] and Fitts and Posner[36] have pointed out that the first stage in motor learning is *cognitive*, that is, the beginner tries to "understand" the overall idea of the task and what it demands; the second stage is *associative*, a period of continuous adjustment and reorganization of motor behavior in which components are tried out and put together; and the third stage, the *autonomous* or

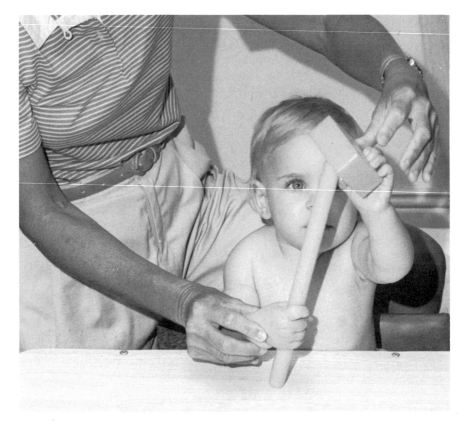

Fig. 5-10. Manual guidance to encourage supination of the right forearm and to ensure the correct forearm alignment for grasping.

automatic stage, is characterized by coordinated execution of the task, requiring little cognitive control and suffering less from distractions. Although there is an increasing lack of conscious awareness during this stage, learning does not cease. It is generally assumed that movement in infants can only be stimulated at an automatic level by play or by "facilitation" of movement. However, even small babies are able to "learn" movement at a cognitive level, that is, by "thinking" about the goal and by reacting to feedback from the therapists and parents about the success or otherwise of their performance. The therapist should not keep the infants practicing any movement for more than a few minutes as they have little ability to concentrate and will resent being held in one position for too long.

It is therefore necessary to think of many different ways for the infant to practice similar movement combinations. It may be that motor training of infants would be more effective if it concentrated on stimulating the infant's cognitive awareness of what he or she must do rather than solely on eliciting an automatic response. One problem with stimulating movement at an automatic level is that it is so often done with insufficient guidance. This results in the infant practicing what, in a sense, he or she can already do, which, without guidance, will frequently be an incorrect movement.

Verbal Feedback and Reinforcement

The infant's correct attempts at using the arm should be rewarded, so that he or she receives feedback as an aid to learning. *Verbal feedback* of successful performance, with reinforcement from tone of voice, smile, and a general attitude of pleasure, seems to have meaning even for small infants, who will usually strive to repeat the performance. The appropriate selection of objects and tasks, the necessary guidance that ensures that the infant is as successful as possible, together with verbal feedback, will mean that therapy sessions are fun and motivating for the infant.

Behavior therapy is also a helpful method of ensuring maximal learning of the desired motor behavior. Behavior therapy involves positive reinforcement by smiling and saying "good boy" or by giving actual rewards, and shaping, which means reinforcing successive approximations of the desired behavior. For example, if the child will not concentrate on practice of a particular activity, he or she is rewarded for practicing for 2 minutes, then for 3 minutes, and so on.

Treatment of Movement Disorganization

Disorganization of scapulohumeral movement is frequently a serious problem evident in the older infant and child (Fig. 5-11). Not only should early therapy aim to prevent contracture of muscles such as subscapularis, which link the scapula and the humerus, it must also aim to stimulate the rhomboids and serratus anterior muscles to contract. Passive movement that ensures the normal range of shoulder abduction and flexion will have no real effect if the muscles that retract, protract, and rotate the scapula are inactive or weak. Figures 5-12 and 5-13 show two ways of ensuring that the scapular retractors have the maximal opportunity to contract. However, once contraction with the arm by the side is possible, these muscles should be encouraged to contract with the arm progressively more and more abducted. Training the serratus anterior muscle is more difficult, but the therapist should stabilize the scapula against the thoracic wall while the infant takes weight through the hands. Therapy should aim to train a more normal relationship both between the protractors and retractors themselves and between these muscles and the muscles for which they act as stabilizers and synergists.

Attempts should be made to elicit activity in the supinators of the forearm, when these are weak or paralyzed, as early as possible in infancy. Unfortunately, an infant in the early months can accomplish much of what he or she wants to do with the forearm in a pronated position (Fig. 5-14), so specific

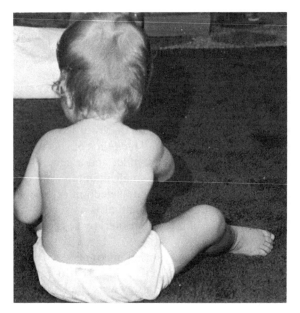

Fig. 5-11. Note the abnormal relationship between the scapula and the humerus on the right side. The scapula is protracted and moves with the humerus instead of adhering to the thoracic wall.

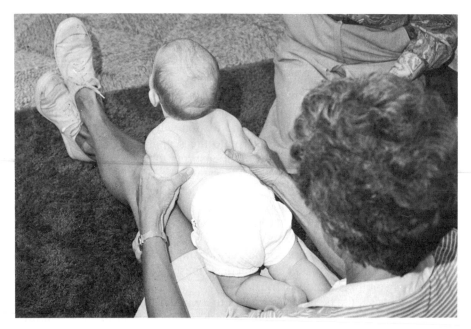

Fig. 5-12. Infant aged 4½ months. One method of encouraging the scapula retractors to contract.

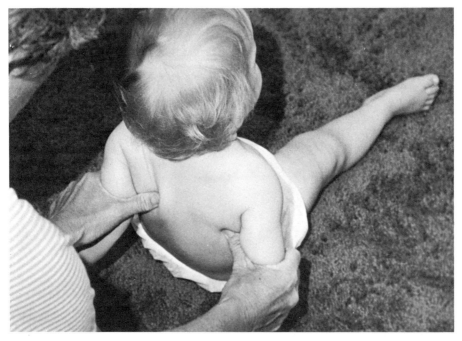

Fig. 5-13. Another method of encouraging the scapular retractors to contract (see Fig. 5-12). The infant's weight is shifted backward onto her hands.

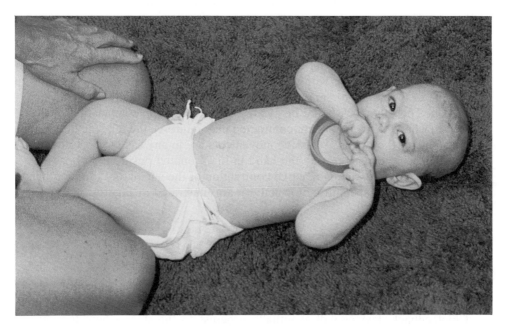

Fig. 5-14. Note the incorrect alignment of the wrist and forearm. If the infant continues practicing without control of his wrist and forearm position, this posturing may become habitual even though recovery of the affected muscle takes place.

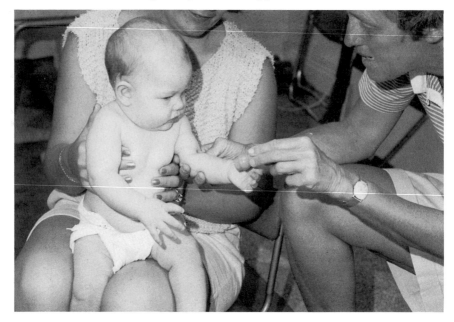

Fig. 5-15.   Holding the elbow in flexion probably makes it easier to activate supination of the forearm.

ways of training active supination must be instituted by the therapist (Figs. 5-15 and 5-16). It is worth noting that active supination is easier to elicit if the elbow and arm are stabilized to prevent other movements (Fig. 5-15). The elbow-flexed position also favors the contraction of biceps brachii, which is the most efficient supinating muscle in this position. Supination is not only more difficult to localize with the elbow extended, it is also less likely to be elicited, as the supinator muscle needs to be of good strength to act in this position. The therapist should be aware that forced passive supination of the forearm when the pronators are contracted may reinforce the tendency toward dislocation of the radius.[17] Passive movements are in any case of no value, as the infant will persist in using the hand in the pronated position, and passive movement will not stimulate active contraction of the supinators. Some other ways to stimulate specific motor activity are illustrated in Figures 5-17 to 5-19.

Biofeedback

Biofeedback or sensory feedback therapy is potentially a means of reinforcing the required motor behavior in infants and children. The development of biofeedback devices will eventually progress to the stage where they are simple and accurate enough to give an irresistible signal to an infant, which will be motivation for further correct practice.

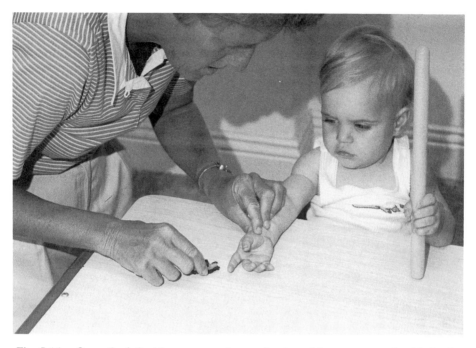

Fig. 5-16. Once the infant has some active supination, this movement should also be encouraged with the elbow extended.

Orthoses

If during training sessions the infant's movements are not guided by the therapist or parent, it is possible that potential improvement in recovering muscles will not take place. Potential improvement may also be inhibited if abnormal alignment of a joint (or joints) is maintained outside of therapy sessions, encouraging the infant to practice only the incorrect muscle activity.

The correct use of splinting or strapping will prevent excessive use of unopposed or relatively unopposed muscles until the child can be trained to contract only those muscles necessary for a movement and to eliminate activity in others not required for the movement. In this way, weak muscles can be forced to contract, the further development of abnormal movement combinations may be prevented, and the child may have a better chance of regaining functional use of the limb.[2,37]

To make it possible for the correct muscle activity to be practiced, a small, light splint may be worn for a significant part of the day. For example, an infant with paralysis of the palmar abductor of the thumb may need a small molded-plastic splint to hold the thumb in palmar abduction, but this should only be worn for periods of the day to help in using the hand effectively and must not interfere with what normal movement the infant has. Similarly, a small wrist

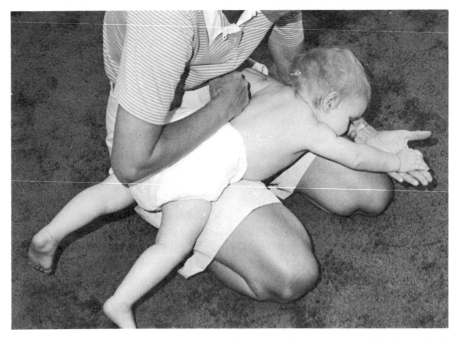

Fig. 5-17. Training the deltoid muscle and the scapular retractors. The therapist is eliciting eccentric contractions by encouraging the infant to lower her hand toward the therapist's hand.

splint may be worn for part of the day to encourage activity in the wrist extensors with the hand in the correct alignment. Dynamic splinting may be useful to reinforce wrist extension in infants with a C7 paralysis.[1]

With increased maturity and ability and inclination to interact with the environment, the infant will practice what he or she likes, whether the movement is correct or not, and at this stage the provision of an orthotic device may be effective in preventing incorrect practicing and in encouraging correct movement. If a splint is used, it must be designed so it does not discourage or impede the movement wanted. Therapy to stimulate activity in particular muscles in the older infant can be combined with the use of a biofeedback training device, which will also make therapy sessions enjoyable and enable appropriate home practice.

Electrical Stimulation

The use of electrical stimulation is controversial and its efficacy has not been adequately tested. Eng and colleagues[1,17] suggested that the use of galvanic current of sufficient intensity to cause a maximum muscle contraction under isometric conditions may prevent wasting of denervated muscle and loss

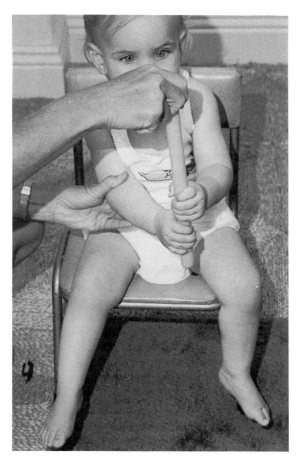

Fig. 5-18. Practicing grasp and release and shoulder flexion by placing hand over hand. The therapist guides the movement by preventing shoulder abduction.

of awareness of the affected limb. Liberson and Terzis[38] also suggest that there is considerable clinical evidence that electrical stimulation of denervated muscle fibers prevents muscle atrophy. However, they are critical of typical physical therapy practice, which they consider grossly inadequate in terms of, for example, length of time allotted to muscle stimulation. These authors have developed a "slow pulse stimulator" that they believe overcomes many of the problems associated with manually operated galvanic stimulation. Functional electrical stimulation can be commenced as soon as active muscle contraction can be obtained, with emphasis at this time on active training of the limb.

Soft Tissue Contracture

Passive Movements

Many authors[1,39] stress the importance of passive movements in preventing soft tissue contracture, particularly scapulohumeral adhesion. Passive movements must, however, be done gently to avoid damage to the unprotected

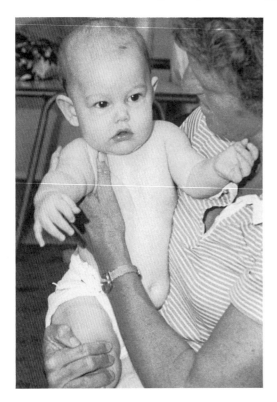

Fig. 5-19. If the parents hold the infant like this, the tendency to abduct instead of flex the shoulder is controlled and the movement of flexion is encouraged.

shoulder joint. Zancolli[40] comments that forceful manipulation is one of the factors that contributes to an alteration in the anatomy of the glenohumeral joint. Although it is important to prevent contracture of the muscles that link scapula to humerus, the normal relationship between scapula and humerus, and the necessity for controlled scapular movement as the glenohumeral joint is abducted or flexed,[41] must be taken into account. The scapula should not be manually restrained once the humerus is moved beyond 30 degrees of range. Elevation of the arm without rotation of the scapula and without lateral rotation at the glenohumeral joint will damage the glenohumeral joint by causing the humerus to impinge on the immobile acromion process. Abduction or flexion of the arm should therefore not take place without associated and appropriate scapular movement, which should be assisted if necessary.

Particular care must also be taken in teaching the infant's parents how to do passive movements. Parents should receive instruction in the anatomy of the shoulder so that they understand the movements they must do and the importance of keeping within the normal range. They should understand the anatomic reasons why they must be careful not to overmobilize and why they must be gentle. They should be warned not to proceed with any movement that causes the infant to cry. Unfortunately, without this knowledge, a parent may severely injure the infant's arm.

However, soft tissue contracture will ultimately be prevented only if activity recovers in the affected muscles. Passive movements will not lead to the restoration of active function. Therapy must therefore concentrate not only on ensuring the optimal position and alignment of joints, but most particularly on the stimulation of active contraction at their lengthened range of those muscles resting persistently at a shortened length.

Splinting

Splinting, particularly when it involves the shoulder, remains a controversial issue.[1,7-9] Although some investigators have recommended it, evidence exists that several of the problems that arise in these infants may be directly related to the type of splinting used.

In the upper arm type, some have suggested that the arm be held in abduction and lateral rotation by pinning the sleeve to the pillow or by a "statue of liberty" splint, or held in abduction and midrotation by an abduction splint. In subsequent articles, some of these investigators, as well as others,[7,9,30,42-44] have pointed out, however, that splinting the arm in this position may lead to "overmobility" of the glenohumeral joint, and that this positioning may be a factor that contributes to pathology in the glenohumeral joint, even to anterior dislocation.[17] Although there seems to be sufficient evidence to discontinue the use of the types of shoulder splinting listed above, when paralysis affects the entire limb it should be possible for therapists and bioengineers to design a means of supporting the humerus in the glenohumeral cavity that will not discourage use of the limb and will not predispose to joint dysfunction.

Neglect of the Arm, or "Learned Nonuse"

Neglect of a paralyzed arm is relatively common in hemiplegic infants and children and in adults following stroke.[32] It appears also to occur in some infants with brachial plexus lesions and may be an important contributing factor to the failure to develop motor control. If initial attempts to use the arm result in failure, the infant may cease trying. Neglect may also be a factor in preventing recovery of muscle function that could potentially have occurred as a result of nerve regeneration. Several reports in the literature mention infants with good return of muscle function who nevertheless ignored the arm and refused to use it.[1,30] Wickstrom[7] attributed this neglect to the lack of development of "functional cerebral motor patterns of coordination." Zalis and colleagues[45] suggested that transitory interruption of peripheral nerve pathways at birth prevented the establishment of normal patterns of movement and the organization of body image. Taub[46] has described what he calls *learned nonuse*, which is demonstrated by monkeys after either deafferentation or brain lesion, and

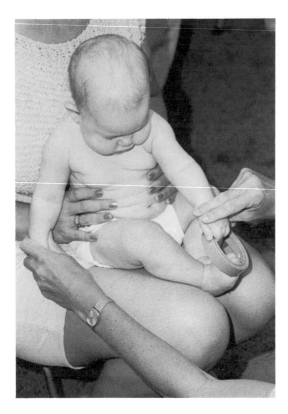

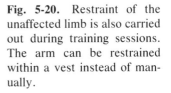

Fig. 5-20. Restraint of the unaffected limb is also carried out during training sessions. The arm can be restrained within a vest instead of manually.

which is primarily due, according to Taub, to a learning phenomenon. The animals learn *not* to use the affected limb because they can perform in a satisfactory manner with the remaining limbs and no motivating factor exists to encourage them to use the affected limb. This habitual nonuse persists so that even when the limb becomes potentially useful, the animal does not seem aware of this possibility. Others[47] have described similar findings. Consequently, motor training procedures for infants with brachial plexus lesions should probably be carried out in conjunction with short periods of restraint of the unaffected arm (Fig. 5-20). One study of two hemiplegic infants[48] involved restraint of the intact arm during the early training sessions for short periods during the day. After 6 months of training, both children were able to successfully use the previously paretic arm and hand.

Sensory Unawareness

Specific attempts should be made in treatment to stimulate sensory awareness, but these can probably only be effective once the infant is old enough to play sensory "games," such as locating certain objects in sand, localizing touch stimuli, and recognizing and naming common objects while blindfolded. When the infant is older, two-point discrimination and stereognosis guessing games can be used in an attempt to improve awareness.

Abnormal Respiratory Function

When diaphragmatic paralysis exists, respiration can be aided by oxygen with continuous positive airway pressure or continuous negative pressure.[49,50] If the nerve lesion is a neurapraxia, there will be eventual recovery of diaphragmatic function, but, during the period of paralysis, it is important to prevent respiratory problems such as atelectasis. Positioning with the paralyzed side underneath should be avoided. Postural drainage in the prone position at a 45-degree angle should be carried out at home for short periods during the day with the objective of preventing retention of secretions in the relatively immobile parts of the lung.

SURGICAL TREATMENT

Surgery is not usually performed in infancy, although some investigators suggest that, with certain lesions, surgical intervention may help in removal of hematomas or neurolysis of adhesions,[10] and others[51] suggest early surgical exploration and repair by nerve graft. In the older child, surgery to stabilize joints, tendon transplantation, and soft tissue elongation are performed with the objective of gaining some improvement in function.[52,53] Zancolli[40] describes surgical techniques aimed at improving function and cosmesis of the shoulder.

CONCLUSION

Brachial plexus injury at birth may be followed by considerable disability involving muscle paralysis and weakness, soft tissue contracture, loss of sensation, and sympathetic changes. The major loss of function is the infant's inability to reach out and to use the hand effectively, and the therapist, sensitive to the child's needs, must set about the task of analyzing treatment approaches to this problem with as much knowledge as can be gathered. Therapists should question whether existing treatment procedures are logical in terms of a biomechanical and anatomic understanding of the dysfunction, and develop more effective ways of training motor control and of preventing habitual substitution movements and "learned nonuse" of the limb. It is probable that most infants could regain better motor function if put on a more specific motor training program than at present appears to exist.

REFERENCES

1. Eng GD: Brachial plexus palsy in newborn infants. Pediatrics 48:18, 1971
2. Draznin E, Maloney FP, Brammell C: Functional strapping for incomplete Erb palsy: a case report. Arch Phys Med Rehabil 65:731, 1984
3. Sjoberg I, Erichs K, Bjerre I: Cause and effect of obstetric (neonatal) brachial plexus palsy. Acta Paediatr Scand 77:357, 1988
4. von Hofsten C: Development of visually directed reaching: the approach phase. J Hum Movement Studies 5:160, 1979
5. Jeannerod M: The timing of natural prehension movements. J Motor Behav 16(3):235, 1984
6. Carr JH, Shepherd RB, Gordon J et al: Movement Science. Foundations for Physical Therapy in Rehabilitation. Aspen, Rockville, MD, 1987
7. Wickstrom J: Birth injuries of the brachial plexus: treatment of defects of the shoulder. Clin Orthop 23:187, 1962
8. Adler JB, Patterson RL: Erb's palsy: long-term results of treatment in eighty-eight cases. J Bone Joint Surg [Am] 49:1052, 1967
9. Johnson EW, Alexander MA, Koenig WC: Infantile Erb's palsy (Smellie's palsy). Arch Phys Med Rehabil 58:175, 1977
10. Swaiman KF, Wright FS: Neuromuscular Diseases of Infancy and Childhood. Charles C Thomas, Springfield, IL, 1970
11. Turner T, Evans J, Brown JK: Monoparesis. Complication of constant positive airways pressure. Arch Dis Child 50:128, 1975
12. Magee KR, DeJong RN: Paralytic brachial neuritis. JAMA 174:1258, 1960
13. Jackson ST, Hoffer MM, Parrish N: Brachial plexus palsy in the newborn. J Bone Joint Surg [Am] 70A 8:1217, 1988
14. Greenwald AG, Schute PC, Shively JL: Brachial plexus birth palsy: a 10-year report on the incidence and prognosis. J Pediatr Orthop 4:689, 1984
15. Specht EE: Brachial plexus palsy in the newborn. Clin Orthop 75(110):32, 1975
16. Davis DH, Onofrio BM, MacCarty CS: Brachial plexus injuries. Mayo Clin Proc 53(12):799, 1978
17. Eng GD, Koch B, Smokvina MD: Brachial plexus palsy in neonates and children. Arch Phys Med Rehabil 59:458, 1978
18. Zverina E, Kredba J: Somatosensory cerebral evoked potentials in diagnosing brachial plexus injuries. Scand J Rehabil Med 19:47, 1977
19. Landi A, Copeland SA, Wynn Parry CB et al: The role of somatosensory evoked potentials and nerve conduction studies in the surgical management of brachial plexus injuries. J Bone Joint Surg [Br] 62B 4:492, 1980
20. Stefanova-Uzunova M, Stamatova L, Gatev V: Dynamic properties of partially denervated muscle in children with brachial plexus birth palsy. J Neurol Neurosurg Psychiatry 44:497, 1981
21. O'Riain S: New and simple test of nerve function in the hand. Br Med J 3:615, 1973
22. Bufalini C, Pescatori G: Posterior cervical electromyography in the diagnosis and prognosis of brachial plexus injuries. J Bone Joint Surg [Br] 51:627, 1969
23. Leffert RD: Brachial plexus injuries. N Engl J Med 291(20):1059, 1974
24. Stanwood JE, Kraft GH: Diagnosis and management of brachial plexus injuries. Arch Phys Med Rehabil 52:52, 1971
25. Gjorup L: Obstetrical lesion of the brachial plexus. Acta Neurol Scand Suppl 18:9, 1966

26. Robinson PK: Associated movements between limb and respiratory muscles as a sequel to brachial plexus birth injury. Johns Hopkins Med J 89:21, 1951

27. Esslen E: Electromyographic findings on two types of misdirection of regenerating axons. Electroencephalogr Clin Neurophysiol 12:738, 1960

28. De Grandis D, Fiaschi A, Michieli G et al: Anomalous reinnervation as a sequel to obstetric brachial plexus palsy. J Neurol Sci 1(43):127, 1979

29. Tada K, Ohshita S, Yonenobu K et al: Experimental study of spinal nerve repair after plexus brachialis injury in newborn rats: a horseradish peroxidase study. Exp Neurol 2(65):301, 1979

30. Rose FC (ed): Paediatric Neurology. Blackwell Scientific Publishers, Oxford, 1979

31. Boome RS, Kaye JC: Obstetric traction injuries of the brachial plexus. J Bone Joint Surg [Br] 70B 4:571, 1988

32. Carr JH, Shepherd RB: A Motor Relearning Programme for Stroke. Ed. 2. Heinemann, London, 1987

33. Gatcheva J: Early diagnosis and long term management of obstetric paralysis. Int Rehabil Med 3(1):126, 1979

34. von Hofsten C: Eye-hand coordination in the newborn. Dev Psychol 18:450, 1982

35. Fitts PM: Perceptual motor skill learning. In Melton AE (ed): Categories of Human Learning. Academic press, San Diego, 1964

36. Fitts PM, Posner MI: Human Performance. Prentice-Hall, London, 1973

37. Perry J, Hsu J, Barber L, Hoffer MM: Orthoses in patients with brachial plexus injuries. Arch Phys Med Rehabil 55:134, 1974

38. Liberson WT, Terzis JK: Some novel techniques of clinical electrophysiology applied to the management of brachial plexus palsy. Electromyogr Clin Neurophysiol 27:371, 1987

39. Shepherd RB: Physiotherapy in Paediatrics. 2nd Ed. Heinemann, London, 1980

40. Zancolli EA: Classification and management of the shoulder in birth palsy. Orthop Clin North Am 12:433, 1981

41. Cailliet R: The Shoulder in Hemiplegia. FA Davis, Philadelphia, 1980

42. Carter S, Gold AP: Neurology of Infancy and Childhood. Appleton-Century-Crofts, East Norwalk, CT, 1974

43. Schut L: Nerve injuries in children. Surg Clin North Am 52:1307, 1972

44. Aitken J: Deformity of elbow joint as sequel to Erb's obstetrical paralysis. J Bone Joint Surg [Br] 34:352, 1952

45. Zalis OS, Zalis AW, Barron KD et al: Motor patterning following transitory sensory-motor deprivation. Arch Neurol 13:487, 1965

46. Taub E: Somato-sensory deafferentation research with monkeys: implications for rehabilitation medicine. p. 371. In Ince LP (ed): Behavioral Psychology in Rehabilitation Medicine: Clinical Applications. Williams & Wilkins, Baltimore, 1980

47. Yu J: Functional recovery with and without training following brain damage in experimental animals: a review. Arch Phys Med Rehabil 57:38, 1976

48. Schwartzman RJ: Rehabilitation of infantile hemiplegia. Am J Phys Med 53:75, 1974

49. Bucci G et al: Phrenic nerve palsy treated by continuous positive pressure breathing by nasal cannula. Arch Dis Child 49:230, 1974

50. Weisman L, Woodall J, Merenstein G: Constant negative pressure in the treatment of diaphragmatic paralysis secondary to birth injury. Birth Defects 12(6):297, 1976

51. Gilbert A, Khouri N, Cartioz H: Exploration chirurgicale du plexus brachial dans la paralysic obstétricale. Rev Chir Orthop 66:33, 1980

52. Hoffer MM, Wickenden R, Roper B: Brachial plexus birth palsies: results of tendon transfers to the rotator cuff. J Bone Joint Surg [Am] 60:691, 1978
53. Manske PR, McCarroll HR, Hale R: Biceps tendon rerouting and percutaneous osteoclasis in the treatment of supination deformity in obstetrical palsy. J Hand Surg 5:153, 1980

6 | Down Syndrome

Susan R. Harris　　　Alice M. Shea

Physical therapy for children with Down syndrome received relatively little attention prior to the early 1970s. Whereas children with more obvious physical handicaps, such as those with cerebral palsy or meningomyelocele, received services from pediatric therapists for many years, children with Down syndrome had been less apt to be the focus of assessment and treatment. Clinical research during the past two decades has demonstrated that there are many aspects of this syndrome that warrant attention from pediatric therapists, such as significant developmental motor delay during infancy and early childhood,[1-3] perceptual–motor deficits,[4] and a variety of orthopedic disorders.[5] This chapter focuses primarily on the physical therapist's assessment and treatment of children with Down syndrome. Other issues addressed are the incidence, etiology, and pathology of this disorder as well as medical, educational, and family involvement for children with Down syndrome.

OCCURRENCE AND ETIOLOGY

Down syndrome has long been recognized as one of the most common causes of mental retardation.[6,7] The current incidence rate of this disorder is estimated at 1.3 per 1,000 live births, with an increased risk occurring with advanced maternal age.[8] Advanced paternal age has also been implicated as a factor contributing to increased risk for giving birth to a child with Down syndrome.[9] Approximately 5,000 infants with Down syndrome are born annually in the United States.[8]

The etiology of Down syndrome is still unknown, but it is generally considered that several developmental errors may exist, any one or a combination of which can produce the alteration in chromosomal pattern that is characteristic of the disorder.[10] The latter was first described by Lejeune and colleagues in 1959, based on chromosome analysis of affected individuals.[11] In 91 percent of Down syndrome cases, there is an extra small chromosome present on the 21st pair of chromosomes. This chromosomal abnormality is labeled more specifically[6] as trisomy 21 and develops as a result of nondisjunction of two homologous chromosomes during either the first or second meiotic division.[12] Approximately 3 to 4 percent of individuals with Down syndrome have a chromosomal abnormality known as translocation in which there is breakage of two nonhomologous chromosomes with subsequent reattachment of the broken pieces to other intact chromosome pairs. Recurrence risk of the birth of a child with Down syndrome to parents who are translocation carriers varies from 2 to 10 percent, a risk that is greater than with the nondisjunction type of trisomy 21.[12] Most of the remaining cases of Down syndrome represent mosaic disorders in which some cells within the individual are normal and some are trisomy 21.

PATHOLOGY

Neuropathology

The neuropathology associated with Down syndrome has been explored by a number of researchers. The overall brain weight of individuals with Down syndrome averages 76 percent of the brain weight of normal individuals with the combined weight of the cerebellum and brain stem being proportionately even smaller, an average of 66 percent of the weight of the cerebellum and brain stem in normal individuals.[13] There is also a reduction in total head circumference.[14] The brain is abnormally rounded and short with a relatively narrow anterior-posterior diameter and relatively wide lateral diameter, a configuration that is termed *microbrachycephaly*.[14,15]

There are also changes in the convolutional pattern of the brain. These include a narrowed superior temporal gyrus that is often bilateral and a reduction of secondary sulci that results in a simplicity of convolutional pattern.[16,17]

In addition to these gross neurologic differences, there are a number of cytologic distinctions that characterize the brains of individuals with Down syndrome. Ross and colleagues noted a paucity of small neurons (postulated to be aspinous stellate cells) and suggested that a migration defect involving small neurons may be related to the neural pathogenesis of Down syndrome as well as to the previously described simplicity of convolutional pattern.[17] Scott and colleagues have also noted reduced synaptogenesis and alterations in synaptic morphology.[18]

Marin-Padilla[19] studied the neuronal organization of the motor cortex of a 19-month-old child with Down syndrome and found various structural abnormalities in the dendritic spines of the pyramidal neurons of the motor cortex. He suggested that these structural differences may underlie the motor incoordination and mental retardation characteristic of individuals with Down syndrome. Loesch-Mdzewska,[20] in his neuropathologic study of 123 brains of individuals with Down syndrome aged 3 to 62 years, also frequently found neurologic abnormalities of the pyramidal system in addition to the reduced brain weight noted by the other researchers cited above.

Benda noted a lack of myelination of the nerve fibers in the precentral areas and frontal lobes of the cerebral cortex and in the cerebella of infants with Down syndrome.[16] A more recent study by Wisniewski and Schmidt-Sidor[21] found myelination delay between 2 months and 6 years in 22.5 percent of the Down syndrome brains studied, with a greater percentage of brains of infants and children with congenital heart disease demonstrating this delay. Some correlation was found between myelination delay and developmental delay; however, details of analysis and of developmental testing were not described.[21]

Another neuropathologic study conducted on the brains of five adults with Down syndrome who died at ages ranging from 21 to 62 years showed a significant decrease in the number of pyramidal neurons in the hippocampus when compared with brains of normal individuals of comparable ages.[22] This finding, combined with a significant increase in neurofibrillary tangles and senile plaques, demonstrated a quantitative similarity to types of neurons found in the brains of adults with Alzheimer's dementia.[23] Research is currently under way to determine the functional consequences of this type of neuropathologic finding in Down syndrome.

In addition to the neuropathologic findings associated with Down syndrome, there are a number of other pathologic characteristics, many of which warrant medical intervention. The following sections discuss a number of these associated deficits and their medical management.

Cardiopulmonary Anomalies

Congenital heart defects are very common in individuals with Down syndrome. These defects are present in approximately 40 percent of individuals with Down syndrome.[24] The two most common cardiac anomalies reported are atrioventricular canal defects and ventriculoseptal defects.[6] Many congenital heart defects can be repaired surgically. It is extremely important that the child's therapist be aware of the presence and extent of any cardiac defects, particularly those severe enough to influence the course of assessment and treatment. A longitudinal study of motor development in infants and children with Down syndrome from birth to 3 years of age indicated that moderate to severe congenital heart disease that had not been corrected is associated with increased delays in achievement of gross motor milestones.[25] Children with heart defects need not be excluded from receiving therapy, but close consultation with the child's physician and careful monitoring of response to treatment is strongly advised.

Sensory Deficits

Another common medical problem that may indirectly influence the child's response to physical therapy is hearing loss. In a study of 107 individuals with Down syndrome, binaural hearing loss was noted in 64 percent of the subjects tested.[26] Otitis media is a frequently recurring medical problem that contributes to hearing deficiencies in individuals with Down syndrome.[6] Visual defects are also much more common in individuals with Down syndrome than in the general population. Strabismus (usually esotropia) was noted in 41.3 percent of a sample of 75 institutionalized individuals with Down syndrome.[27] Nystagmus, cataracts, and myopia were frequently found.[27] Other ocular findings of less clinical significance were the presence of Brushfield spots in the iris and the characteristic upward and outward slanting of the palpebral fissures. Interestingly, the presence of epicanthal folds—a classic clinical diagnostic feature of Down syndrome—was noted in only 17.3 percent of this institutionalized sample.[27]

With regard to visual perception, a frequent area of deficit in all handicapped populations, a recent study examining the ability of school-age children with Down syndrome to replicate and match block structures concluded that the inability to replicate the structures was due to a perceptual–motor deficit rather than to a defect in visual perception, since the subjects were able to correctly match like structures. The author concluded that visual perception was intact in this sample of children.[4]

Musculoskeletal Differences

Of particular interest to physical therapists are the number and types of musculoskeletal differences associated with Down syndrome, due in part to the generalized hypotonia and ligamentous laxity characteristic of this disorder. Diamond and colleagues[5] evaluated the prevalence of orthopedic deformities among a sample of 265 persons with Down syndrome, 107 of whom were institutionalized patients, with the remainder being outpatients. A much greater prevalence of major orthopedic problems existed among the institutionalized sample. The two major foot deformities noted were metatarsus primus varus and pes planus (secondary to severe ligamentous laxity). Both of these disorders frequently required the prescription of special shoes and, occasionally, surgical intervention. Patellar instability resulting in subluxation or dislocation was present in 23 percent of the subjects and usually was managed surgically. Hip subluxation or dislocation occurred in 10 percent and also required surgical intervention.[5]

While thoracolumbar scoliosis was present in 52 percent of individuals in this sample, most of the curves were defined as "mild to moderate," and only one case required surgery.[5] Physical therapists who work with children with Down syndrome should be aware of their propensity for developing such orthopedic deformities and should provide periodic musculoskeletal assessments such as posture screening and range of motion (ROM) evaluation of hips and knees.

One of the most serious orthopedic problems associated with Down syndrome is the risk for atlantoaxial dislocation. Because of the laxity of the transverse odontoid ligament,[28] there may be "excessive motion of C1 on C2,"[29] which can result in subluxation or dislocation of the atlantoaxial joint. Andrews[30] reported in 1981 that 33 cases of atlantoaxial dislocation in individuals with Down syndrome had been cited in the medical literature. Radiologic examination of various samples of persons with Down syndrome has demonstrated atlantoaxial dislocation in 12 to 20 percent of subjects.[31] Although the majority of cases with dislocation have been clinically asymptomatic, a small number of individuals have shown myelopathy, including spastic quadriplegia.

Early symptoms associated with atlantoaxial dislocation include gait changes (ankle instability and increased difficulty in walking),[29] urinary retention,[29] torticollis,[4,28] reluctance in moving the neck, and increased deep tendon reflexes.[31] Posterior arthrodesis of C1 to C2 is recommended in cases of atlantoaxial dislocation without neurologic symptomatology, whereas posterior stabilization and fusion of C1 to C2 are recommended for cases with early neurologic involvement.[29] The Committee on Sports Medicine of the American Academy of Pediatrics recommends an initial set of cervical spine radiographs at 2 years of age with follow-up radiographs in grade school, adolescence, and adulthood.[32]

Physical therapists who work with children with Down syndrome should be acutely aware of the increased risk for atlantoaxial dislocation. While every effort should be made to mainstream the handicapped child into recreational activities engaged in by their nonhandicapped peers, particular caution should be exercised when involving the child with Down syndrome in strenuous gymnastics and tumbling or contact sports, such as football and wrestling, since the ligamentous laxity of the atlantoaxial joint makes it "less resistant to superimposed flexion trauma."[29]

In addition to the skeletal differences noted above, anatomic research on cadavers of five individuals with Down syndrome revealed a number of muscle variations including frequent absence of certain muscles, such as palmaris longus; extra muscles, including supernumerary forearm flexors; and variations of muscles.[33] According to Bersu,[33] the "most striking variation" appeared among the muscles of facial expression with lack of differentiation of distinct muscle bellies for zygomaticus major and minor and levator labii superioris. This aberration was present in all five cadavers and "may contribute to the characteristic expressions of the DS individual."[33]

Hypotonia

In addition to the foregoing complications associated with Down syndrome that frequently warrant medical or surgical management, there are several other characteristic features of this disorder that indicate the need for assessment and treatment by qualified developmental therapists. One of the hallmarks of Down syndrome and, in fact, one of the most characteristic diagnostic features at birth is generalized hypotonia.[34] Particularly evident during the early years,[1,35] the hypotonia is probably a major contributing factor to the significant motor delay characterizing the period of infancy and early childhood in children with Down syndrome. These characteristics are discussed in more detail in the following sections, which address the physical therapist's role in the assessment and treatment of children with this disorder.

Finally, other medical problems appearing with greater frequency among individuals with Down syndrome than among those in the normal population include seizure disorders (5 to 6 percent), duodenal stenosis, leukemia, and senile dementia.

PHYSICAL THERAPY ASSESSMENT

The physical therapist who participates in the evaluation of a child with Down syndrome should be cognizant of the medical problems associated with this disorder and aware of recent research reports that have explored the degree of motor delay, the interrelationship of mental and motor delay, and the effects of the generalized hypotonia on other aspects of development. The first part of this section provides a review of recent literature examining these concerns, with the latter part of the section directed at specific evaluation strategies based on these research findings.

Review of Motor Differences Associated with Down Syndrome

The most common motor difference associated with Down syndrome is hypotonia or low muscle tone.[7,15,36] Estimates vary as to the percentage of infants with Down syndrome who display hypotonia and the degree to which it is present.[37-40] McIntire and coworkers[41] described hypotonia as the most frequently observed characteristic and also indicated that it was found in all major muscle groups including neck, trunk, and extremities for 98 percent of the population tested.

A number of researchers have demonstrated a relationship between low muscle tone and delayed motor development. Crome and colleagues,[42] in their neuropathologic study of the brains of individuals with Down syndrome, speculated that the lower weight of the cerebellum and brain stem characteristic of this population may account for the muscular hypotonia, which in turn is probably a major influence on early motor development. In their descriptive retrospective report on the developmental data of 612 noninstitutionalized children with Down syndrome ranging in age from birth to 16 years, Melyn and White[43] found a wide range of development in every attribute they tested, including motor and speech milestones derived from the norms of Gesell and Amatruda.[44]

These researchers suggest that one of the most influential characteristics affecting early motor development is degree of hypotonia. They further implicate hypotonia of the speech musculature as a contributing factor in the delayed speech development that characterizes children with Down syndrome.[43]

LaVeck and LaVeck,[2] in their administration of the mental and motor scales of the Bayley Scales of Infant Development[45] to 20 female and 20 male infants with Down syndrome ranging in age from 12 to 36 months, found that the mean mental quotients were significantly higher than the mean motor quotients and that the average motor age lagged 2.86 months behind the average mental age. These investigators suggested that this significantly greater delay in motor development may be related to the hypotonia associated with Down syndrome and not solely to the mental retardation, since a comparison group of developmentally delayed non-Down syndrome infants, many of them with known or suspected neurologic deficits, were not as severely delayed in psychomotor functioning as were the infants with Down syndrome. In replicating this study with younger infants with Down syndrome (2.7 to 21.5 months), Harris[3] reported similar findings in that significantly greater delays were noted in motor development than in mental development as measured on the Bayley scales.

Not only has hypotonia been implicated as a contributing factor in delayed motor development and delayed speech acquisition in infants and young children with Down syndrome, but it has also been shown to be correlated with lags in affective and cognitive development. Cicchetti and Sroufe,[46] in their longitudinal study of 14 infants with Down syndrome ranging in age from 4 to 24 months, demonstrated that the four most hypotonic infants were not only the most delayed in affective expression, but also scored the lowest on measures of cognitive development as shown by the mental portion of the Bayley scales[45] and the Uzgiris-Hunt scales of cognitive development.[47] Cowie, in her neurologic study of 79 infants with Down syndrome from birth to 10 months, also noted a correlation between extreme hypotonia and poor performance on the Bayley scales.[35]

The lowered muscle tone characteristic of Down syndrome has also been shown to contribute to slower reaction time and depressed kinesthetic feedback. O'Connor and Hermelin[48] compared reaction time on a task between a group of children with Down syndrome and a comparable group of children with mental retardation who did not have Down syndrome. They theorized that the slower reaction time that characterized the group of children with Down syndrome was due, in part, to the marked hypotonia. They also hypothesized that the hypotonia contributed to a lessened degree of kinesthetic feedback, another sensory difference characteristic of individuals with Down syndrome.[48]

In a more recent study, the relationship of muscle tone (as evaluated during the first 3 years of life in 89 infants with Down syndrome) with later outcome variables was assessed. The researchers reported that muscle tone "was a powerful predictor of all of the outcome variables including language acquisition, motor and social development, and mental functioning."[49] One of the most important findings of the previous study was that of marked variability in muscle tone (as measured by resistance to passive movement) that was present in the study group. This increased variability is comparable to that which prevails in many aspects of Down syndrome.[38]

Although hypotonia is the neuromotor deficit most frequently mentioned in describing the characteristics of infants and young children with Down syndrome, a number of additional problems also have been noted. In her longitudinal study of 79 infants with Down syndrome from birth to 10 months, Cowie[35] administered comprehensive neurologic examinations during the neonatal period, at 6 months, and at 10 months. In addition to the universal finding of marked hypotonia, Cowie also noted a persistence of primitive reflexes past the time when they should normally disappear. These reflexes included the palmar and plantar grasp reflexes, the stepping reflex, and the Moro reflex.[35] Haley[50] noted a slower rate of development of postural reactions in infants with Down syndrome, with the association between postural reactions and motor milestones similar to that which is seen in normal children. Rast and Harris,[51] using the Movement Assessment of Infants (MAI),[52] examined qualitative differences in head righting and active hip movement between 3- to 4-month-old infants with Down syndrome and an age-matched comparison group. They found the infants with Down syndrome "to have difficulty in adjusting their heads in space against the pull of gravity and they showed less antigravity control of lower extremities."[51] The infants with Down syndrome tended to use compensatory movement strategies in their efforts to stabilize themselves. The authors cautioned against reinforcing the use of these strategies in treatment because they do not represent qualitatively normal postures or movements.

In a study of preschool children with Down syndrome, Shumway-Cook and Woollacott[53] found deficits in postural response synergies when balance perturbations were introduced. These investigators argued that the balance deficits are more important than hypotonia in understanding the movement problems of Down syndrome.[53] Grip strength and isometric muscle contractions have been shown to be deficient in school-aged children with Down syndrome[54]; another study involving school-aged children reported that ankle strength was reduced in the children with Down syndrome and contributed to the typical posture of squatting with heels down.[55]

Because of the multiplicity of medical, cognitive, and motor problems associated with Down syndrome, evaluation by the physical therapist must be comprehensive and must reflect information from members of the interdisciplinary assessment team. In light of the frequency of major medical problems associated with this disorder, the therapist should work in close consultation with the child's physician. Prior to performing an evaluation, the therapist should obtain current medical information about the child's cardiac status, risk for atlantoaxial dislocation, any history of seizures, and results of visual and auditory examinations. Information from the child's teacher concerning IQ, any behavioral problems, and known reinforcers for positive behavior should also be gleaned. The parents' goals and expectations about the evaluation process should also be derived. Reports from psychologists, speech therapists, nurses, and nutritionists may also be available and should be examined prior to conducting the evaluation.

Qualitative Assessment

The physical therapist's examination should be directed at a qualitative assessment of the child's movement patterns as well as a developmental assessment of the child's gross motor and fine motor functional skills. For example, it has been our experience that a number of young infants with Down syndrome may roll from prone to supine as early as 1 to 2 months of age, a developmental motor milestone that is first performed by normal infants at approximately 4 months of age. A qualitative evaluation of this "precocious" motor skill in infants with Down syndrome reveals that their ability to move out of prone into supine is accomplished because of a lack of cocontraction of muscles in the trunk and an inability to grade movement so that any initiation of rolling results in a marked "flip over" into supine rather than a graded ability to smoothly execute the transition. Delayed righting reactions in the head and trunk also appear to contribute to this early ability to flip over from prone to supine (Fig. 6-1).

Another motor milestone that frequently appears in developmental assessment tools is the ability to rise to sitting independently from a prone or supine-lying position.[45] Lydic and Steele[56] have noted an important qualitative difference in the manner in which infants with Down syndrome accomplish this motor skill as compared with the manner in which normal infants rise to sitting: "Advancing from a prone to a sitting posture, the child with Down syndrome who has received no therapeutic intervention characteristically spreads his legs until he is in full-split position with his legs 180 degrees from each other and then uses his hands (or his head) to push up into the sitting position with the legs still in partial- to full-split position or tailor style" (Fig. 6-2). These authors suggest that this qualitative difference may be due in part to the hypermobility of the hip joints as well as the lack of active trunk rotation.[56]

While a number of qualitative differences in movement patterns may be observed during administration of a developmental assessment tool, it is optimal to conduct a separate qualitative assessment as well. The MAI[52] is a suggested evaluation instrument for examining qualitative aspects of movement in infants with Down syndrome, since it assesses four different components of movement: postural tone, primitive reflexes, automatic reactions, and volitional movement (see Ch. 3 for a review of this test). Since research has suggested that the generalized hypotonia, delayed integration of primitive reflexes, and delayed development of automatic reactions characteristic of infants with Down syndrome[35] may all contribute to the documented delays in achieving motor milestones, it is important for physical therapists to examine these qualitative aspects of movement as well as to assess the child's developmental motor level (Fig. 6-3).

Qualitative assessment of older children with Down syndrome should in-

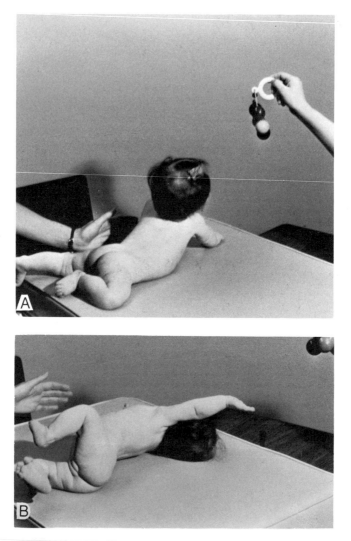

Fig. 6-1.   Rolling prone to supine (4 months of age).

clude analysis of the manner in which they perform functional activities such as gait[57] and task analysis of fine motor activities, such as shoe tying or prevocational skills. In light of the frequency of associated orthopedic problems,[5] posture screening and ROM evaluation of hips and knees should also be included as part of the global physical therapy assessment.

Assessment of developmental motor level is also an integral part of the physical therapist's evaluation of the child with Down syndrome. Whenever possible, a standardized norm-referenced motor assessment tool should be used. Documentation of degree of developmental motor delay is important for

Coventry University
Lanchester Library
Tel 02476 887575

Borrowed Items 05/11/2017 19:27
XXXXX2507

Item Title	Due Date
38001005351485	26/11/2017
* Handbook of pediatric physical therapy	
38001001116528	26/11/2017
* Pediatric neurologic physical therapy	
38001002771271	26/11/2017
* Decision making in pediatric neurologic physical therapy	
38001004610386	20/11/2017
Reflective practice for healthcare professionals : a practical guide	

* Indicates items borrowed today
Thankyou for using this unit
www.coventry.ac.uk

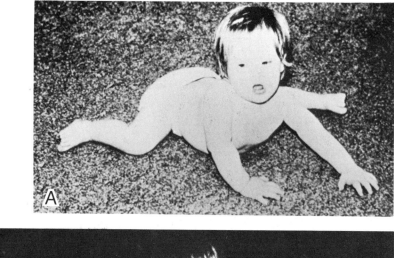

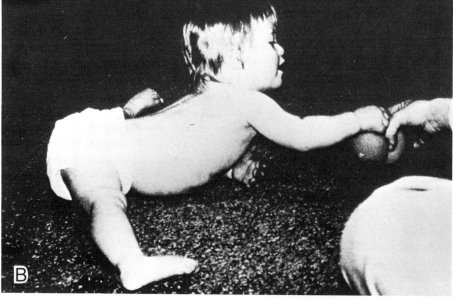

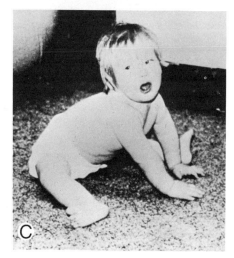

Fig. 6-2. Advancing from prone to sitting posture without trunk rotation. (From Lydic and Steele,[56] with permission.)

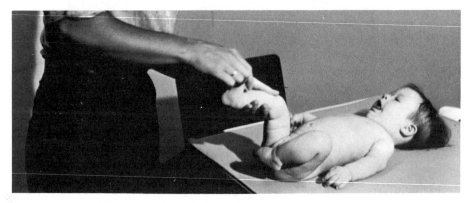

Fig. 6-3. Administering the MAI to a 4-month-old infant. (Item 2 in Muscle Tone: extensibility of heelcords.)

several reasons: (1) to qualify the child for placement in a special education or developmental disabilities program, (2) to justify the receipt of physical therapy services, and (3) to serve as a baseline measurement in documenting change as a result of intervention.

Developmental Assessment

Physical therapists are limited in their choice of developmental motor assessment tools that are both standardized and norm-referenced. A standardized tool uses consistent or standardized assessment procedures and frequently utilizes standardized equipment in the form of a test kit. For an assessment instrument to reflect the degree of motor delay of the child with Down syndrome as compared with normal chronologic age mates (a norm-referenced tool), normative data must have been collected on samples of children from a cross-section of ethnic and socioeconomic strata for each age level represented on the test. The availability of acceptable reliability and validity data also contributes to the utility of a particular test.

To assess developmental motor levels of infants and young children with Down syndrome, therapists may choose from among several standardized tests. The Bayley Scales of Infant Development[45] have been used to assess developmental motor levels of infants with Down syndrome in a number of research studies.[1-3,58,59] Both Mental and Motor Scales are available as part of the Bayley, but there is no differentiation of gross and fine motor skills. The Motor Scale consists primarily of gross motor items but also includes some fine motor items, particularly at the younger age levels. A number of items on the Mental Scale also require fine motor abilities.

Although the upper limit of the age range for the Bayley is 30 months, many preschoolers with Down syndrome are functioning at or below this level.

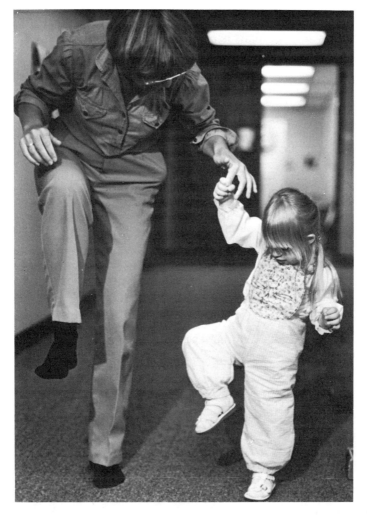

Fig. 6-4.   Administering the Bayley Motor Scale to a 3-year-old. (Item 52: stands on left foot with help.)

Because it is possible to derive an age-equivalent score for both the Mental and Motor Scales, it is frequently possible to continue to use the Bayley for assessing developmental levels in 3-, 4-, and even some 5-year-old children with Down syndrome. Figure 6-4 shows the Bayley Motor Scale being administered to a 3-year-old child with Down syndrome.

The Gesell and Amatruda Developmental Examination, another standardized assessment instrument, was renormed between 1975 and 1977 on a sample of 1,053 children ranging in age from 4 weeks to 36 months.[60] Five fields of behavior are assessed on the Gesell: adaptive, gross motor, fine motor, language, and personal–social. In each field of behavior, the child's "maturity level'' can be derived, although it is impossible to determine a specific age level if a wide scatter of items is passed and failed. A developmental quotient is derived by using the following formula:

$$DQ = \frac{\text{maturity age}}{\text{chronologic age}} \times 100$$

In assessing young children with Down syndrome, the Gesell has an advantage over the Bayley in that both a gross motor and a fine motor quotient can be derived. Eipper and Azen,[61] in a comparison of the Gesell based on earlier norms (1940s) and the current version of the Bayley administered to a sample of children with Down syndrome, concluded that the Gesell is more appropriate for clinical use because of its ease and speed of administration and the Bayley is more applicable for research purposes because it more reliably estimates developmental age.

The Peabody Developmental Motor Scales, published in 1983, cover an age span from birth to 7 years and include both Gross Motor and Fine Motor Scales.[62] Normative data were collected between 1981 and 1982 on a stratified sample of 617 children.[62] This test has the advantage of having more recent normative data than either the Bayley Scales or the Gesell. Individual developmental quotients, z scores, and age equivalent scores can be obtained for both the Gross Motor and Fine Motor Scales.

Despite the advantages of the Peabody Scales, therapists should be aware that a number of concerns were identified recently by a group of developmental therapists who have used the Peabody.[63] These include the poor quality of some of the materials in the test kit, the failure to place certain items in the correct developmental sequence, unequal representation of the five skill categories at different age levels, and discrepancies in correspondence between z scores and age equivalent scores.[63]

For assessing motor development in older children with Down syndrome, there are two available instruments that are both standardized and norm referenced: the Bruininks-Oseretsky Test of Motor Proficiency[64] and the Test of Motor Impairment by Stott and colleagues.[65] Normed in 1973, the Bruininks-Oseretsky consists of 46 items that examine running speeding and agility, balance, bilateral coordination, strength, upper limb coordination, response speed, visual motor control, and upper limb speed and dexterity.[66] This test is appropriate for children with motor ages between 4.5 and 14.5 years. The complete battery can be administered in 45 to 60 minutes with the additional option of using a 15- to 20-minute short form; both gross motor and fine motor ages can be derived. A limitation in using the Bruininks-Oseretsky with children with Down syndrome is the complexity of the verbal directions for administering each item. Since young children of normal intellect frequently have difficulty interpreting the directions on the Bruininks-Oseretsky, any child with a mental age of less than 5 years would also have difficulty trying to comply with the complex instructions.

The Test of Motor Impairment, although normed and standardized for ages

5 to 13 years, is oriented toward assessing children with more subtle forms of neural dysfunction such as the child with "minimal brain damage."[65] For this reason, this test is probably inappropriate for assessing motor development of the child with Down syndrome.

Self-Care Assessment

In addition to assessing the general developmental motor level of the child with Down syndrome, the physical therapist may also be called on to assess the child's abilities in the areas of self-help or daily living skills. Campbell[67] has suggested a problem-oriented approach to the evaluation of self-care skills in which the therapist assesses the child's abilities in a particular self-care area and then hypothesizes about the possible factors that may be interfering with the achievement of age-appropriate skills. Possible interfering problems may include neuromotor deficits or inappropriate behaviors. One goal of programming, then, is to minimize the effects of the interfering behaviors by developing alternative strategies for treatment.[67] For example, in the child with Down syndrome who is having difficulty drinking from a cup, two hypothesized causes of interfering problems might be the generalized hypotonia affecting the oral musculature resulting in inadequate lip closure (neuromotor deficit) or the existence of inappropriate behaviors such as throwing or dropping the cup. By observing the child during feeding time, the therapist can hypothesize about which type of behavior is interfering with the achievement of independent drinking and then develop appropriate alternative strategies. If the failure to drink successfully is due to poor lip closure, a program designed to increase tone in the oral muscles through such activities as vibration or chin tapping might be recommended. Hypotonia of the jaw muscles probably contributes to the inability to close the lips.

If inappropriate behaviors, such as dropping or throwing the cup, are interfering with the achievement of independent drinking, rather than a true neuromotor deficit, a behavioral program of systematically ignoring the inappropriate behavior or of modeling appropriate cup drinking with an empty cup might be preferred alternative strategies.

Feeding is, in fact, one of the most important self-care areas to be evaluated by the physical therapist who works with infants and children with Down syndrome. Neuromotor deficits such as hypotonia of the oral muscles and delayed appearance of oral reflexes are frequent concerns in working with this population.[68] Of particular concern is the hypoactive gag reflex, which may contribute to aspiration or choking during feeding. Palmer has identified five specific feeding problems commonly seen in children with Down syndrome: (1) poor suck and swallow in early infancy, (2) drooling secondary to poor tongue and lip control from hypotonia, (3) presence of the protrusion reflex of the tongue, (4) chewing difficulties, and (5) xerostomia or dry mouth leading to swallowing difficulties.[68] The underdeveloped bones of the facial skeleton contribute to a smaller oral cavity[69] and create the illusion that the tongue is abnormally large.

Specific eating problems identified by mothers of children with Down syndrome include difficulty in using utensils, difficulty in chewing foods (particularly meat), difficulty in drinking from a cup, and regurgitation of food.[70] Pipes and Holm,[71] in a review of medical charts of 49 children with Down syndrome seen at an interdisciplinary diagnostic center, reported feeding practices that were developmentally inappropriate for more than half of the children in the sample. These included failure to offer table food when appropriate, failure to encourage self-feeding, and persistence of bottle feeding.[71] Part of the evaluation role of the physical therapist is to determine the child's developmental readiness for certain foods and feeding practices and to encourage parents and teachers to provide foods that are developmentally appropriate.

Avoidance of foods that are particularly difficult to chew, swallow, and digest should also be advised. Pomeranz[72] has cautioned that celery, carrots, popcorn, and peanuts should not be given to any child under the age of 6 years. Since many older children with Down syndrome continue to exhibit developmentally delayed oral motor patterns, caution should be exercised in allowing them to eat such difficult to handle foods.

While eating difficulties are particularly prevalent among younger children with Down syndrome, excessive caloric intake and resultant obesity were found to be problems in 50 percent of the children over the age of 5 years in the study of Pipes and Holm.[71] Cronk[73] reported excessive weight as compared with length in 30 percent of a sample of children with Down syndrome ranging in age from birth to 3 years. The physical therapist who works with children with Down syndrome should be cognizant of this risk for obesity and should encourage exercise programs that will facilitate caloric expenditure as well as being developmentally appropriate.

In assessing the feeding and oral motor development of the child with Down syndrome, the physical therapist should work closely with other members of the interdisciplinary team, particularly the nutritionist, speech therapist, and pediatrician. Pipes and Holm[71] suggest the use of a developmental feeding table, modified from Gesell and Ilg,[74] for the evaluation of feeding skills in children with Down syndrome (Table 6-1). Palmer[68] advises using the prespeech evaluation schedule developed by Mueller[75] to assess feeding problems in children with Down syndrome that may result from neuromotor dysfunction.

Summary

Three general strategies have been suggested when conducting physical therapy assessment of a child with Down syndrome: qualitative assessment of movement patterns, developmental assessment of gross and fine motor skills, and assessment of self-care skills, particularly feeding. One of the primary goals in conducting a physical therapy assessment is to establish programming objectives that will serve as the framework for the plan of treatment. The following

Table 6-1. Progression of Feeding Behavior in Normal Children

Developmental Stage	Approximate Age (mo)	Food Introduced	Observed Behavior
Sucking or suckling (reflexive at birth)		Bottle	Nipple grasped with slight tongue curling and lip seal
Head erect in supported sitting	4	Strained fruit	Tongue protrudes before swallowing; food ejected; mouth poises to receive spoon
Looks at objects in hands; beginning bilateral reaching	5	Crackers; piece of cheese	Food grasped in a squeeze and brought to mouth; munching movements; lips close on swallowing
Bites (nipple, fingers); grasps large objects with palmar grasp; hands to mouth	6		
Pincer grasp (inferior); pokes with index finger	9–10	Peas and carrots	Interested in feel of food; finger-feeds
Uses spoon to scoop (e.g., sand); empties spoon to mouth upside down or sideways	15	Custard; macaroni and cheese	Fills spoon by pushing into food; tongue licks food on lips
Turns pages in books; builds two-block tower	18	Hamburger in gravy; ice cream	Begins to inhibit spoon turning; skilled finger-feeding

(Adapted from Pipes and Holm,[71] with permission.)

section discusses an objective-oriented approach to developing an appropriate treatment plan for the child with Down syndrome. A review of treatment strategies previously reported in the literature is also provided.

PHYSICAL THERAPY INTERVENTION

The goals of this section on intervention are to provide an overview of research examining the efficacy of specific treatment techniques for infants and young children with Down syndrome, and to outline an objective-oriented approach to treatment that can be used in measuring change in the clinical setting. A case study of an infant with Down syndrome will be presented to exemplify the objective-oriented approach to treatment. A case study of an older child with Down syndrome will be used to highlight the physical therapist's role as a consultant.

Review of Research Evaluating the Efficacy of Treatment

In spite of the well-documented motor problems associated with Down syndrome, relatively few intervention programs reported in the medical and educational literature have been aimed specifically at remediating these problems. A search of the Down syndrome literature from the past two decades reveals only a handful of descriptive articles specifically pertaining to physical therapy for infants and children with Down syndrome.[76-79]

Similarly lacking in the published literature are studies examining the effectiveness of different types of physical therapy intervention strategies for these children. Five such studies published since 1976 are described briefly.

One of the first reported studies on the effects of physical therapy on the improvement of motor performance in infants with Down syndrome was reported by Kantner and associates.[80] The intervention technique used was vestibular stimulation of the horizontal and vertical canals for a period of 10 days. Infants were placed in the laps of volunteers who were seated in a hand-operated rotary chair. Two infants with Down syndrome received treatment and two others were used as controls. Motor performance as measured by an assessment scale developed for use in the study was one of the two dependent variables examined. Since one of the treatment group subjects failed to cooperate during post-testing, the reported results are based solely on the post-test measurements of the one treatment subject remaining and of the two control subjects. Since the experimental group subject gained 16 points on the motor scale and the mean gain for the control group subjects was 0.75 point, the researchers concluded that the treatment was responsible for the 15.25-point difference in mean gain. The extremely small number of subjects used in the study as well as the lack of mention of random assignment to groups makes the investigators' strong concluding statement that the treatment was effective highly questionable.

In 1980, Piper and Pless[81] published the results of a study that evaluated the effects of a biweekly developmental therapy program on the improvement of mental development in a sample of infants with Down syndrome. Infants in the experimental group received 2 hours of developmental programming each week for a period of 6 months, while infants in the control group received no intervention services during this same period. No significant between-group differences were found on any of the change scores on the Griffiths Mental Developmental Scales. A number of limitations, such as the relatively short duration and limited intensity of the intervention program, were discussed in analyzing the differences in the results of this study to those of several earlier studies.

In a controlled experimental study designed to assess the effects of neurodevelopmental therapy on improving motor performance in a group of infants with Down syndrome, Harris[59] reported that although there were no significant differences between groups on either the Bayley Scales of Infant Development[45] or the Peabody Developmental Motor Scales,[82] there was a significant difference in favor of the treatment group in the achievement of specific individualized therapy objectives, such as "S. will correct her head to vertical and display a C-curve in trunk when tipped laterally to left and to right three out of four times in each direction" (Fig. 6-5). This finding lends support to the importance of early motor intervention for infants with Down syndrome. However, as Harris points out, there is certainly an urgent need for further

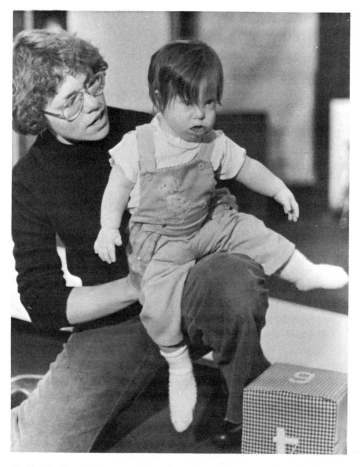

Fig. 6-5. Individualized therapy objective. S. will correct her head to vertical and display a C-curve in trunk when tipped laterally to left and to right (13-month-old infant).

studies designed to examine the efficacy of various treatment approaches on improving motor abilities in children with Down syndrome.

Another early intervention program for children with Down syndrome has been described by Connolly and Russell.[83] Their article describes an interdisciplinary program at the University of Tennessee Child Development Center in which 40 children with Down syndrome, from birth to 3 years of age, were included. Physical therapy consisted of gross motor activities including "muscle strengthening, range of motion, sensory and gross motor stimulation."[83] The use of vibrators for the stimulation of weak extensor muscles as well as for oral facilitation and sensory stimulation was also included as part of the intervention. Equipment included beach balls, which were used for facilitation of righting reflexes and neck and back extension.

In an effort to measure the success of their intervention strategies, Connolly and Russell[83] compared the achievement of gross motor milestones for their group of infants with those achieved by the infants with Down syndrome in a descriptive study of untreated infants by Fishler and colleagues[84] using the Gesell Developmental Scales.[85] The investigators reported that all gross motor milestones were achieved at an earlier age by the children in the study group. In a follow-up study with 20 of these same children,[86] Connolly et al. showed that there was earlier acquisition of both motor and self-help skills among the children who received early intervention as well as statistically significant differences in terms of intelligence and social quotients in favor of the group of treated children as compared with a similar group of noninstitutionalized children with Down syndrome who had not received early intervention.

A second follow-up study, when the children were 7 to 10 years of age,[87] included 15 members of the original sample. Gross motor composite scores on the Bruininks-Oseretsky Test of Motor Proficiency[64] had a mean of 4.7 years; the mean fine motor composite score was 4.9 years. No comparison group was available for motor scores, but adaptive and cognitive functioning levels were significantly higher than those of a comparison group of children with Down syndrome of similar age.[87]

In 1987, a single–subject study was published by Purdy and colleagues that examined the efficacy of two treatment approaches to reduce tongue protrusion of children with Down syndrome.[88] Using a single-subject withdrawal design (A-B-A), three children received oral–motor treatment as the intervention and two children received behavior modification. Tongue protrusion decreased for all three children receiving the oral–motor program; however, the improvement leveled off for two of the children during the final return-to-baseline phase, but continued to improve for the third child. One of the children receiving the behavior modification treatment showed decreased tongue protrusion during treatment and maintained that improvement even when the treatment was withdrawn. For the second child receiving behavior modification, data points were insufficient to draw definite conclusions about the efficacy of the treatment.

Although experimental research with large numbers of children is beyond the scope of most clinical settings, single-subject methodology is a promising research tool that can be used by practicing clinicians to examine the efficacy of their treatment strategies for children with Down syndrome as well as children with other developmental disabilities.[89,90] It is incumbent on the clinicians in our profession to develop strategies for the systematic documentation of individual changes as the result of their therapeutic intervention. Through an objective-oriented approach to treatment, such changes can be monitored and those facets of the treatment program that are most successful can be maximized.[91]

Treatment by Objectives

One of the primary goals of conducting a comprehensive evaluation for a child with Down syndrome is to develop a treatment plan that includes objectives aimed at improving the child's motor abilities. Through the qualitative assessment of the child's movement patterns, postural tone, primitive reflexes, and automatic reactions, the therapist can ascertain which aspects of movement may be interfering with the achievement of age-appropriate motor milestones. The results of a standardized developmental assessment will provide the therapist with additional information about which specific milestones the child is lacking. In addition to evaluating the general levels of gross and fine motor development, specific evaluation of self-care areas, such as feeding, will provide further information for developing a comprehensive treatment plan. Finally, the therapist should collect observational data of the child in the educational or home environment to determine if there are any interfering problems, such as specific neuromotor deficits or attentional deficits, that are preventing the acquisition of functional skills.[67] All information gleaned from such a comprehensive evaluation is then used by the therapist to develop treatment objectives that are both functional and developmentally appropriate for the particular child.

Input from other professionals on the interdisciplinary team and from the child's parents should also be used to develop objectives that are relevant to their overall goals for the child. When developing a treatment plan for older children with Down syndrome, input from the child as to what aspects of motor performance the child would like to improve should also be sought. Perhaps learning to tie shoelaces independently is a very important goal for a school-age child with Down syndrome, in which case this goal should become a part of the overall treatment plan.

The following case studies illustrate the development of a treatment plan based on specific evaluation data. One study is of an infant with Down syndrome for whom direct treatment is indicated, and the other is of a 12-year-old girl with Down syndrome for whom specific consultation and outside referral is warranted. Both of these case summaries demonstrate that children with Down syndrome have very special needs that frequently require consultation, evaluation, and treatment by a physical therapist. While portions of these case summaries are fictitious, they both represent examples of children with Down syndrome with whom the senior author has been involved in both evaluation and treatment. The breadth of associated physical, medical, and nutritional problems that frequently accompany a diagnosis of Down syndrome should not be overlooked by physical therapists concerned with evaluation and treatment of the "whole child."

Case Study: Patrick

Patrick is a 17-month-old infant with Down syndrome who lives at home with his parents and is enrolled in a developmental infant intervention program. Chromosome analysis shortly after birth revealed that Patrick has the standard trisomy-21 nondisjunction type of Down syndrome. In addition, he has a severe congenital heart defect for which the risks of surgical intervention are so great that surgery is inadvisable. Patrick exhibits bilateral esotropia that has been conservatively treated by alternate eye patching with no observable improvement. Patrick's pediatrician, after consultation with his cardiologist, has recommended evaluation and treatment by a physical therapist with the advice that excessive fatigue should be avoided.

Patrick's initial physical therapy assessment was conducted on two separate occasions to minimize the chance of fatiguing him. During the first phase of the evaluation, the MAI and Bayley Motor Scale were administered, since there is some overlap of items on these two tools. Administration of the postural tone section of the MAI revealed that Patrick was severely hypotonic, as measured by items evaluating extensibility of joints, consistency of muscles, passivity of hands and feet (amplitude and duration of flapping of a distal extremity when it is shaken by the examiner), and ability to assume antigravity postures in prone, supine, and prone suspension. Evaluation of primitive reflexes indicated there was no retention of early reflexes that would interfere with motor progress. Assessment of automatic reactions revealed immaturities in lateral head righting and head righting into flexion during pull-to-sit. Although head righting into extension could be accomplished when Patrick was in the prone position, it was observed that he needed to hyperextend his neck and rest his head back on his upper trunk in order to maintain this posture. Prone equilibrium reactions were absent, although beginning truncal equilibrium reactions were elicited in ventral suspension and supported sitting. Forward and sideways protective extension reactions in the arms were present inconsistently.

The volitional movement section of the MAI was administered concurrently with the Bayley Motor Scale. Patrick was able to sit independently when placed and was able to free his hands to play with toys, although he frequently propped forward on extended arms as probable compensation for his low trunk tone and trunk weakness. He was unable to get into or out of sitting independently, nor was he able to pull to standing. Patrick could progress forward on his abdomen and could rock in the quadruped position; he was unable to creep in quadruped. Fine motor skills included the ability to grasp cubes using a radial digital grasp, to scoop or rake the pellet, and to combine two cubes. On the Bayley Motor Scale. Patrick achieved a raw score of 35, which converted to an age equivalent of 7 to 8 months at chronologic age (CA) 17 months.

During the second evaluation session, the Bayley Mental Scale was administered to Patrick and an oral motor assessment and feeding inventory were conducted. Patrick achieved a basal level of 6 months on the Bayley Mental Scale with his highest pass at 12 months (turns pages of book). He received a raw score of 83, which converted to an age equivalent of 7 to 8 months, identical to his age equivalent on the Bayley Motor Scale. The oral motor assessment revealed no interfering influence of primitive oral reflexes; however, the gag reflex was hypoactive. In spite of the severe generalized hypotonia, Patrick maintained his tongue in his mouth and his mouth closed more than 50 percent of the evaluation time. Delayed dental development was apparent because of the absence of canine teeth. Patrick chewed using an up-and-down munching pattern. Patrick's mother was questioned about his feeding habits, and it was learned that he was eating some table foods as well as finger-feeding crackers and cookies, but not yet using a spoon. He was beginning to drink from a cup with assistance.

A summary of the physical therapy evaluation results for Patrick (CA = 17 months) is as follows:

Test	Developmental Level/Findings
Movement Assessment of Infants	Severe hypotonia, appropriate absence of primitive reflexes, delayed development of automatic reactions (6-month level)
Bayley Motor Scale	7–8 mo
Bayley Mental Scale	7–8 mo
Feeding Inventory	6–10 mo

Patrick's greatest area of delay appears to be in the development of age-appropriate automatic reactions. According to Fiorentino,[92] prone equilibrium reactions and forward protective extension should appear between 6 and 8 months in the normal infant. Patrick's absence of prone equilibrium reactions and the inconsistent appearance of forward protective responses would suggest that automatic reactions are significantly delayed. It could also be hypothesized that the severe truncal hypotonia and weakness might contribute to the failure to elicit age-appropriate equilibrium responses. The results of Patrick's oral motor assessment (see Table 6-1 for reference) indicate that his skills in this self-care area are certainly in line with his general mental and motor development as measured by the Bayley.

In developing a comprehensive treatment plan for Patrick, it is suggested that the problem-oriented approach described by Campbell[67] be utilized. Based on the foregoing evaluation, it could be hypothesized that Patrick's severe hypotonia and weakness of trunk muscles are interfering with his attainment of age-appropriate motor skills. This hypothesis is based, in part, on two observations: (1) there were no obvious inappropriate behaviors, such as throwing, refusal to comply, or self-stimulatory mannerisms, that appeared to interfere with Patrick's achievement of various items and (2) recent studies examining the relationship of hypotonia in Down syndrome to delays in affective, cognitive,[46] motor,[2] and feeding development[93] show a high level of consistency between the degree of hypotonia and the degree of delay in these other domains. Severe congenital heart disease in young children with Down syndrome has also been shown to contribute to greater delays in feeding and social development.[93]

Based on these observations, it would appear that Patrick's truncal weakness and severe hypotonia are interfering with his achievement of more age-appropriate developmental milestones. Using Campbell's problem-oriented approach[67] the first goal of treatment, therefore, would be to increase functional strength of trunk muscles. Specific developmental motor objectives would include Patrick's ability (1) to rise to sitting independently using trunk rotation and (2) to get out of sitting independently using trunk rotation. Each of these

Table 6-2. Developing an Instructional Sequence

NAME: *Patrick*   CHRONOLOGIC AGE: *17 months*

Goal: To increase functional strength of trunk muscles.
Objective 1: Patrick will get into sitting independently using trunk rotation by January 1, 1992.

Instructional Sequence:

1.1 P. will roll from supine to sidelying with therapist assist at hips, to right and to left, 3 out of 4 times, for 3 consecutive therapy sessions.

1.2 P. will roll from supine to sidelying with therapist prompt at hip, to right and to left, 3 out of 4 times, for 3 consecutive therapy sessions.

1.3 P will roll from supine to sidelying independently, to right and to left, 3 out of 4 times, for 3 consecutive therapy sessions.

1.4 P. will push up from sidelying to position halfway between sidelying and sitting using both hands, with therapist assist at hips, to right and to left, 3 out of 4 times, for 3 consecutive therapy sessions.

1.5 P. will push up from sidelying to position halfway between sidelying and sitting using both hands, with therapist prompt at hip, to right and to left, 3 out of 4 times, for 3 consecutive therapy sessions.

1.6 P. will push up from sidelying to position halfway between sidelying and sitting using both hands, independently to right and to left, 3 out of 4 times, for 3 consecutive therapy sessions.

1.7 P. will push up from sidelying into sitting position with therapist assist at hips, to right and to left, 3 out of 4 times, for 3 consecutive therapy sessions.

1.8 P. will push up from sidelying into sitting position with therapist prompt at hip, to right and to left, 3 out of 4 times, for 3 consecutive therapy sessions.

1.9 P. will push up from sidelying to sitting position independently, to right and to left, 3 out of 4 times, for 3 consecutive therapy sessions.

Therapist Activities Directed Toward Goal:

1.   Joint approximation down through shoulders in sitting.
2.   Joint approximation upward through buttocks while bouncing on therapy ball.
3.   Joint approximation through shoulders and hips while in quadruped.
4.   Facilitation of trunk righting while sitting on ball in 6 planes of motion: forward, backward, right, left, right diagonal, and left diagonal.
5.   Manual resistance to shoulders and hips during rolling: supine to prone and prone to supine.
6.   Manual facilitation at hip of supine $\rightarrow$ sitting: to right and to left.

objectives should then be further task analyzed, and an instructional sequence should be developed (Table 6-2). Objectives should always be written in terms of child-achievement,[91] such as "Patrick will get into sitting independently using trunk rotation." In addition, the therapist's activities directed at the achievement of the objective may also be specified as part of the treatment plan for each goal and objective (Table 6-2).

Based on the results of Patrick's evaluation, another important goal would be to improve automatic reactions. An example of an objective that would work toward this goal would be as follows: "When placed in prone on the therapy ball, Patrick will display a C-curve in the trunk when tipped laterally to left and to right, two out of three times to each side." Examination of the evaluation data in the areas of feeding and fine motor skills shows that Patrick is beginning to finger-feed crackers and cookies and is able to scoop or rake the pellet used in Bayley testing. A combined feeding/fine motor objective that is both developmentally and functionally appropriate is as follows: "Patrick will pick up two out of three Cheerios presented to him at the table using an inferior pincer grasp.''

In developing an objective-oriented treatment plan for Patrick, the therapist should include ideas from his parents, teachers, and any other professionals who are working with him. Certain objectives may be more appropriate than others based on environmental factors in the home or classroom, parental desires for the achievement of specific skills, nutritional needs, and so on. Treatment planning should be interdisciplinary and treatment delivery, particularly when working with young infants, should be transdiciplinary with the parent serving as the primary caregiver. Harris[79] has suggested that in light of the severe motor problems that characterize infants with Down syndrome, the physical or occupational therapist may be the most appropriate coordinator of the intervention services.

Case Study: Carole

Carole is a 12-year-old girl with Down syndrome and moderate mental retardation who was referred to the physical therapist by her special education teacher for posture screening. Her teacher had noted an increasing propensity by Carole to tilt her head toward the right while sitting at her desk and during recess activities. Carole is in a self-contained classroom in a junior high school. She was recently evaluated on the Peabody Developmental Motor Scales by her adaptive physical education teacher; her gross motor age equivalent was 4 years 9 months. Both her classroom and physical education teacher are also concerned about her recent weight gain, which has caused moderate obesity.

In this instance, the physical therapist has been called on to serve as a consultant in evaluating two specific concerns: the head tilt to the right and the recent weight gain. Since Carole has recently had a developmental motor examination and is participating in a developmentally oriented physical education program, there is no need to further assess her level of gross motor skills. In Carole's case, the physical therapy assessment consisted of ROM measurements of the neck and posture screening. Neck ranges were within normal limits, but Carole complained of pain in her neck during lateral flexion to the left. The therapist also questioned Carole about any numbness or tingling in her arms and legs, neither of which she reported. Posture screening demonstrated a mild thoracic scoliosis with convexity toward the left in standing, which disappeared during forward trunk flexion. No prominence of the left posterior rib cage was noted.

With the assistance of the school nurse, Carole's height and weight measurements were taken and plotted on a growth grid. Her height was below the 5th percentile for her age and sex; her weight was at the 30th percentile. On the basis of these findings, the therapist called Carole's parents to share the results and to suggest that Carole's pediatrician be contacted. At the parents' request, the therapist called Carole's pediatrician to discuss the postural and weight gain concerns. Cognizant of the risk of atlantoaxial instability, particularly in light of the clinical symptoms of neck pain and torticollis, the therapist and pediatrician discussed an orthopedic referral to rule out the possibility of subluxation or dislocation and to evaluate the spinal curve as well. The pediatrician also ordered laboratory tests to evaluate thyroid function in light of the recent weight gain and discrepant growth measurements and referred Carole to a nutritionist.

In this instance, the physical therapist served primarily as a consultant in evaluating two specific areas of concern. Because of the grave risks associated with atlantoxial dislocation, discussion with the pediatrician was the important first course of action. Establishing an exercise program for weight reduction or for treatment of the scoliosis would be inappropriate goals until the more immediate concerns were addressed. The therapist also advised Carole's classroom and physical education teachers to limit her involvement in strenuous physical activities until receiving the assessment results from the orthopedist.

Measuring Change as a Result of Treatment

One of the purposes of the objective-oriented approach to treatment is to provide a system for measuring progress or change as a result of therapy. By using measurable therapy objectives in treating the child with Down syndrome, the therapist can establish a baseline for each objective and then systematically monitor the child's progress toward the achievement of that objective by collecting data during each treatment session. O'Neill and Harris[91] have outlined procedures for developing goals and objectives for handicapped children and have emphasized the importance of measuring the child's ongoing performance in meeting those objectives. Table 6-3 shows a typical data sheet that could be used for measuring Patrick's progress toward the achievement of the objective presented in his case study summary.

By using measurable objectives in the treatment of the child with Down syndrome, the therapist can also establish the methodology for incorporating

Table 6-3. Daily Data Sheet

Student's Name: Patrick
Objective: Patrick will get into sitting independently using trunk rotation by January 1, 1992.
Steps 1. P. will roll from supine to sidelying with assist at hips.   Criterion 75% for 3 sessions
       2. P. will roll from supine to sidelying with prompt at hips.   Criterion 75% for 3 sessions
       3. P. will roll from supine to sidelying independently.   Criterion 75% for 3 sessions

Date	Data Taker	Trials 1	2	3	4	5	Crit. reach *	Step #	Comments
11/15/91	SH	+	−	+	+		*	1	
11/16/91	SH	+	+	+	+		*	1	
11/17/91	SH	+	+	+	+		*	1	Proceed to Step 2 at next PT session.

a single-subject research design into the clinical setting. Martin and Epstein[90] have described procedures for using single-subject research in the treatment of the child with cerebral palsy. Such procedures are also applicable for conducting clinical research on children with Down syndrome. Wolery and Harris[94] have presented strategies for the interpretation of single-subject research designs that include visual analysis of graphed data, which is the simplest method for use in the typical clinical setting. Readers are referred to Ottenbacher's excellent text on single-subject methodology.[89]

Summary

The foregoing section has presented a review of the recent research literature examining the efficacy of physical therapy for the child with Down syndrome as well as an objective-oriented approach to treatment. Case studies of an infant and an older child with Down syndrome were used to exemplify the therapist's role in assessment, treatment, and consultation. The importance of using a data system to monitor the child's progress toward the achievement of therapy objectives was also discussed.

The role of the physical therapist in working with the child with Down syndrome should not be limited solely to assessment and treatment. As was emphasized in this section previously, the therapist must also be concerned with the involvement of the child's family as well as with other professionals on the interdisciplinary team in the assessment and treatment of the child. The following section will discuss the therapist's role in interacting with family members and other professionals with the goal of ensuring the best services for the "whole child."

PARENT/CLIENT EDUCATION

Because infants with Down syndrome are usually diagnosed at birth, based on typical clinical signs and symptoms,[34] and because this diagnosis is usually confirmed within a few weeks through chromosome analysis, their parents are confronted very early on with the realization that their child has a disability, even though its extent cannot be determined. Mourning the loss of the expected normal infant has been described as being parallel to the stages of grief associated with the permanent loss of a loved one.[95] In addition, parents of children with mental retardation are confronted with "chronic sorrow"[96] based on the realization that their child may never be able to live totally independent of them and may remain at least partially their responsibility throughout their lives.

Because of the availability of early diagnosis, intervention for the infant with Down syndrome may begin as early as 2 to 3 weeks of age. The therapist, who, with the pediatrician, may serve as a primary professional contact for the family during the early months of the infant's life, must be cognizant of the mourning process described by Solnit and Stark.[95] By relating positively to the infant, but within realistic developmental goals, the therapist can promote attachment and adjustment by the parents toward their child with Down syndrome.[97]

In addition, support groups made up of parents of infants with Down syndrome and other disabilities may provide a valuable adjunct to early treatment and may help promote early acceptance of the child through the realization that they are not the only ones dealing with this dilemma.[97] Several excellent references are now available for parents of infants and children with Down syndrome of which the therapist should be aware.[98–101] Suggested periodicals for parents are *Down's Syndrome News*, a publication of the National Down Syndrome Congress, an organization of parents and professionals (Telephone: 1-800-NDSC), and *Sharing Our Caring*, a newsletter written by parents with practical advice on raising the child with Down syndrome (Caring, Box 400, Milton, WA 98354).

Education of parents and other family members of individuals with Down syndrome should include genetic counseling about the nature of the occurrence of the chromosome abnormality as well as risks of recurrence. Based on the infant's karyotype and the age of the parents, the risks of giving birth to another child with Down syndrome can be estimated. Parents should be counseled that although Down syndrome is a genetic disorder, it does not tend to ''run in families,'' except for the translocation type, in which the risk of recurrence is between 2 and 10 percent.[12] Physical therapists should be aware of the location and availability of genetic counseling services within their geographic area.

Recent federal legislation (Public Law 99-457) has mandated programs for infants and toddlers with handicaps, which will be administered by states, to provide multidisciplinary, interagency early intervention programs with a strong family component.[102] Intervention for the preschool and school-age child is frequently interdisciplinary, utilizing the talents of the special education teacher, the speech therapist, the physical therapist, the occupational therapist, and the adaptive physical educator. Consultation as needed should be available from other specialists, including the physician, psychologist, nurse, and audiologist. It is important to recognize that intelligence quotients of individuals with Down syndrome vary widely, with most individuals functioning in the mild and moderate ranges and a small percentage at the borderline, severe, and profound levels of retardation. School placement options may range from an integrated classroom or resource room for the child with mild mental retardation to a self-contained classroom for the child with a severe degree of involvement. Every effort should be made to place the child in the ''least restrictive environment'' as mandated by Public Law 94-142.[103]

Educational and family concerns surrounding the adolescent with Down syndrome may include the need for prevocational and vocational training as well as eventual placement in a setting that will maximize opportunities for independent or semi-independent living, such as a group home or supervised apartment setting. The therapist who works in a job setting where there are teenagers with Down syndrome may become involved in the assessment and training of independent living skills for the purpose of enhancing the clients' opportunities for placement in semi-independent living situations (see Ch. 11).

RECENT TRENDS IN MANAGEMENT

In addition to the medical and therapy management strategies discussed earlier in this chapter, several other management strategies directed at improving the well-being of children with Down syndrome have been reported in the recent research literature. A number of these are highly controversial.

Drug and Vitamin Treatments

In 1980, the effects of the administration of 5-hydroxytryptophan and pyridoxine on the motor, social, intellectual, and language development of young children with Down syndrome were examined in a double-blind study by a group of investigators who had encountered mixed results in previous studies that had evaluated these forms of therapy.[104] Administration of 5-hydroxytryptophan is directed at raising the blood levels of serotonin, a neurotransmitter that has been found to be present in decreased levels in children with Down syndrome. Pyridoxine has been reported to act in a similar fashion.[105] The primary goal of these modes of therapy is to increase muscle tone with secondary aims of enhancing motor, mental, and social skills.

Shortly after birth, 89 children with Down syndrome were randomly assigned to one of four treatment groups and were evaluated in this study during their first 3 years of life.[104] One group received 5-hydroxytryptophan, the second group received pyridoxine, the third group received a combination of 5-hydroxytryptophan and pyridoxine, and the fourth group received a placebo. There were no significant differences among the groups on muscle tone ratings, Bayley Mental or Motor Scales, or on the Receptive-Expressive Emergent Language Scale.[106] The investigators concluded that their generally negative findings were in agreement with several previously published studies.[105,107,108]

In 1981, a controversial study was published examining the effects of vitamins and nutritional supplements on improving IQ in a group of 16 children with mental retardation, five of whom were children with Down syndrome.[109] Statistically significant IQ gains were noted in the group of children who received the vitamins and nutritional supplements as compared with a control group who received placebos during the first 4 months of the study. Other changes reported in the children who received the supplements were improvements in visual acuity and a decrease in hyperactive behavior.

Several replications or partial replications of this study were conducted during the early 1980s.[110-114] According to a recent position statement by the National Down Syndrome Congress, "All of these studies have been unable to verify any of the claims which had been advanced regarding the benefits of the so-called megavitamin therapy."[115] The position statement proceeds to declare that no vitamin or nutritional supplements are supported by the National Down Syndrome Congress, and that certain vitamin supplements may, in fact, be toxic. Physical therapists should be aware of this position statement and should be ready to share it with parents of children with Down syndrome who are considering megavitamin therapy for their children.

Cell Therapy

Of even greater potential danger than megavitamin or nutritional therapy is the subcutaneous injection of freeze-dried cells from fetal tissues of sheep and rabbits into children with Down syndrome with the promise of improvement in characteristics as diverse as physical appearance, height, language, and memory.[116] Not only has this procedure been questioned because of its potential for introducing dangerous animal viruses into humans,[117] but a recent retrospective study of 190 individuals with Down syndrome, 21 of whom had received cell therapy, revealed no differences between the cell-treated group and a matched control group on 18 different variables in the areas of growth, cognitive development, motor development, and adaptive/social status.[118]

Although cell therapy is illegal in the United States, we have known of families of children with Down syndrome who have flown to Germany to have their children injected. Physical therapists must be prepared to alert parents to the potential dangers of this treatment. Not only has it been shown to have no positive value, but the potential dangers of introducing animal viruses into humans cannot be overlooked. A 1986 statement by the National Down Syndrome Congress warned parents that this form of treatment may be "life threatening."[116]

Patterning Therapy

Another controversial type of therapy that has been advocated for children with Down syndrome as well as for children with more severe brain damage is the Doman-Delacato approach to treatment, otherwise known as "patterning therapy."[119] Based on the assumption that passive manipulation of the limbs and head can affect brain development,[120] the goal of this approach to therapy is to achieve neurologic organization, or "the process whereby the organism, subject to environmental forces, achieves the potential inherent in its genetic endowments."[120] In a study conducted by investigators at Yale University, 45 seriously retarded youngsters were assigned to one of three treatment groups: one group received a modified sensorimotor patterning treatment, the second group received additional individualized attention from foster grandparents, and the third group received no treatment and served as controls.[121] The researchers used 22 different dependent measures in analyzing the effects of treatment, including scores on the neurologic profile developed by the Institute for the Achievement of Human Potential where the patterning method is taught.

No significant differences were noted between the two treatment groups on any of the measures following the 1-year interventions. The investigators concluded that "no evidence was found that treatment resulted in an improvement of the children's performance over what would be expected on the basis of attention (as assessed by the performance of the motivational group) and maturation."[121] Physical therapists who work with children with Down syndrome should be familiar with such studies, since their opinions of alternative forms of therapy may be sought out by the parents of the children with whom they work. For a recent critique of patterning therapy, readers are referred to a report by Harris and colleagues.[122]

Surgery

A relatively new and controversial type of surgical management for individuals with Down syndrome is the use of facial reconstructive surgery to "normalize" their facial characteristics (Fig. 6-6).[123] The plastic surgery has been aimed at correcting six features: (1) the epicanthal folds, (2) the oblique eyelid axes, (3) the saddle nose, (4) the macroglossia (large tongue), (5) hy-

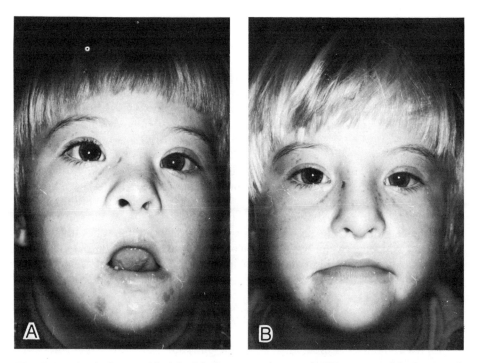

Fig. 6-6. (A) A 6-year-old girl with Down syndrome. (B) The same girl after nasal augmentation and tongue reduction. (From Lemperle and Radu,[123] with permission.)

potonia of the lower lip, and (6) the receding chin (micrognathia).[123] In reviewing a 1980 report of this new form of management, a leading medical researcher in Down syndrome commented that several of these features tend to improve with age (the epicanthal folds and macroglossia) and that such treatment should be highly individualized depending on the needs and feelings of the child, the family, and the school or community in which the child is involved.[124]

In spite of the radical nature of this surgery and the increasing popularity of its use in a number of different countries, few well-controlled studies have been published that have attempted to examine its efficacy. A recent literature review[125] examining the effectiveness of facial plastic surgery for persons with Down syndrome showed mixed results. Those studies in which parents or surgeons were questioned on the effectiveness of the surgery tended to support improvements, whereas more rigorously designed studies that include ratings by professionals less involved in the treatment were not as supportive of positive outcomes. In the conclusion of their review on the surgery's effectiveness, the authors stated, "A final and comprehensive conclusion as to its effectiveness in achieving its goals will require systematic and scientific assessment of longitudinal studies; only through such research will professionals be able to reach conclusions as to its effectiveness in improving the quality of life of persons with Down syndrome."[125]

Physical therapists who work with children with Down syndrome and their families should keep abreast of the research on these controversial treatments so that they can assist families in critically analyzing such interventions.

CONCLUSION

The goal of this chapter has been to describe the role of physical therapy in the management of children with Down syndrome. A review of the recent literature has demonstrated increasing involvement by physical therapists in providing descriptive approaches to therapy for this population as well as in providing controlled research studies to examine the effects of therapy on improving various aspects of development. An urgent need exists for continued involvement by physical therapists in both the treatment of individuals with Down syndrome as well as involvement in clinical research studies, including the documenting of individual gains made in the typical clinical setting through systematic monitoring of objective-oriented progress. Our own involvement in the management of children with Down syndrome and in interaction with their families has been extremely rewarding and positive, and it is our personal wish that this chapter will stimulate similar interest and involvement on the part of other pediatric therapists.

DEDICATION

This chapter is dedicated to all of the children with Down syndrome who have helped us to grow and learn.

REFERENCES

1. Carr J: Mental and motor development in young mongol children. J Ment Defic Res 14:205, 1970
2. LaVeck B, LaVeck GD: Sex differences in development among young children with Down syndrome. J Pediatr 91:767, 1977
3. Harris SR: Relationship of mental and motor development in Down's syndrome infants. Phys Occup Ther Pediatr 1:13, 1981
4. Stratford B: Perception and perceptual-motor processes in children with Down's syndrome. J Psychol 104:139, 1980
5. Diamond LS, Lynne D, Sigman B: Orthopedic disorders in patients with Down's syndrome. Orthop Clin North Am 12:57, 1981
6. Coleman M: Down's syndrome. Pediatr Ann 7:90, 1978
7. Kirman BH: Genetic errors: chromosome anomalies. p. 121. In Kirman BH, Bicknell J (eds): Mental Handicap. Churchill Livingstone, Edinburgh, 1975
8. Huether C: Demographic projections for Down syndrome. p. 105. In Pueschel SM, Tingey C, Rynders CE et al (eds): New Perspectives on Down Syndrome. Paul H Brookes Publishing, Baltimore, 1987
9. Sasaki M: Paternal origin of the extra chromosome in Down's syndrome. Lancet 2:1257, 1973
10. Jagiello GM, Fang Y, Ducayen MB et al: Etiology of human trisomy 21. p. 23. In Pueschel SM, Tingey C, Rynders CE et al (eds): New Perspectives on Down Syndrome. Paul H. Brookes Publishing, Baltimore, 1987
11. Lejeune J, Gauthier M, Turpin R: Les chromosomes humain en culture de tissus. C R Acad Sci [D] (Paris) 248:602, 1959
12. Novitski E: Human Genetics. Macmillan, New York, 1977
13. Crome L: The pathology of certain syndromes. p. 225. In Hilliard LT, Kirman BH (eds): Mental Deficiency. 2nd Ed. Little, Brown, Boston, 1965
14. Roche AF: The cranium in mongolism. Acta Neurol 42:62, 1966
15. Penrose LS, Smith GF: Down's Anomaly. Churchill Livingstone, London, 1966
16. Benda CE: The Child with Mongolism (Congenital Acromicria). Grune & Stratton, Orlando, FL, 1960
17. Ross MH, Galaburda AM, Kemper TL: Down's syndrome: is there a decreased population of neurons? Neurology 34:909, 1984
18. Scott BS, Becker LE, Petit TL: Neurobiology of Down's syndrome. Prog Neurobiol 21:199, 1983
19. Marin-Padilla M: Pyramidal cell abnormalities in the motor cortex of a child with Down's syndrome: a Golgi study. J Comp Neurol 167:63, 1976
20. Loesch-Mdzewska D: Some aspects of the neurology of Down's syndrome. J Ment Defic Res 12:237, 1968
21. Wisniewski KE, Schmidt-Sidor B: Postnatal delay of myelin formation in brains from Down syndrome infants and children. Clin Neuropathol 6(2):55, 1989
22. Gath A: Cerebral degeneration in Down's syndrome. Dev Med Child Neurol 23:814, 1981
23. Ball MJ, Nuttall K: Neurofibrillary tangles, granulovacuolar degeneration, and neuron loss in Down syndrome: quantitative comparison with Alzheimer dementia. Ann Neurol 7:462, 1980
24. Spicer RL: Cardiovascular disease in Down syndrome. Pediatr Clin North Am 31:1331, 1984

25. Zausmer EF, Shea AM: Motor development. p. 143. In Pueschel SM (ed): The Young Child with Down Syndrome. Human Sciences Press, New York, 1984
26. Balkany TJ, Downs MP, Balkany DJ et al: Hearing problems in children with Down's syndrome. Down Syndr Pap Abstr Profess 2:5, 1979
27. Jaeger EA: Ocular findings in Down's syndrome. Trans Am Ophthalmol Soc 78:808, 1980
28. Curtis BH, Blank S, Fisher RL: Atlantoaxial dislocation in Down's syndrome: report of two patients requiring surgical correction. JAMA 205:464, 1968
29. Giblin PE, Micheli LJ: The management of atlanto-axial subluxation with neurologic involvement in Down's syndrome: a report of two cases and review of the literature. Clin Orthop 140:66, 1979
30. Andrews LG: Myelopathy due to atlanto-axial dislocation in a patient with Down's syndrome and rheumatoid arthritis. Dev Med Child Neurol 23:356, 1981
31. Whaley WJ, Gray WD: Atlantoaxial dislocation and Down's syndrome. Can Med Assoc J 123:35, 1980
32. American Academy of Pediatrics, Committee on Sports Medicine: Atlantoaxial instability in Down syndrome. Pediatrics 74:152, 1984
33. Bersu ET: Anatomical analysis of the developmental effects of aneuploidy in man: the Down syndrome. Am J Med Genet 5:399, 1980
34. Hall B: Mongolism in newborns: a clinical and cytogenetic study. Acta Paedriatr Scand, Suppl 154, 1964
35. Cowie VA: A Study of the Early Development of Mongols. Pergamon Press, Oxford, 1970
36. Benda CE: Mongolism: a comprehensive review. Arch Pediatr 73:391, 1956
37. Cummins H, Talley C, Platou RV: Palmar dermatoglyphics in mongolism. Pediatrics 5:241, 1950
38. Levinson A, Friedman A, Stamps F: Variability of mongolism. Pediatrics 16:43, 1955
39. McIntire MS, Dutch SJ: Mongolism and generalized hypotonia. Am J Ment Defic 68:669, 1964
40. Wagner HR: Mongolism in orientals. Am J Dis Child 103:706, 1962
41. McIntire MS, Menolascino FJ, Wiley JH: Mongolism—some clinical aspects. Am J Ment Defic 69:794, 1965
42. Crome L, Cowie V, Slater E: A statistical note on cerebellar and brainstem weight in mongolism. J Ment Defic Res 10:69, 1966
43. Melyn MA, White DT: Mental and developmental milestones of noninstitutionalized Down's syndrome children. Pediatrics 52:542, 1973
44. Gesell A, Amatruda C: Developmental Diagnosis: Normal and Abnormal Child Development. 2nd Ed. Hoeber, New York, 1947
45. Bayley N: Bayley Scales of Infant Development. Psychological Corporation, New York, 1969
46. Cicchetti D, Sroufe LA: The relationship between affective and cognitive development in Down's syndrome infants. Child Dev 47:920, 1976
47. Uzgiris IC, Hunt JM: Assessment in infancy: ordinal scales of psychological development. University of Illinois Press, Urbana, 1975
48. O'Connor N, Hermelin B: Speech and Thought in Severe Subnormality. Pergamon Press, Oxford, 1963
49. Reed RB, Pueschel SM, Schnell RR et al: Interrelationships of biological, environmental and competency variables in young children with Down syndrome. Appl Res Ment Retard 1:161, 1980

50. Haley SM: Postural reactions in infants with Down syndrome. Phys Ther 66:(1):17, 1986
51. Rast MM, Harris SR: Motor control in infants with Down syndrome. Dev Med Child Neurol 27:675, 1985
52. Chandler LS, Andrews MS, Swanson MW: Movement Assessment of Infants: A Manual. Rolling Bay, WA, 1980
53. Shumway-Cook A, Woollacott M: Dynamics of postural control in the child with Down syndrome. Phys Ther 65:1315, 1985
54. Morris AF, Vaughn SE, Vaccaro P: Measurements of neuromuscular tone and strength in Down syndrome children. J Ment Defic Res 26:41, 1982
55. MacNeill-Shea SH, Mezzomo JM: Relationship of ankle strength and hypermobility to squatting skills of children with Down syndrome. Phys Ther 65:1658, 1985
56. Lydic JS, Steele C: Assessment of the quality of sitting and gait patterns in children with Down's syndrome. Phys Ther 59:1489, 1979
57. Parker AW, Bronks R: Gait of children with Down syndrome. Arch Phys Med Rehabil 61:345, 1980
58. Dameron LE: Development of intelligence of infants with mongolism. Child Dev 34:733, 1963
59. Harris SR: Effects of neurodevelopmental therapy on motor performance of infants with Down's syndrome. Dev Med Child Neurol 23:477, 1981
60. Knobloch H, Stevens F, Malone AF: Manual of Developmental Diagnosis: The Administration and Interpretation of the Revised Gesell and Amatruda Developmental and Neurologic Examination. Harper & Row, Hagerstown, MD, 1980
61. Eipper DS, Azen SP: A comparison of two developmental instruments in evaluating children with Down's syndrome. Phys Ther 58:1066, 1978
62. Folio M, Fewell R: Peabody Developmental Motor Scales and Activity Cards. DLM Teaching Resources, Hingham, MA, 1983
63. Hinderer KA, Richardson PK, Atwater SA: Clinical implications of the Peabody Developmental Motor Scales: a constructive review. Phys Occup Ther Pediatr 9:81, 1989
64. Bruininks RH: Bruininks-Oseretsky Test of Motor Proficiency. American Guidance Service, Circle Pines, MN, 1978
65. Stott DH, Moyes FA, Henderson SE: Test of Motor Impairment. Brook Educational Publishing, Guelph, Ontario, 1972
66. Connolly B: Bruininks-Oseretsky tests of motor proficiency. Totline 8(1):21, 1982
67. Campbell P: Daily living skills. In Haring NG (ed): Developing Effective Individualized Education Programs for Severely Handicapped Children and Youth. Bureau of Education for the Handicapped, Washington, DC, 1977
68. Palmer S: Down's syndrome. p. 25. In Palmer S, Ekvall S (eds): Pediatric Nutrition in Developmental Disorders. Charles C Thomas, Springfield, IL, 1978
69. Hunt PJ: Oral motor dysfunction in Down's syndrome: contributing factors and interventions. Phys Occup Ther Pediatr 1(4):69, 1981
70. Calvert SD, Vivian VM, Calvert GP: Dietary adequacy, feeding practices and eating behavior of children with Down's syndrome. J Am Diet Assoc 69:152, 1976
71. Pipes PL, Holm VA: Feeding children with Down's syndrome. J Am Diet Assoc. 77:277, 1980
72. Pomeranz VE: Choking: the best cure is prevention. Parents 57:76, 1982
73. Cronk CE: Growth of children with Down's syndrome: birth to age 3 years. Pediatrics 61:564, 1978
74. Gesell A, Ilg FL: Feeding Behavior of Infants: A Pediatric Approach to the Mental Hygiene of Early Life. JB Lippincott, Philadelphia, 1937

75. Mueller H: Pre-speech Evaluation and Therapy. Paper presented at the Bobath Course at Sussex Rehabilitation Center, Long Island, NY, 1973. Cited in Palmer S, Horn S: Feeding problems in children. In Palmer S, Ekvall S (eds): Pediatric Nutrition in Developmental Disorders. Charles C Thomas, Springfield, IL, 1976

76. Kugel RB: Combatting retardation in infants with Down's syndrome. Child Today 17:188, 1970

77. Hughes NAS: Developmental physiotherapy for developmentally handicapped babies. Physiotherapy 57:399, 1971

78. York-Moore R: Physiotherapy management of Down's syndrome. Physiotherapy 62:16, 1976

79. Harris SR: Transdisciplinary therapy model for the infant with Down's syndrome. Phys Ther 60:420, 1980

80. Kantner RM, Clark DL, Allen LC et al: Effects of vestibular stimulation on nystagmus response and motor performance in the developmentally delayed infant. Phys Ther 56:414, 1976

81. Piper MC, Pless IB: Early intervention for infants with Down syndrome: a controlled trial. Pediatrics 65:463, 1980

82. Folio R, DuBose RF: Peabody Developmental Motor Scales. IMRID Behavioral Science Monograph No. 25. George Peabody College, Nashville, TN, 1974

83. Connolly B, Russell F: Interdisciplinary early intervention program. Phys Ther 56:155, 1976

84. Fishler K, Share J, Koch R: Adaptation of Gesell Developmental Scales for evaluation of development in children with Down's syndrome (mongolism). Am J Ment Defic 68:642, 1964.

85. Gesell A, Amatruda C: Developmental Diagnosis. Hoeber, New York, 1941

86. Connolly B, Morgan S, Russell FF et al: Early intervention with Down syndrome children: follow-up report. Phys Ther 60:1405, 1980

87. Connolly B, Morgan S, Russell F: Evaluation of children with Down syndrome who participated in an early intervention program. Phys Ther 64:151, 1984

88. Purdy AH, Deitz JC, Harris SR: Efficacy of two treatment approaches to reduce tongue protrusion of children with Down syndrome. Dev Med Child Neurol 29:469, 1987

89. Ottenbacher KJ: Evaluating Clinical Change: Strategies for Occupational and Physical Therapists. Williams & Wilkins, Baltimore, 1986

90. Martin JE, Epstein LH: Evaluating treatment effectiveness in cerebral palsy: single-subject designs. Phys Ther 56:285, 1976

91. O'Neill DL, Harris SR: Developing goals and objectives for handicapped children. Phys Ther 62:295, 1982

92. Fiorentino MR: Reflex Testing Methods for Evaluating C.N.S. Development. 2nd Ed. Charles C Thomas, Springfield, IL, 1973

93. Cullen SM, Cronk CE, Pueschel SM et al: Social development and feeding milestones of young Down syndrome children. Am J Ment Defic 85:410, 1981

94. Wolery M, Harris SR: Interpreting results of single-subject research designs. Phys Ther 62:445, 1982

95. Solnit A, Stark M: Mourning and the birth of a defective child. Psychoanal Study Child 16:523, 1961

96. Olshansky S: Chronic sorrow: a response to having a mental defective child. Soc Casework 43:190, 1962

97. Irvin NA, Kennell JH, Klaus MH: Caring for parents of an infant with a congenital malformation. p. 167. In Klaus MH, Kennell JH (eds): Maternal-Infant Bonding. CV Mosby, St. Louis, 1976

98. Horrobin JM, Rynders JE: To Give an Edge. Colwell Press, Minneapolis, 1974

99. Stray-Gundersen K (ed): Babies with Down Syndrome: A New Parent's Guide. Woodbine House, Kensington, MD, 1986

100. Hanson MJ: Teaching the Infant With Down Syndrome. 2nd Ed. Pro Ed, Austin, TX, 1987

101. Pueschel SM (ed): A Parent's Guide to Down Syndrome: Toward a Better Future. Paul H Brookes Publishing Co., Baltimore, 1990

102. Public Law 99-457. Education of the Handicapped Act Amendments of 1986. 99th Congress, 2nd Session, 1986

103. Public Law 94-142. Education For All Handicapped Children Act of 1975 (S.6). 94th Congress, 1st Session, 1975

104. Pueschel SM, Reed RB, Cronk CE et al: 5-Hydroxytryptophan and pyridoxine. Am J Dis Child 134:838, 1980

105. Coleman M, Steinberg L: A double blind trial of 5-hydroxytryptophan in trisomy-21 patients. In Coleman M (ed): Serotonin in Down's Syndrome. American Elsevier, New York, 1973

106. Bzoch KR, League R: The Receptive-Expressive Emergent Language Scale for the Measurement of Language Skills in Infancy. The Tree of Life Press, Gainesville, FL, 1970

107. Partington MW, MacDonald MRA, Tu JB: 5-Hydroxytryptophan (5-HTP) in Down's syndrome. Dev Med Child Neurol 13:362, 1971

108. Weise P, Koch R, Shaw KNF, Rosenfeld MJ: The use of 5-HTP in the treatment of Down's syndrome. Pediatrics 54:165, 1974

109. Harrell RF, Capp RH, Davis DR et al: Can nutritional supplements help mentally retarded children? An exploratory study. Proc Natl Acad Sci USA 78:574, 1981

110. Bennett FC, McClelland S, Kriegsmann EA et al: Vitamin and mineral supplementation in Down's syndrome. Pediatrics 72:707, 1983

111. Ellis NR, Tomporowski PD: Vitamin/mineral supplements and intelligence of institutionalized mentally retarded adults. Am J Ment Defic 88:211, 1983

112. Weathers C: Effects of nutritional supplementation on IQ and certain other variables associated with Down syndrome. Am J Med Defic 88:214, 1983

113. Ellman G, Silverstein CI, Zingarelli G et al: Vitamin-mineral supplement fails to improve IQ of mentally retarded young adults. Am J Ment Defic 88:688, 1984

114. Smith GF, Spiker D, Peterson CP et al: Use of megadoses of vitamins with minerals in Down syndrome. J Pediatr 105:228, 1984

115. National Down Syndrome Congress Megavitamin Therapy Position Statement. Down Syndrome Pap Abstr Profess 12(4):3, 1989

116. Fackelmann K: New Hope or false promise? Science News 137:168, 1990

117. Bird T, Harris S: New hope for the retarded? (letter) Am J Med Genet 18:183, 1984

118. VanDyke DC, Long DJ, van Duyne S et al: Cell therapy in children with Down syndrome. a retrospective study. Pediatrics 85:79, 1990

119. Chapanis NP: The patterning method of therapy: a critique. p. 265. In Black P (ed): Brain Dysfunction in Children. Raven Press, New York, 1981

120. LeWinn EB: Human Neurological Organization. Charles C Thomas, Springfield, IL, 1969

121. Sparrow S, Zigler E: Evaluation of a patterning treatment for retarded children. Pediatrics 62:137, 1978

122. Harris SR, Atwater SW, Crowe TK: Accepted and controversial neuromotor therapies for infants at high risk for cerebral palsy. J Perinatal 8(1):3, 1988.

123. Lemperle G, Radu D: Facial plastic surgery in children with Down's syndrome. Plast Reconstr Surg 66:337, 1980
124. Coleman M: Current papers of special interest. Down Syndr Pap Abstr Profess 4(4):2, 1981
125. Katz S, Kravetz S: Facial plastic surgery for persons with Down syndrome: research findings and their professional and social implications. Am J Ment Retard 94:101, 1989

7 | Myelodysplasia

June Bridgford Garber

Myelodysplasia is one of the most complex congenital anomalies compatible with life. Commonly accompanied by hydrocephalus, the anatomic complexity of the primary nervous and skeletal system defects belies the conventional thinking that simply equates myelodysplasia with traumatic paraplegia. In addition to the medical and surgical procedures needed to treat the anomalies present at birth effectively, the secondary problems that occur and recur present a significant challenge to all the health care professions.

ETIOLOGY AND PATHOLOGY

Terminology

Considering the multifaceted nature of neural tube defects, it is not surprising to find a vast and varied nomenclature associated with them. The term *spina bifida* is defined here as a congenital vertebral defect characterized by lack of dorsal arch fusion. The term *melodysplasia* refers to the wide variety of congenital spinal cord and nerve root abnormalities generally associated with spina bifida and characterized by varying degrees of spinal cord function.[1]

Open myelomeningocele is a general label used by Sharrad[2] to describe the spinal cord and vertebral defects associated with approximately 85 percent of surviving spina bifida births. The deficiencies in lower extremity sensation and motor control characteristic of this group have been specifically delineated into different patterns by several investigators.[2-4] Based on the extent of intact spinal cord reflex activity, Stark and Baker[4] have developed one of the more frequently used methods of labeling these patterns. They define four types (I to IV) with two subtypes (a,b).

From 65 to 100 percent of infants born with open myelomeningoceles are reported to have varying degrees of central nervous system abnormalities that lead to hydrocephalus.[5-7] The primary abnormality responsible for the hydrocephalic condition is commonly called an Arnold-Chiari malformation. The levels of severity of the malformation have been classified into types I to III (or IV).[3] This classification system is unrelated to that of spinal cord function described in the previous paragraph.

PATHOGENESIS AND EPIDEMIOLOGY

Although investigated for over 300 years, the pathogenesis and etiology of spina bifida, myelodysplasia, and Arnold-Chiari malformation are still not clearly understood. Several hypotheses of failed neuropore closure and occlusion of the neural tube lumen continue to be explored.[5,8-14] More specifically, the effect of teratogenic agents on cell adhesion and recognition mechanisms during primary neural tube fusion are being studied.[15] The role of a posterior shift in the brain–spinal cord transition zone of the neural plate has been proposed as an event common to anencephaly, myelogeningocele, and Arnold-Chiari malformation.[16] The etiology of this complex of defects is still believed to be multifactorial.[12] Numerous environmental factors[17-21] and genetic patterns[21-27] have been investigated. The roles of poor maternal nutrition and, more specifically, folic acid deficiency or the presence of folate antagonists are still not clarified.[21] The relationship between prevalence of myelodysplasia at birth, lower socioeconomic status, and limited access to health care has been confirmed but not explained.[28] While the incidence of spina bifida births across the United States has remained between 0.30 and 0.90 per 1,000 births during the past 10 years, specific factors leading to this stability or causing previous fluctuations remain unknown.[13,29,30]

DIAGNOSIS AND MANAGEMENT

Prenatal Diagnosis

During the 1980s, methods for prenatal diagnosis of myelodysplasia came into general use in the United States. Elevated levels of alpha-fetoprotein within amniotic fluid as well as maternal serum between 16 and 18 weeks of pregnancy have proven predictive of open neural tube defects.[31-35] Standard values as early as 11 to 15 weeks' and as late as 18 to 22 weeks' gestation have been validated.[36,37] The growing use of ultrasonography to monitor fetal status and structure has aided in the screening process as well as avoidance of abortion in cases of repeated false-positive laboratory results. Although only one state, California, legally requires the testing, screening for aberrant maternal alpha-fetoprotein is becoming an expected part of obstetrical care.[37,38] Initial attempts at intrauterine treatment of congenital hydrocephalus have been disappointing, but may prove helpful in the future for prenatal management of myelodys-plasia.[39]

Advances in Medical and Surgical Management

During the past decade, significant progress has been made in the medical and surgical management of myelodysplastic and hydrocephalic children. Although long-term follow-up information is not yet available, the techniques for neonatal closure of myelodysplasic defects have improved. The surgical microscope has paved the way for development of microneurosurgical methods that facilitate anatomic reconstruction of the open spinal cord as well as improved preservation of functional neural tissue.[40] Increased understanding of the dynamics of shunt obstruction and infection resulted from the use of radiologic methods such as computed tomography and radioisotope ventriculography. Children with nonfunctioning shunts in place who were thought, because of absence of clinical symptoms, to have arrested hydrocephalus, were found to have significantly dilated ventricles or compensating hydromyelia. This insidious level of brain damage has been proposed as the cause of gradual loss of upper and/or lower extremity function, an increase in scoliosis, and/or a decrease in cognitive function.[41] More frequent evaluation of hydrocephalic status is now safer and more easily done than a decade ago. Cranial ultrasound for infants with open fontanelles and computed tomography or magnetic resonance imaging for older individuals allow for improved management. These technologic advances combined with the use of prophylactic antibiotics have decreased the shunt-related infection rate to approximately 2 percent in many centers.[42] Use of clean intermittent catheterization techniques continues to provide more effective management of urinary incontinence than surgical diversion methods.[43–47] Follow-up studies of sphincter-impaired children using intermittent catheterization, bowel training techniques, dietary planning, and neurohormonal medications have shown a frustrating pattern of delayed independence and adolescent rebellion that was not anticipated in most clinical settings. In most cases, psychosocial factors emerge from these studies as more significant limiting factors than physical disability. This seems to indicate a need for ongoing, accessible family and client counseling rather than increasingly complex medical procedures.[48,49]

Advances in the orthopedic management of myelodysplasia patients reflect an increased understanding of criteria that identify those most likely to benefit from various procedures. Several follow-up studies now support the use of iliopsoas transfers and acetabuloplasties with only those children demonstrating essentially normal quadriceps function and high potential for adult ambulation.[50,52] For the individual who may be with bilateral long leg braces or dependent on a wheelchair for mobility, soft tissue release, femoral osteotomy, and tendon division or excision of the iliopsoas and adductor muscle groups are recommended to manage hip flexion deformities. Thus, the recent changes made in orthopedic management of the hips of myelodysplasia patients reflect a consensus that fewer and less complex procedures need to be done rather than the development of additional procedures. The potentially adverse effects of immobilization following surgery include fractures and decreased mobility that may not be recovered.[53,54] One evaluation of factors predicting a loss of ambulatory skill among young adolescents revealed that a period of immobilization marked the beginning of the ambulatory decline for the majority.[54]

The changes in orthopedic management of spinal deformities, however, reflect the development and refinement of surgical techniques. Controversy persists concerning the optimal surgical technique for correction of myelomeningocele-related spinal deformity. A frequently used method for stabilization of many scoliosis and lordoscoliosis deformities is now a two-stage combination of anterior and posterior spinal fusion. The anterior fusion, stabilized by Dwyer or Zielke instrumentation, precedes by 2 weeks the posterior fusion stabilized by Harrington rod or Luque instrumentation. The type of instrumentation has not proven to be a significant determinant of fusion or correction rates.[55-57] With both anterior and posterior fusion completed, however, 83 to 100 percent fusion and 45 to 68 percent correction rates are reported, in vivid contrast to results of single anterior or posterior fusion.[57] Unfortunately, prolonged immobilization is still required following these procedures.

Delineation of Associated Problems

Progress has been made in understanding the multiple complex problems associated with myelodysplasia and hydrocephalus. The extent to which the upper extremities of these children can be affected by central nervous system dysfunction is more clearly appreciated.[58-67] The educational disadvantage implicit in the limited hand-writing skill of most children with hydrocephalus and myelodysplasia is receiving more attention.[65-67] Numerous investigators have reported studies that delineate the variety of ways in which the perceptual motor dysfunction of myelomeningocele hydrocephalic patients can be manifested.[68-72] The incidence and pathogenesis of strabismus and visual tracking disturbances are understood better than they were a decade ago.[73,74] Understanding of the relationship between cognitive skills, language development, and Cocktail Party Syndrome in this population has increased.[75-77] Awareness of the effects of myelodysplasia and the multiple hospitalization periods required for its management on psychosocial development, as well as family interaction patterns, has increased.[78-81] While these associated problems require further investigation to be thoroughly understood, the studies that have been reported focus attention on aspects of the function and development of myelodysplasia children that warrant consideration during physical therapy evaluation and habilitation.

PHYSICAL THERAPY EVALUATION

Since the primary and secondary problems resulting from myelodysplasia defects are so numerous and interrelated, it is obviously important that the physical therapist focus on a primary purpose of that evaluation. The lengthy, detailed evaluation of clinical symptoms that either have little to do with actual treatment planning or duplicate the evaluations of other health care providers are pitfalls to be avoided. In general terms, the primary purpose of physical therapy evaluation, for this population, is to define each individual's current and potential secondary neuromusculoskeletal problems that are amenable to treatment provided by physical therapists. The secondary problems of decreased joint mobility, skin ulceration, lack of independent mobility, lack of self-care skills, and delayed development of fine and perceptual motor skills can be prevented or ameliorated by physical therapy. Clearly, the depth in which these functions are evaluated is dictated by the setting or circumstances in which the evaluation occurs. In multidisciplinary clinics, the physical therapist is more likely to be screening in order to identify aspects that require more detailed, diagnostic attention and/or treatment at a later time. In outpatient or inpatient treatment settings, the therapist is more likely to be screening all functions while fully assessing some specific areas.

Joint Contractures and Deformities

In screening patients with myelodysplasia for joint contractures and deformities, the presence of malaligned body segments and decreased passive joint range of motion must be documented. Problem areas can be identified by observing spontaneously assumed postures in supine lying and sitting as well as standing in braces. These observations, in combination with a gross assessment of passive range of motion, can be used to identify the presence of clinically significant torticollis, scoliosis, kyphosis, lordosis, pelvic obliquity, and apparent leg length discrepancy. Problems such as genu valgus, talipes calcaneovalgus, as well as other hip, knee, and ankle contractures can also be identified in brief screening

Once malalignment and/or contractures are identified, they should be documented by goniometry. Next, the extent to which their presence or progression can be altered by positioning and therapeutic exercise needs to be determined. Of the numerous joint deformities that occur secondary to myelodysplasia defects, only certain types are amenable to nonsurgical treatment.

The deformities that characterize myelodysplasia can be divided into static and dynamic types.[82] Static joint deformities develop as a result of prolonged positioning, while dynamic joint deformities are caused by imbalanced muscular forces. Both types of deformity are initially supple; however, both become fixed or rigid as skeletal and connective tissue structures change in response to prolonged abnormal positioning.

Dynamic joint deformities can be caused by unopposed force from either voluntarily controlled muscle groups or nonfunctional groups with spinal reflex activity intact. One of the most common dynamic deformities associated with unopposed voluntary muscle function is hip dislocation. Equinus deformity of the ankle is frequently caused by reflex activity in nonfunctional gastrocnemius-soleus muscles unopposed by anterior tibialis function.

Static joint deformities can be caused by prolonged intrauterine positioning of the relatively inactive fetus with myelodysplasia. Although they may be supple, soft tissue contractures at some point during intrauterine development, these deformities often involve skeletal change by the time the infant is born. Static joint deformities also can be caused by habitually assumed postures of initially normal joints without muscular imbalance. One of the most commonly occurring static deformity patterns associated with thoracolumbar level myelodysplasia is flexion contracture of the nonfunctional hips and knees. The supine lying and sitting postures assumed by the essentially flaccid lower extremities for prolonged periods of time are responsible for the eventual loss of extension in these joints.

Prolonged joint malalignment during weight bearing can also produce static deformities. Another commonly occurring deformity pattern that can be considered static in nature is the external tibial torsion and genu valgum associated with lower lumbar level myelodysplasia. When an ankle valgus deformity is present, the lack of appropriate orthotic alignment and support of the knee can gradually produce these skeletal changes.[83,84] It is these static joint deformities, developed after birth, that can be prevented by frequent passive range of motion and positioning incorporated into daily activity patterns.[85]

The ideal means of treating dynamic joint deformities is surgical redistribution of the available muscle force before skeletal and capsular structures become significantly altered.[85] Although positioning, splinting, and passive exercise can delay the progressive effect of muscle imbalance, they are ultimately unsuccessful. Once mobility of the joint is lost, these nonsurgical methods can prevent or delay further progression of deformity, but they are not effective corrective measures of static or dynamic deformities. The use of braces or splints to decrease joint deformity is contraindicated by the presence of anesthetic skin. Necrosis of that skin is likely to occur before joint mobility is affected.

If full passive range of motion and normal body alignment in recumbent and antigravity positions are found to be present, further evaluation can determine the likelihood of the persistence of this desirable situation. Through discussion with the patient and caregivers, the variety and distribution of postures or positions used during each day can be determined. A variety of sitting, supine lying, prone lying, and standing positions clearly has more potential than less variability for maintaining the ideal state.

If compromised joint range of motion and/or postural nonalignment are found to be present, more detailed evaluation needs to focus on determination of the cause. After identifying the specific joints with decreased mobility or inappropriate alignment in certain postures, the therapist needs to identify imbalanced voluntary or involuntary muscular forces associated with those joints. This can be accomplished by manual muscle testing or by facilitating similar movements through play. Movements observed to occur spontaneously or in response to tactile stimulation of the face, neck, arms, or clearly innervated chest area are thought to demonstrate, with fair consistency, use of voluntarily controlled muscle groups. Tactile or painful stimulation to the feet and lower legs are thought to facilitate reflexive, withdrawal movement patterns that can be qualitatively differentiated from controlled, voluntary movement.[1,2] Comparison of spontaneously assumed postures of specific joints in gravity-eliminated positions to those in antigravity positions can help determine the role of extremity weight or weight bearing in the deformity.

Pressure Sores

When screening patients with myelodysplasia for pressure sores, the presence of various stages of anesthetic skin breakdown needs to be identified and documented. The earliest signs of prolonged pressure are redness with, as well as without, swelling. Signs of blistering may precede actual evidence of open sores with partial or full-thickness epithelial loss.[85] In screening these patients, all these signs need to be looked for within areas of anesthetic skin. Generally, the areas at high risk for breakdown are those that either bear body weight for prolonged periods or that bear unequally distributed pressure. Activity level, joint mobility, and joint deformity are major factors determining the location of this prolonged or asymmetric pressure distribution. Infants are likely to develop skin breakdown in the area of their original spinal defect. Particularly in cases of lumbar kyphoses, the prolonged recumbent and supported sitting periods they experience make this a susceptible area.

Children attending school are particularly vulnerable to ischial and sacral skin breakdown if they are functionally limited to wheelchair mobility.[85] The prolonged sitting periods dictated by many school settings, as well as the extended periods required for transportation to and from school, increase the vulnerability of these areas. Prolonged periods of wetness with resultant skin maceration, due to ineffective management of incontinence, facilitate the development and subsequent infection of these pressure sores. The presence of a pelvic obliquity in association with scoliosis or a unilaterally dislocated hip further increases the vulnerability of sacral and ischial areas by shifting the majority of the upper body's weight to one side.

Braces, splints, and casts can create focused pressure on bony prominences, which is amplified or diminished by body positioning. When lower extremity casts are removed, evidence of pressure on the heel is commonly found as a result of supine lying or straight leg sitting posture that focused pressure to that area. Among children wearing braces, shoes are a common source of pressure that leads to skin breakdown. The inappropriate fit of shoes or malalignment of braces is a recurring source of problems. The small, muscularly imbalanced feet of many ambulatory individuals, however, create an unequal, focused weight distribution that is difficult to accommodate by orthotic adjustments.

If no areas of erythema or skin necrosis are found in screening, further evaluative effort can be directed toward the identification of areas still at risk for this problem. Based on the patient's activity level, means of functional mobility, and the significance of joint contractures or deformity, these areas can be determined. If danger areas are identified, it is necessary to find out the extent to which the patient and caregivers are engaged in preventive measures.

Lack of Independent Mobility and Self-Care Skills

The spinal cord dysfunction characteristic of myelodysplasia dictates the extent to which normal patterns of mobility and self-care skills can develop. Patterns adapted to the upper and lower extremity function available have to be learned so that independence in mobility, bathing, dressing, and toileting can be achieved. On screening for the presence or emergence of these adaptive patterns, the evaluator observes the patient's mobility within the clinic and solicits additional information through questioning.

Functional, age-appropriate mobility can be accomplished by a variety of methods. While upright ambulation with braces and crutches is the goal sought for many, mobility in a wheelchair or prone scooter, as well as by means of an adaptive creeping pattern, may also be considered functional relative to the patient's age and environment.

If space and equipment are available, a child is likely to use the most functional, preferred means of mobility in the clinic or department waiting area. If spontaneous mobility is not observed, the patient can be encouraged to get to and from the examination area with as little assistance as possible. While observing mobility, energy cost and quality should be grossly evaluated. Observation of changes in respiratory rate, face coloration, and perspiration can be used to analyze energy expenditure subjectively. Speed and consistency of performance are other factors reflecting endurance relative to energy demands. An individual's control over speed and direction, the smoothness of their movements, and their equilibrium control can all be observed as measures of quality. Through questioning and observation, the extent to which the patient can get into and out of this position or means of mobility needs to be determined. If a wheelchair is used, the ability to transfer between it and a bed, toilet, and the floor should be noted. If a 2-year-old uses an adaptive creeping pattern as the functional means of exploratory play, the ability to safely get in and out of that creeping position as well as down to the floor needs to be noted.

By discussion with the patient and, if appropriate, the caregiver, the extent to which the following skills have developed needs to be determined: (1) taking off and putting on upper body garments, (2) taking off and putting on lower body garments, (3) taking off and putting on braces and shoes, (4) transferring into and out of the bathtub, (5) bathing and drying, and (6) skin inspection.

Depending on the method of bowel and bladder control used, the extent to which the patient accepts responsibility for assisting with or performing stages of the process needs to be determined. The age means and ranges for achievement of these self-care skills among physically normal children cannot be reasonably applied to the myelodysplasia population. The adaptive patterns learned by children with myelodysplasia generally require more mature levels of cognitive and upper extremity function than their counterparts in normal development. While some developmental information has been reported,[49,81] the age means and ranges for achievement of adaptive mobility and self-care skills are essentially unknown. Based on knowledge of normal development, individual abilities, and environmental requirements, the therapist needs to make a judgment regarding the age-appropriateness of each patient's adaptive abilities.

If the mobility and self-care skills, which are demonstrated and reported, are determined to be appropriate for age and environmental requirements, the purpose of further evaluation is to determine the extent to which abilities prerequisite for higher levels of skill are being developed. A young child who is independently mobile within the home by use of a prone scooter is not necessarily developing the upright equilibrium responses or upper extremity function that will be needed for upright ambulation or wheelchair transfers. The upper extremity gross motor skills required for most of these adaptive patterns can be evaluated through analysis of the child's ability to perform pull-up and push-up movements in a sitting position. From a stable sitting position, the ability to grasp an overhead support and lift hips off the sitting surface can be observed. The child's ability to lift the body upward using shoulder depression can also be evaluated. From the suspended position, as well as the push-up position, observation of the ability to swing forward and backward can be a source of evaluative information.

During observation of a child's attempts to perform these activities, the evaluator's attention needs to be directed toward the rate and smoothness of movement, the length of time the hip elevation can be maintained, the amount of extraneous movement present, and the symmetry of the upper extremity efforts. If not evident during these activities, identification of the level to which postural reactions have developed is worthwhile. Postural adjustment and protective upper extremity responses in sitting should be specifically evaluated. If appropriate to the child's level of function, they should be evaluated in standing with braces and crutches.

If the mobility and self-care skills identified are determined to be inadequate for age or environmental requirements, the purpose of further evaluation is determination of the limiting factors. The gross upper extremity function prerequisite for most of these activities can be determined as described in the above paragraph. The child's attempt to perform the mobility or self-care tasks of concern should be observed to isolate specific problem areas. Causes of inadequate function are commonly found in the method or movement pattern used by the child. For example, hand placement used for sliding board transfers may be such that weight shifting is made more difficult than necessary. Erroneous learning of hand placement can simply be corrected and remediated by practice in an appropriate position. Problems with motor planning, however, can be present and should be anticipated. The inability to shift or advance body weight can reflect lack of upper extremity strength or inability to coordinate use of neck and shoulder musculature to move the trunk. Poorly developed equilibrium responses often account for inadequate mobility skills. Lack of sensory input from the lower extremities as well as lack of lower extremity participation in the movement response significantly alter the development of upright postural control.

Joint contractures or deformities may also be a limiting factor. The limitations created by assistive devices need to be considered. Wheelchairs that are ill-fitting or without removable arm rests can hinder transfer function, as can braces that are malaligned or with debris-clogged ankle joints. Other factors relative to adaptive mobility and self-care skills that need to be considered are motivation and opportunity for practice.

Deficient Development of Fine Motor and Perceptual– Motor Skills

This area of concern in evaluation encompasses the wide range of skills for which children with myelodysplasia generally use normal upper extremity movement patterns. These skills include such basic movements as directed reaching and pincer grasping, as well as complex patterns such as cutting with scissors and writing. They include functional skills such as self-feeding, buttoning, and snapping upper body garments. This group of skills is in contrast to the self-care skills, such as applying braces, which involve complex, sensorimotor abilities that are not required of physically normal children.

The primary focus of screening for deficient development of fine and perceptual motor skills is documentation of the presence or absence of age-appropriate milestones in these areas. Unfortunately, a standardized, norm-referenced measure designed to validly screen this range of skills in the myelodysplasia population does not exist. To avoid the time required for use of detailed diagnostic tests and to obtain the reliability afforded by use of standardized tests, the Denver Developmental Screening Test (DDST) can be used.[86] Although intended for use with "apparently well" children, the DDST can be used to monitor the apparently normal development of skills that do not involve the lower extremities. The standardized administration and scoring criteria can be implemented without modification in the personal–social, fine motor–adaptive, and language sections of the test. As stated in the manual, an evaluation that reveals a DDST section with two or more delayed test items, in addition to the gross motor section, should be classified as "abnormal." An evaluation that reveals a section with one delayed item and no age-appropriate items passed, in addition to the gross motor section, should be classified as "questionable." An evaluation that reveals no delays in any of the sections, other than the gross motor, should be classified as "normal." Clearly, the

DDST needs to be administered to this population, with consideration given to the quality of their responses. The labels of "abnormal," "questionable," and "normal" should be used only to help determine the need for further evaluation and not for literal interpretation.

One element of quality that can be easily observed while administering the DDST is hand preference. The age at which hand preference or dominance is established within the neurologically normal population is relative to specific skills and is a topic of continued debate.[87] It can, nevertheless, be a revealing area to use in screening 4- to 6-year-olds for upper extremity dysfunction. In two studies of myelodysplastic, hydrocephalic children from 6 to 10 years of age, 30 percent were found to demonstrate mixed handedness, in contrast to 2 to 5 percent in control groups.[88] While no significant link has been established between lack of hand preference and low IQ or neurologic dysfunction, its relationship to delayed manual skill development seems apparent.[88] Absolute dependence on one upper extremity for skilled activity, however, is significantly predictive of neurologic dysfunction.

After the age of 6 years, use of the DDST for screening becomes inappropriate.[87] There is no single valid standardized screening test that samples the full range of complex fine and perceptual motor skills in the school-age population. Portions of standardized, norm-referenced tests can, however, be useful as objective screening measures if interpreted judiciously.

Although in need of further validation, Cornish[89] has described an 11-item screening test for age-appropriate motor planning ability from 6 to 12 years of age. Of the 11 items, only 5 can be uniformly administered to children with myelodysplasia because of lower extremity function requirements. Those five items that can be used are (1) a vertical throw, hand clap, and catch sequence repeated as rapidly as possible with a tennis ball for 30 seconds, (2 and 3) a peg placement test using dominant and nondominant hands, and (4 and 5) a grip strength measurement using dominant and nondominant hands. Mean scores and standard deviations for these five items, which are based on their administration to 210 normal children, are reported. Failure of a child with myelodysplasia to score within the ranges reported for his or her age on these test items can be cautiously interpreted as an indication for further diagnostic evaluation.

Another screening measurement can be adopted from a study comparing the performance of 8-year-olds with and without diagnosed learning disabilities on measures of fine motor activity speed. After analyzing the responses of 50 children (25 control subjects and 25 with learning disabilities), Kendrick and Hanter[90] reported that rapid sequence opposition between the thumb and index finger differentiated between the two groups. During a second testing period, the normal children touched 38.4 ± 3.8 times in comparison to the learning disabled children's 30.6 ± 4.5 ($P < .01$). Keeping in mind that predictive validity of this item remains to be proven, it could be administered to 8-year-old patients with myelodysplasia and interpreted in terms of speed within the normal range, smoothness, rhythm consistency, and elimination of extraneous movement. Lack of speed within the normal limits or subjectively poor response quality could be used as indications for further evaluation.

If no deficiency is suggested by screening test items, no deficiency perceived by the quality of responses, and no significant frustrations expressed by the child or caregivers, further evaluation of perceptual and fine motor skills may be deemed unnecessary or of low priority. From a preventive perspective, however, further evaluation can be directed toward determination of the experiential opportunities available to the child for further expansion of these abilities. Of specific concern with the infant and young toddler are opportunities for independent exploration of space and for two-handed play in a stable upright posture.[91]

If deficiency is suggested by screening test items, by diminished quality of performance perceived by the examiner, or by concerns expressed in caregiver–child interviews, further diagnostic evaluation can branch out in several directions. When concerns are based primarily on screening test results, those tests need to be readministered at a later date to determine whether the pattern of delay persists. Delayed development specific to the language section of the DDST is appropriately investigated further by a speech pathologist. Consistently delayed development throughout all sections of the DDST may be indicative of mental retardation. This is further appropriately evaluated by individuals skilled in the administration of standardized, norm-referenced tests of learning potential or intelligence. Although not highly predictive of later scores on the Stanford-Binet Intelligence Test, the Bayley Scales of Infant Development (BSID) Mental Scale is a well-standardized test that can reliably describe a child's learning or developmental level relative to the general population.[92] Due to the gross motor nature of the items throughout the Psychomotor Scale of the BSID, this portion of the test is inappropriate for use with the myelodysplasia population. The Mental Scale of the BSID, however, can describe learning level as well as basic fine and perceptual motor skill development among this group.

Delays in development of fine motor and/or personal–social abilities identified on the DDST or by other screening methods require further evaluation of upper extremity functional abilities as well as refined coordination capacity. To explore upper extremity functional activities in detail, relevant sections from the numerous standardized developmental profiles can be used for preschool levels. The Callier-Azusa Scale is one such profile that has subscales for fine motor, visual motor, feeding skills, and perceptual abilities.[93] The perceptual abilities subscale is further divided into responses to visual, auditory, and tactile input.

Four of the eight subtests that make up the Bruininks-Oseretsky Test of Motor Proficiency (BOTMP) are appropriate for administration to 4.5- through 14.5-year-olds affected by myelodysplasia.[94] For evaluation of refined visual motor coordination skills of the upper extremities, three subtests from the BOTMP can be helpful, as can subtests from Touwen's protocol for evaluation of children with minor neurologic dysfunction.[87,94] Seven of the nine test items Touwen includes in his assessment of coordination and associated movements can be administered to this group, the only modification being the use of a sitting rather than a standing posture. Administration, recording, and interpretation criteria are explained for each of these items, which are thought by Touwen to reflect central nervous system maturation and "proprioceptive system" function.[87] Visual pursuit, scanning, and fixation limitations may appear to be a source of visual motor problems. If this is the case, the relatively quick assessment of these factors outlined by Touwen can be helpful.

Neonatal Assessment

Physical therapy evaluation of a neonate with myelodysplasia should serve the same primary purpose as assessment of a child or adolescent. The limited response capacity of neonates, however, places assessment of their problems in a distinct category. Differentiating between voluntary and involuntary lower extremity movement responses for purposes of anticipatory management can be quite a challenge. Voluntary movement is more likely to be observed in the lower extremities when the infant is alert and actively moving the arms.[2] Lower extremity movement responses to stimulation around the face, chest, and shoulders are likely to be voluntary in nature.[2,4] The reflexive character and stimulus dependency of involuntary muscle responses help to distinguish them from voluntary movement. Tactile stimulation of skin over the hip flexor, knee flexor, and all ankle and toe musculature can produce contractile responses in physically normal neonates.[95] These same responses can be elicited when only segmental spinal cord function is present. Consequently, they alone should not be interpreted as evidence of corticospinal tract integrity.[4] While one to two beats of ankle clonus is within normal limits for the immature central nervous system of any neonate, sustained or easily elicited ankle clonus is suggestive of involuntary function of the gastrocnemius-soleus muscles. Similar clonic responses as well as resistance to quick lengthening may also be detected in the lateral hamstrings and toe flexors. If quick stretching of a muscle group on one leg elicits not only a contraction response of that muscle, but of the same muscle(s) on the other leg as well, a crossed stretch reflex has been elicited. This is characteristic of isolated spinal cord segment function and should not be confused with spontaneous, voluntary movement.[4] Stimulus-dependent flexor withdrawal is a primary pattern associated with involuntary movement. The time span between stimulus and onset of movement as well as between onset and completion of withdrawal movement is reported to vary within a wide range.[3,4] Consequently, a smooth, slow, but stimulus-dependent flexor withdrawal movement is no more indicative of spinal cord integrity than a jerky, brisk withdrawal to stimulation. Stark and Baker[4] reported that crossed extensor reflexes are seldom present when corticospinal tract function is not present; however, Brocklehurst[3] includes this response among those that can be elicited when no voluntary control of the extensor muscle groups is present. Electrical stimulation of muscle groups has been used by Sharrard[2] as a means of confirming lower motoneuron innervation; however, the usefulness of the process has been described as minimal by several other researchers.[85,96]

Determination of the level of intact sensation is probably more difficult and subjective than determination of motor function, but is important for preventive management. When an infant is in a drowsy or quiet state, noxious stimulation can be administered to the areas of skin innervated by the sacral and distal lumbar cord segments. By progressing from most distal to proximal segments, the examiner can usually determine which areas produce cry, grimace, or startle responses distinguishable from spinal cord level withdrawal responses.[2,3]

The primary functional skill to be evaluated in neonates with myelodysplasia is nipple-feeding ability. Since these neonates are at risk for cranial nerve damage from an Arnold-Chiari malformation, a feeding evaluation should focus on components of suck, swallow, and respiration, as well as the function of each cranial nerve. The neonatal assessment of sensorimotor function should provide a basis for planning treatment measures that prevent or improve joint contractures, pressure sores, and oral motor dysfunction.[97]

Observation of Complications

Therapists caring for myelodysplastic–hydrocephalic patients should be well aware of the signs of shunt malfunction and neuropathic fractures. These signs should not only be considered during designated evaluation periods, they should also be monitored in any treatment setting. The initial signs of acute shunt obstruction and/or infection mimic those of a viral illness. They are headache, irritability, lethargy, and vomiting.[3] The initial sign of a fracture is often a fever.[98] As is often the case, no traumatic event can be recalled, and the fever is logically attributed to a urinary tract infection.

PHYSICAL THERAPY

The facilitation of both the development and maintenance of as optimal a level of independent function as possible is the general goal shared by the medical team members involved in the care of each individual with myelodysplasia. More specifically, the overall goals of physical therapy for an individual with myelodysplasia are to facilitate as normal a sequence of sensorimotor development as possible and to prevent the development of secondary joint deformities and skin ulceration. These goals are ideally pursued through a combination of direct, therapist-provided patient care coordinated with an ongoing home care program. The specific methods for adaptive function and developmental facilitation appropriate for each patient's age and ability need to be taught by the therapist to that patient and caregivers. Once these methods are correctly learned, they should be incorporated into the daily care routines or play within the home environment. The actual refinement of adaptive self-care and mobility skills should be the result of practice that meets the caretaking and play activity needs of the child and family. A recent study has confirmed the beneficial role of adequately trained parents in initial gait training.[99] The parents or primary caregivers of a physically normal child generally feel competent to provide for the needs of that child. For the caregiver of a child with myelodysplasia, however, this sense of competence needs to be fostered rather than diminished by the treatment-related activities carried out at home.

Joint Contractures and Deformities

Physical therapy is directed toward the goals of preventing static joint deformities, resolving minor static joint deformities, preventing the rapid deterioration of dynamic deformities, and minimizing the risk of neuropathic fractures. The primary methods for accomplishing these goals are passive range of motion (ROM) exercises, positioning, and splinting.

Full passive joint mobility throughout the body is ideally the goal of treatment. Mobility that allows stable joint alignment for standing, sitting, and transfers, however, is often accepted as a more realistic guide for both physical therapy and orthopedic management. In an upright position, the cervical and upper thoracic spine need to be centered over the pelvis. The pelvis must be level for equal weight distribution in sitting. Hips and knees should flex to at least 90 degrees for sitting and transferring without increasing the risk of neuropathic fractures. For standing, the hips should extend to neutral without significant rotation or adduction. If this hip range is not present, development of knee flexion contractures and lumbar lordosis can be facilitated. When standing with hip flexion contractures, tightened iliopsoas muscles can exert an amplified dislocating force on the hip joint.[96] Standing and, especially, ambulation are limited in their functional value if hip extension to neutral or beyond is not present. With locked long leg braces in place, hip flexion tightness precludes sufficient shifting of the center of gravity over the feet to produce a balanced stance and allow upper extremity freedom from weight bearing. Knees should reach essentially full extension for functional dressing skills, if not for standing and ambulation. In standing, the presence of knee flexion contractures dictates positions of hip flexion and ankle dorsiflexion if balance is to be achieved. Lack of essentially complete hip and knee extension limit bed mobility and the variety of lying positions that are comfortable. In standing, the joints of the ankle and foot should provide a plantigrade surface across which body weight can be equally distributed. While a neutral ankle is adequate for standing, approximately 10 degrees of ankle dorsiflexion is needed for forward progression. In the absence of gastrocnemius-soleus muscle function, dorsiflexion of approximately 10 degrees may be all that is desirable. Dias has noted that 20 to 30 degrees dorsiflexion, in the absence of plantarflexion control, facilitates development of ankle valgus, external tibial torsion, and genu valgum.[84] If not for standing purposes, the ankle and foot should have unrestricted passive mobility into a neutral position so that shoes and wheelchair pedals do not create pressure sores.

Passive ROM can be performed for patients with myelodysplasia using any of the methods appropriate for soft tissue tightness. Since the risk of neuropathic fractures is present, considerable attention should be directed toward secure stabilization both proximal and distal to the joint being treated. The range of single joints should be attended to before two-joint muscle groups receive passive stretching. While maintenance of joint mobility in the lower extremities is a ubiquitous component of physical therapy for patients with myelodysplasia, neck mobility is often overlooked in hydrocephalic patients until torticollis is evident. Neither the incidence nor the etiology of this problem has been investigated. Habitual prone positioning, shunt tubing adhesions, irritation of cervical soft tissue by tubing, and/or compensation for spinal deformity, however, are possibilities. As with torticollis in otherwise normal children, neck mobility and facial symmetry can be maintained and restored by exercise and positioning if initiated soon enough.[100]

The amount of time that should be invested in range of motion exercises for torticollis or other contractures, or for preventive purposes, has not been established by clinical research. Kopits[96] recommends that all joints without complete sensorimotor function receive full range two to four times each day. Menelaus,[85] on the other hand, considers it "improper to impose on the parents" the responsibility of passive range of motion exercises. Perhaps the number of variables that complicate each individual situation will cause this to remain an intuitive decision mutually agreeable to the child, parent, and therapist.

Although maximum available range can be achieved for brief periods during passive exercise, positioning can be used to maintain functional ranges for longer periods of time. Prone lying and standing are the two positions most frequently used to counteract the hip and knee flexion postures characteristic of supine lying and sitting. One position, recommended by Drennan,[101] consists of prone lying with placement of the feet off the end of a mattress or cushion and swaddling of the legs together. The foot position eliminates pressure from their dorsal aspect and allows them to assume a relatively plantigrade position. By use of a towel, diaper, or, as Menelaus[85] recommends, a section of "Tubigrip," the legs are held together, preventing hip abduction and later rotation. While this position is designed to prevent tightening of the iliotibial bands, it may be contraindicated for children having unstable hips with muscular imbalance. Lack of mobility in the hips or knees may also preclude the use of a flat, prone position.

When hip, knee, and ankle mobility are sufficient, periods of standing can be used to maintain lower extremity joint ranges. Obviously, orthoses of appropriate fit and sufficient support are required for this. For the individual without ambulation skill, standing in braces can be a frightening, as well as boring, situation. A standing table that provides additional external stability and a play surface can resolve this problem. Various forms of supervised standing play can be used to encourage functional upper extremity skills.

Regardless of the specific position used to maintain mobility, anesthetic joints should not be forced to their maximum range in that position. To prevent joint damage, fractures, and skin breakdown, these joints should be maintained in positions within the limits of free mobility.

The splints used for treatment of myelodysplasia generally serve the purposes of slowing the progression of dynamic deformities, halting the progression of static deformities, or preventing the recurrence of deformities after surgical correction. The role of lower extremity splints in the early management of hips at risk for dislocation due to muscle imbalance is still a topic of debate among orthopedists. McKibon,[102] who originally proposed their use, considers a splint that holds both hips in extension, abduction, and slight medial rotation to be useful in maintaining hip reduction and preventing hip flexion contracture development. Various heat and vacuum-formed plastic splints have been designed to serve this purpose. While avoiding the cost and pressure-point problems associated with these rigid splints, Jaeger[103] has reported successful use of a foam wedge splint placed between the legs and held in place by foam straps that control hip rotation.

The recurrent nature of knee flexion contractures and equinovarus deformities have made them a focus of splinting efforts. The dynamic nature of most of these knee or ankle contractures limits the initial preventive role of splints. After soft tissue release, however, posterior splints for use during sleep are considered appropriate preventive measures by Menelaus.[85] The creation of splints that cover areas of anesthetic skin is clearly a refined skill that has to be developed through experience. Basically, however, the splint must conform closely to the body in order to distribute pressure evenly rather than focus it on high-risk areas. To avoid shearing forces on the skin, the splints should fit tightly enough to prevent slipping movement. Thin cotton stockinette is frequently used to separate the splint from direct contact with the skin. Splint use should be completely discontinued when redness is noted from pressure. Once the erythema has completely resolved and the splint has been altered, splint use can be gradually resumed if the signs of pressure do not return. Pressure sore development is such a common complication of splint use over anesthetic skin that their use is considered altogether inappropriate by some physicians.[2] As with range of motion exercises and position, no valid formula exists for determination of how long splints should be worn each day or how long daily use should be continued. Even if there was such a formula, it would have to accommodate the same factors of tolerance level and individual motivation currently guiding these decisions.

Approximately 20 percent of individuals with myelodysplasia experience neuropathic fractures.[85,53] A high percentage of these fractures follow postoperative cast immobilization. Avoiding prolonged immobilization periods is one preventive method that is being implemented more frequently by surgeons. The use of bulky "Webril" dressings for immobilization has been reported to support healing metaphyseal and diaphyseal fractures as well as a plaster cast, with fewer complications.[53] After a fracture itself or corrective orthopedic surgery, initiation of weight bearing as soon as stability is confirmed is another measure thought to prevent fractures.[85,96] Lack of proper stabilization during transfers and too vigorous an effort during therapeutic exercise are possible causes of neuropathic fractures. While whirlpools are very useful in skin care after cast removal, the poorly controlled movement of buoyant legs needs to be minimized. Bivalved casts or supportive splints can be used to cradle the vulnerable leg(s) during transfers until functional joint mobility has been gently reestablished.[85]

Pressure Sores

Whether treating pressure sores that have already developed or designing a program to prevent their occurrence, physical therapy is directed at controlling the factors that facilitate skin breakdown. These factors are sustained local pressure, friction, shearing force, skin maceration, and infection.[104] Once skin necrosis has developed, the effects of these factors need to be eliminated for complete healing to occur. Since total elimination of those factors is not conducive to a functional lifestyle, preventive programs are directed toward minimizing and counteracting their effects.

Sustained local pressure over ischial or sacral areas of skin breakdown can only be eliminated for healing purposes by discontinuing wheelchair use and sitting. This requires a closely followed program of prone lying, sidelying, and, if appropriate, standing to allow for healing while preventing the development of skin breakdown in other areas. If standing with braces is not feasible, prone standing devices can be used.

In theory, the location of focused pressure can be changed by increasing the area over which force is distributed or increasing the distance between points of force.[104] One treatment method that applies this theory to the treatment of pressure sores on the feet is total contact plastering. Positioning the foot and ankle in as functional a position as possible, plaster is applied to conform closely to lower extremity contours. This method of casting can prevent further shearing and friction injury, distribute pressure, and facilitate deep tissue healing. Sharrard[2] reports complete healing of significant sores on the feet of myelodysplasia patients within 6 weeks by use of this below-knee casting technique.

Although costly and supported primarily by uncontrolled clinical trials, hyperbaric oxygen therapy is another means of treating pressure sores that may prove to be a valuable addition for the care of patients with myelodysplasia. Fischer[105] reports complete healing of 26 cases of previously ''resistant'' pressure sores following this type of treatment.

Because of poor healing with conservative treatment and loss of ambulatory function following prolonged immobilization, some treatment centers now advocate early surgical closure of pressure sores.[106] The benefits of surgically rotated skin and muscle flaps to high-risk anesthetic areas remain a source of debate.[106–108]

Once healing has occurred or prior to the ulceration of skin in anesthetic areas, programs for alternating body positions during the day need to be developed in collaboration with the patient and caregivers. These positioning periods correspond with those already discussed as needed for the prevention of flexion contractures. Particular attention needs to be directed toward the school-age patient who spends long periods of time in a wheelchair. The ongoing facilitation of prone or standing periods for primarily wheelchair-limited children during school hours can be a very worthwhile, preventive role for school-system therapists to fulfill. Teaching and encouraging these individuals to do push-ups and shift their weight from side to side in the wheelchair are commonly implemented preventive measures. These practices, however, do not seem to preclude the need for periods when pressure is totally removed from the ischial-sacral area. Clinical research validating the usefulness of wheelchair push-ups and lateral weight shifting in terms of temperature or circulatory changes in the posterior skin is lacking.

Particular attention needs to be directed toward the individual with ambulatory skill sufficient for community mobility. Periods that provide for complete elimination of weight bearing and prevention of venous stasis should be planned within daily routines. Correctly fitting shoes and braces are crucial to these individuals. With varying degrees of success, numerous modifications of shoes, such as cut-outs and shoes that unlace their entire length, have been tried in order to distribute pressure as well as ensure that the foot is positioned correctly.

Wheelchair cushions are one of the primary means of distributing body weight away from the sacral and ischial areas during sitting. Because of its availability and relatively low cost, polyurethane foam is one of the most commonly used materials for wheelchair cushions. Loss of load-bearing capacity is one of the factors that limits the useful life-span of these cushions. Through static and dynamic fatigue testing, McFadyen and Stoner[109] have confirmed that a patient's weight and the duration of sitting periods are prime factors determining the length of time a polyurethane foam pad can serve a protective function. They also determined that during 24-hour periods without compression, these pads recovered an average of 80 percent of their indentation load deflection capacity. Consequently, they recommend the purchase of two cushions that can be used on alternate days.

Investigating the heat and humidity-dissipation capacity of various types of padding, Stewart and associates[110] noted a moisture-absorbing ability relatively unique to polyurethane. The heat-absorbing capacity of this type of pad, however, was found to be poor and a cause of increased local skin temperature among subjects. On the other hand, they found that humidity remained at a relatively low level during use as long as the pad was covered with a porous material. This humidity-controlling effect was lost when vinyl covered the foam.

Because of their increased load-bearing capacity, wheelchair cushions made of gel materials are generally thought to be superior to foam cushions. Results from the investigation of Stewart and associates[110] point out the limitations of gel cushions in controlling heat and humidity. They found that gel material had very little, if any, capacity for dissipating moisture. They found that this material was effective for approximately 2 hours in controlling skin temperature because of its capacity to absorb heat. Due to an apparent loss of heat-absorbing ability and the presence of high humidity, these researchers recommended that gel cushions be used for no more than 3 hours without permitting them to cool. Similarly, water flotation cushions were found to reduce skin temperature, at least initially. Due to their nonporous structure, flotation pads were found to control humidity poorly.[110]

Clearly, the ideal wheelchair cushion capable of compensating for lack of sensation and mobility under all circumstances has not been developed. When programs for the prevention of pressure sores are being outlined, these load-bearing, heat, and humidity-dissipating characteristics of cushions need to be considered. The cost, availability, and durability need to be considered in light of the limit capacity of any wheelchair cushion to provide protection when used all day every day.

Friction and shearing forces need to be controlled in addition to static pressure in order for pressure sores to heal or be prevented. Friction is primarily a force abrading superficial epithelial tissue. Shearing, however, refers to the tangential force caused by gliding of superficial over deeper tissues, which results in obstructed circulation and relatively deep trauma.[111] Skin damage due to friction is controlled in the lower extremities by eliminating significant movement within shoes and braces during ambulation and standing transfers. When pressure sores are on the feet, even the abrasion produced by bed sheets may have to be eliminated.[85] Sitting transfers are a main source of friction and shearing to the ischial-sacral area. Moist skin, clothing, or wheelchair cushions are sources of friction that complicate sliding transfers. Shoulder depression ability that is insufficient to shift weight off the ischial-sacral area during transfers is another factor contributing to skin breakdown. To prevent skin breakdown, measures should be taken to improve the quality of these sitting transfers. A tightly fitting pelvic band that pulls sacral area skin upward during stationary sitting or sitting transfers can be a source of shearing damage to the sacral area. A tightly fitting calf band that pulls skin upward as ankle dorsiflexion occurs during standing or ambulation can be a source of shearing damage to the heel area. Such situations can be altered by proper fitting of braces and the use of long socks or other thin, conforming articles of clothing between braces and skin.

The effects of maceration and infection also need to be eliminated for ulceration healing and controlled for prevention.[111] Maceration describes the damage to superficial skin that occurs when an area is kept moist for a prolonged period by excessive perspiration or incontinence. In the absence of open sores, hair follicles and pores can become infected due to poor circulation and incontinence. Maceration and infection facilitate the presence of each other, as well as make skin more vulnerable to the effects of prolonged pressure, shearing, and friction. To free open sores of infectious organisms and necrotic tissue, whirlpools are frequently used in conjunction with topical or systemic antibiotics. Of particular importance to both preventive and corrective treatment is an effective bowel and bladder management pattern that is appropriate for home as well as school.

In summary, the prevention or healing of pressure sores requires the development of positioning programs and effective management of incontinence. It can require the modification of brace, wheelchairs, and their accessories, as well as techniques used for ambulation and transfers. Programs for preventive care are incomplete without the establishment of a routine skin inspection method.

Lack of Independent Mobility and Self-Care Skills

Numerous studies of the mobility skills achieved by patients with myelodysplasia lesions at varying levels have provided information on which predictions of functional mobility in child and adulthood can be based.[54,112-114] From these results, the goal of therapeutic ambulation for any myelodysplasia patient without major brain damage is justified as realistic during childhood. While therapeutic ambulation serves many purposes, it often does not meet the child's need for mobility during the preschool or school years. The therapist must keep a realistic perspective on the potential for ambulation to actually fulfill each child's need for functional mobility. When time, teaching, and financial resources are applied only to the development of walking skill in early childhood, the unfortunate result can be a 5-year-old child with ability to independently walk 100 feet in 10 minutes, but lack of the transfer and wheelchair mobility skills needed for a school setting.

Longitudinal studies of mobility skills among people with myelodysplasia defects use the terms *community, household, therapeutic,* and *wheelchair* to describe levels of skill. *Community ambulation* describes the ability to walk with or without braces and other assistive devices indoors and outdoors as well as to negotiate most natural and architectural barriers.[114] Ability to functionally ambulate within a community implies that the person has endurance sufficient to the energy demands presented by their gait pattern and environment. *Household ambulation* describes the ability to walk with or without assistive devices and braces on level surfaces of varying textures as well as negotiate doorway and other minor architectural barriers found indoors.[114] While household ambulation imposes lower endurance demands than community ambulation, both require the ability to transfer independently between sitting and standing positions. *Therapeutic* and *exercise ambulation* are terms used interchangeably with nonfunctional ambulation. While a therapeutic ambulator may be able to ambulate independently with braces and assistive devices, assistance is required to transfer between sitting and standing.[114] The energy demands of the gait pattern often limit the range of their ambulation to relatively short distances. *Wheelchair mobility* describes the ability to independently propel from one point to a destination. The label of functional wheelchair mobility implies the ability to transfer in and out of the chair and to negotiate doorways and other minor barriers.

These studies of mobility skill achievement consistently demonstrate an eventual transition from ambulation to wheelchair mobility among all but the population with L5 and S1 lesion levels.[112–114] Individuals with loss of function below the T2–T12 level are able, as a general rule, to develop therapeutic ambulation skill in childhood. The majority, however, use a wheelchair as their primary means of mobility throughout childhood and adulthood. Children born with a loss of sensorimotor function below L1 and L2 generally develop therapeutic or household ambulation skills. Their primary means of mobility, however, remains the wheelchair throughout childhood and adulthood. Loss of sensorimotor function below L3 or L4 generally predicts the ability to develop household ambulation skills, if not community-wide skill, in childhood. During adolescence, these individuals generally convert to use of a wheelchair for community and household mobility. This is due, in part, to the energy demands of ambulation, which rise in proportion to increases in their height and weight. The majority of people with L5 and S1 levels of sensorimotor function develop community ambulation skill in childhood and maintain that ability throughout adulthood.

Investigations of ambulation velocity and physical activity capacity for children with myelodysplasia provide data that can be helpful in treatment planning. After 6 to 7 years of age, the achievement of functional household or community ambulation becomes statistically unlikely.[54,81] The ability to independently engage in community ambulation at this age predicts functional adolescent ambulation in more than 85 percent of cases.[54] Simple clinically useful methods for calculation of oxygen consumption during ambulation or wheelchair propulsion provide insight into the energy demands and, therefore, the functionality of these forms of mobility.[115,116] Studies have demonstrated that maximum ambulatory speed greater than 150 m/min predicts functional ambulation into adolescence while less than 90 m/min predicts early adolescent reliance on a wheelchair for mobility.[115]

Horizontal mobility is normally achieved between 8 and 10 months of age by a child's development of the ability to crawl on the abdomen and creep on the hands and knees.[92] With this horizontal mobility, the child explores the surrounding environment and begins to delight in a sense of emerging independence. This activity also provides opportunities for development of upper body strength, coordination, endurance, and equilibrium responses. Horizontal mobility must be facilitated among infants with myelodysplasia to provide similar experience in preparation for other mobility skills. Although many children with partially functioning lower extremities are able to learn adaptive creeping patterns (side-hitching and rabbit hopping), these patterns may reinforce imbalanced muscle control or joint deformities already present. Before facilitating the development of adaptive creeping skill, therapists and caregivers should determine the extent to which that skill will contribute to hip and knee flexion contractures, equinus foot deformities, scoliosis, and increased lumbar lordosis or kyphosis. If introduced before a child learns an adaptive creeping pattern, prone scooter boards and hand-propelled sitting carts (chariots) can provide less-deforming alternatives.

Hand-propelled carts that support the child in a long sitting position are generally more popular with young children than prone scooters. Although they provide household mobility and are simple to operate, they have disadvantages that should be considered. The more complex upper extremity movement patterns required for ambulation and transfers are not well facilitated during use of these carts. Prolonged periods of hip flexion and ischial-sacral pressure occur as the child becomes adept with its use. While prone scooters have none of these disadvantages, the determined resistance of some myelodysplasia children to them is a commonly encountered problem. Whether this is due to lack of experience, to a feeling of helplessness in prone, or to some type of vestibular system dysfunction, the benefits of prone scooter mobility make consistent, patient teaching efforts worthwhile. The prone scooter should be introduced to a child when he or she has the ability to roll and pivot in prone lying as well as support weight and balance on one extended arm in prone while reaching with the other. To make initial encounters with the scooter positive, the child can be encouraged to play with it while not on it. The child can put toys on it and move the scooter about in order to feel its motion. Seeing other children scooting in prone on it is helpful. When the child is on the scooter, he or she can be reinforced for staying on it for periods of stationary prone play or for periods of back and forth rocking. Once the child enjoys this, slow rides on the scooter can be provided to familiarize the child with the motion.

As with ambulation, progression on smooth, polished surfaces should be achieved prior to textured surfaces. As in the normal prone progression sequence, backward movement on the scooter is more quickly learned than forward. As an initial step, the child on the scooter, supporting weight on extended arms, can be slowly rocked back and forth by another person. The child can be assisted in pushing backward in order to obtain a toy placed under the scooter. A play partner sitting in front of the child on the scooter can hold hands with that child and encourage pushing and pulling movements. With this activity, as well as backward, pivoting, and forward movement, the amount of assistance provided can be decreased as the child gains control.

Prone scooters are available through many medical equipment companies; however, parents and staff in institutions often choose to build their own. Detailed plans for a prone scooter suitable for use by any child with myelodysplasia, but designed for a 5-year-old child in a double spica cast, are presented in an article by Streissguth and Streissguth.[117]

The ability of most patients with myelodysplasia to achieve at least a therapeutic level of ambulation skill is supported by studies of relatively large populations; however, the value of this ability has been and continues to be questioned.[112-116] In response to this questioning, the following list of beneficial effects directly related to childhood ambulation and standing has been proposed in current literature[3,85,96,117-119]:

1. Improved bowel and bladder drainage
2. Prevention of osteoporosis and facilitation of osteoblastic activity
3. Improved cardiopulmonary endurance

4. Prevention of ischial-sacral pressure sores
5. Maintenance of hip and knee joint extension and ankle dorsiflexion
6. Improved interaction with the environment
7. Improved upper extremity strength, coordination, and endurance

Clinical studies supporting these proposed benefits are still lacking. If these effects do occur, they clearly facilitate the development of functional wheelchair skills as well as ambulatory capacity.

Although some people with low lumbar level lesions are able to ambulate without braces in adolescence and adulthood, bracing is required in at least the initial stages of gait training for the majority of children with myelodysplasia. Double upright, metal braces with hinged joints are still the most common type of orthosis used for individuals with myelodysplasia. The ankle joints of long and short leg orthoses should have their free motion limited to approximately 10 degrees.[84,118] Dorsiflexion or anterior ankle stops, in combination with rigid sole plates extending to the metatarsophalangeal joints, should counteract the knee flexion tendency imposed by lack of or weakened gastrocnemius-soleus function.[120,121] If functional dorsiflexion is not present, a posterior or plantar flexion stop should simulate toe pick-up and prevent a foot drop pattern from interfering with forward progression.[120] Posterior calf bands of short or long braces should be located as high on the calf as possible without interfering with knee movement or creating pressure on the neural or vascular structures.[122] High placement decreases the amount of pressure exerted on the calf by this band, as it helps control ankle plantar flexion during swing phase. This band should also prevent the lower leg and knee from moving posteriorly in the brace and should play a significant role in maintaining the brace aligned with the leg when a long leg brace is unlocked and flexed during sitting.[120] For long leg braces, the knee-straightening force supplied by knee pads or straps should be applied as close to the knee as possible, with greater force applied below the knee than above. Ideally, the force should be carried by two straps applied over the suprapatellar and patellar tendon areas, rather than a single wide knee pad that allows focused pressure on the patella itself.[120] The posterior upper thigh band is appropriately located 1 to 1.5 inches from the ischium during standing and walking.

All orthotic joints should be matched with their anatomic or functional counterparts on the legs. Correct alignment of the orthotic knee and the functional knee joint axis of the person is important for prevention of pressure, friction, and shearing points during ambulation. As children grow and minor lengthening adjustments are made on their braces, the knee joint is easily displaced. Since the functional axis of the human knee changes during movement from full extension to full flexion, the functional axis of the knee in extension is usually the starting point for orthotic knee joint alignment. When the orthotic knee axis is posterior to or behind the human knee axis in extension, flexion of the knee will increase pressure from the posterior thigh and calf bands as well as shift the entire brace distally.[123] Each time the child sits down, the heels will tend to come out of the shoes and pressure will be increased over the dorsum of the foot. Location of the axis anterior to or in front of the extended knee's functional axis produces the opposite effect.[123] This problem can produce the groin pressure that occurs when some children sit from standing. Location of the axis distally or below the knee's functional joint in extension creates a similar shifting of the brace into the groin. The pressure of the calf band against the posterior lower leg is increased and a shearing force affecting the calf and heel areas can result. The opposite effect occurs when the orthotic knee axis is proximal to or above the extended knee axis in standing.[123] Orthotic uprights and knee joints may be deliberately aligned in lateral or medial rotation relative to the anatomic knee in order to counteract slight genu valgus or varus. If excessive rotation is present, however, pressure from the uprights against the thigh can occur in standing or sitting. These uprights not only create static pressure points but also rotational shearing forces. Consequently, this is not a situation that should be allowed to persist.

The use of pelvic bands and lockable orthotic hip joints with paraplegics is a subject of controversy. Electrogoniometric studies have shown that posterior pelvic tilt is not maintained and lumbar movement is actually increased in the presence of locked orthotic hips and a pelvic band.[118,120] Unless extension force is applied at the sternum by more elaborate thoracic bracing methods, hip flexion and lumbar lordosis will probably persist with orthotic hip joints locked. If present, however, a pelvic band with hip joint locks should significantly limit the amount of hip rotation or lateral movement that can occur. The additional bracing should also increase the child's sense of security and balance.

While these standard, double upright, metal braces are the most commonly used orthoses with the myelodysplasia population, numerous other types have been developed as a result of improvement efforts. The parapodium, introduced by Motlock, is one of the more frequently used orthoses developed for the specific problems associated with myelodysplasia.[85] This brace succeeds in providing such a stable base of support that children with thoracic and lumbar lesions can stand without assistive devices. Although not the ideal situation, the parapodium has been modified to accommodate joint contractures and deformities more safely than conventional long leg braces.

Taylor and Sand[124] report favorable gait training results using a modification of the parapodium called the Verlo brace or vertical loading orthosis. With this orthosis, the angle the base or standing plate makes with the uprights supporting the legs can be adjusted to vary the child's ankle position and projection of the center of gravity. With placement of the ankles in slight dorsiflexion with the center of gravity forward, locomotion is made less laborious than with a fixed baseplace that maintains neutral ankle position. These investigators report that 16 patients from 3 to 10 years of age, with lesions from T8 to L3, were fitted with a Verlo brace.[124] Of those 16, only one 3-year-old child failed to learn either a pivot or swing-to gait pattern. Lack of gait training opportunities, illness, and central nervous system dysfunction accounted for the four children that were unable to progress from a pivot to a swing-to gait pattern. Another adaptation of the parapodium, called a "swivel walker," has been designed to require less energy output during maneuvering.[125,126]

Rose and associates[126,127] report favorable gait training results using a "hip guidance orthosis" with 27 myelodysplasia patients between the ages of 5 years 8 months and 15 years 7 months. The rigid bilateral long leg braces are attached to an essentially rigid thoracic support with a specific type of orthotic hip joint that permits no more than 5 degrees of adduction. As the child shifts weight off one lower extremity by a lateral movement, that free extremity moves forward under the influence of gravity. Of the 27 myelodysplasia patients fitted with this hip guidance orthosis, 13 improved from therapeutic to household, or household to community, ambulation status. In comparison with their previous bracing, the 27 subjects had a mean increase in ambulation speed of 87.3 percent. A reciprocating gait orthosis has been developed in an effort to provide additional assistance to the swing phase of gait.[126]

The parapodium and hip guidance orthoses are primarily designed to assist patients with thoracic and high lumbar lesions. Methods of bracing reported by Lindseth and Glancy[128] and by Nuzzo[129] are of particular use among patients with L3 to L5 function. A polypropylene ankle-foot orthosis based on the principles of the SACH foot prosthesis is described by Lindseth and Glancy.[128] Using the solid ankle of this molded orthosis to facilitate knee extension control, these investigators report significantly improved gait quality for 43 of 74 subjects. Nuzzo[129] describes the use of ankle-foot orthoses connected to a pelvic belt by elastic strapping that is wrapped around the thigh in various helical patterns. By variation in the location of the strap's attachments and their circumferential wrapping patterns, hip extension and abduction can be assisted in combination with knee flexion, knee extension, and hip medial or lateral rotation.

Regardless of the type of orthosis used, tolerance to wearing it for both nonweight-bearing and weight-bearing periods must be gradually developed. The need for families beginning brace-wearing programs to be taught a correct and safe method of putting them on and taking them off should be clear. Methods for safe use of standing tables or simply providing support in standing should also be carefully taught. The child's initial experiences wearing braces and standing should be well planned to emphasize their positive aspects. If the child has developed the ability to roll, sit, and come to a sitting position, the accommodation of these skills to the weight of braces should be facilitated. Through play on the floor, the caregiver can assist and encourage these movements. By development of mobility in braces, the child not only improves upper body strength and control, but also decreases the helpless or trapped perception many of them experience. While standing in the braces, the child can be introduced to activities that necessitate standing. Playing in upper level drawers, looking out windows, and playing with water in a sink are examples of such activities.

In preparation for gait training or the learning of transfer techniques, children with myelodysplasia lesions need to develop trunk control and strength in their arms. Development of these general prerequisites clearly makes the initial learning period less frustrating and more enjoyable for everyone involved. A child's directed reaching efforts can be used in play to challenge their postural adjustment abilities as the center of gravity is altered. These balance activities can be initiated when the child is in a stable sitting position using the surfaces of low tables or the floor for play. Once mastered in sitting, activities can be pursued on the surface of a standing table or at a table that is approximately at the child's waist level. Trunk equilibrium responses in sitting can be further challenged on tilting boards or large therapeutic balls. "Bucking broncho" rides while sitting on an adult's lap can provide a similar challenge to the child's postural control responses.

To have sufficient upper extremity strength and endurance for successful ambulation and transfers, development of the upper extremities must begin at a young age. Learning to maneuver a prone scooter or sitting cart as well as use an adaptive creeping pattern contributes to this developmental process. Pull-up and push-up arm activities can be incorporated into home routines in numerous ways to develop these movement patterns. Using the hands of an adult, a child can be encouraged to pull up from supine lying into sitting. From a sitting position, the child can lift the hips off the floor or bed in a similar manner. The difficulty of sitting pull-ups can be increased by replacing the adult's hands with a vertically held broom handle or knotted rope, encouraging use of one arm only, or by positioning the handle or rope off to one side. Children who are able to do sitting pull-ups usually enjoy swinging from that position while holding onto an adult's hands. The amount of swinging provided by the adult can be gradually decreased as the child learns to control it by upper body movements. Once mastered in a sitting position, these same pull-up and swinging patterns can be encouraged in standing during brace-wearing periods.

As is the case in the developmental sequence of physically normal children, push-up movement patterns in the upper extremities need to develop in prone lying before sitting. An adult can assist prone push-up patterns by supporting a child at the hips and lower trunk while reducing the amount of body weight the child supports with the arms. While the child pushes the body upward, trucks or balls can be rolled through the space under the elevated chest to add an element of play. From a prone position, wheelbarrow or hand walking can be facilitated by an adult supporting the lower extremities and, if necessary, the trunk. Forward, backward, and lateral hand walking can be encouraged, as well as "races" with playmates.

While a child is learning to do sitting push-ups, the body lifting component needs to be assisted. Once the child is able to control a degree of upward movement, the adult can help move the pelvis backward in order to produce a backward scooting movement pattern. This backward scooting movement is generally mastered by children with myelodysplasia before forward and lateral scooting. The learning of all these scooting patterns is facilitated in a bathtub or inflatable wading pool. The slick surface and buoyancy provided by waist-deep water can decrease the energy requirements and increase the element of play involved in developing these skills. Scooting on a smooth floor is more easily learned with braces off and clothing covering the legs. As soon as the movement pattern is learned, however, it should be practiced with braces on. While this requires more strength, and may initially shorten play periods in this position, braces protect the legs from abrasions and fracture-producing forces. The alignment maintained by braces can improve the efficiency of forward scooting once sufficient upper extremity strength is developed.

Concensus is lacking among physical therapists concerning an optimal sequence or protocol for gait training of patients with myelodysplasia. General agreement does seem to exist, however, on some main principles. First, gait training is ideally begun as soon as the child is maturationally ready in terms of prerequisite skills. Second, the sequence of gait training should represent a progressive increase in requisite energy expenditures, as well as in upper extremity and trunk coordination and equilibrium responses. And third, once a child becomes skilled at any method of ambulation, a preference for that method and resistance to other methods naturally develops.

Determining that a child is maturationally ready to begin gait training remains a fairly intuitive matter. Menelaus[85] recommends that a child's attempts to pull up into a standing position be used as a criterion for beginning a standing and gait training program. Others use the age of 1 year as a time to begin standing programs and 18 months for gait training.[96] Many therapists use the presence of head and trunk control while standing in braces, as well as protective equilibrium responses in sitting, as prerequisite skills or criteria for initiation of gait training. Very helpful information is provided by Taylor and Sand's[130] study designed to determine the chronologic age at which normal children could learn to ambulate independently in a Verlo brace with a minimal number of training sessions. These investigators found 24 months to be the age or developmental level at which independent ambulation with a "walkerette" could be achieved within a reasonable period of training. After 22 months, however, they found that more children were strongly resistant to putting on the brace. The youngest children, between 11 and 15 months, were the group that most readily accepted the brace's confinement. For these reasons, they recommend that braces be provided to children for standing purposes when they are 11 to 15 months old, or of that developmental equivalent, in order to avoid the risk of brace rejection.

In general, a progression of difficulty is reflected in the range of gait patterns, which begins with a swivel movement and progresses to a four-point or swing-to pattern. The swing-to pattern is followed by the actual swing-through pattern. In the progression of difficulty, a four-point pattern with locked orthotic knees is followed by the unlocking of one side, then the unlocking of both. This ideally precedes the introduction of short leg braces unless full knee function is present. The swivel gait, used with parapodiums or hip-knee-ankle-foot orthoses, requires primarily weight shifting and trunk rotation ability when used with various assistive devices. While a four-point gait pattern requires that both hip joints move freely, a modified gait that requires only one unlocked hip can be taught as an intermediate step. The modified four-point pattern requires unilateral hip flexion with pelvic-hip stability assisted by the locked orthotic hip joint. Alternating hip flexion, with no anterior-posterior hip stability assistance provided by the braces, is required for the conventional four-point pattern. The swing-to pattern and, to a greater extent, the swing-through pattern, require strength in the upper extremities sufficient to support body plus brace weight, as well as equilibrium and coordination sufficient to produce a swinging movement. While the upper extremity demands of four-point patterns are less, the extent to which they perpetuate hip dislocation by strengthening the deforming hip flexors should be considered before these patterns are taught.

A progression of increasing difficulty, or decreasing support, is also reflected in the range of assistive devices used for gait training. The sequence begins with parallel bars, progresses to a walker with front wheels or other means of assisting forward progression, then to a standard walker, to "quad" canes, and, finally, to forearm crutches.

Obviously, the gait patterns taught and the assistive devices used with myelodysplasia patients should be chosen and changed on the basis of the individual's current ability and projected level of achievement. The transition from one assistive device to a less supportive device should not be concurrent with a transition from one gait pattern to a more demanding one.

A significant determinant of gait training success appears to be the type of reinforcement received by a child for his or her efforts. Frequently, a logical explanation of treatment goals to a child is the initial method of persuasion used by therapists. Once resistance or actual negative behavior patterns develop in response to the prospect of practicing ambulation, these negative responses may become the focus of considerable reinforcing attention. Hester[131] has demonstrated with a profoundly retarded child, and Manella and Varni[132] with a myelodysplasic child, the benefits of the incorporation of behavior modification techniques into gait training. Within a period of 3 weeks, the transition from nonambulatory status and temper tantrums at the prospect of gait training, to independent assumption of standing and walking for 300 feet is reported by Manella and Varni.[132] Before "tantrum" patterns of behavior develop, it is obviously important to provide children with reinforcement that they comprehend as a reward rather than logical adult explanations. Once these disruptive patterns occur, however, behavior modification techniques appear to be a means of reversing them.

A variety of guidelines are used among physical therapists and orthopedists concerning the optimal time to provide a child with a wheelchair. Once a child masters the ability to propel a wheelchair, interest in gait training declines in direct proportion to the laboriousness of that child's ambulation. One guideline that can aid this decision-making process stems from the goal to facilitate as normal a sequence of development as possible. When a child's continued cognitive and psychosocial development is limited by that child's lack of efficient independent community mobility, the learning of functional wheelchair skills becomes more important than maintenance of marginally functional ambulation skills. In addition to providing a means of independent mobility, the advantages of wheelchair use are believed to be (1) provision of a less energy-consuming means of mobility than their ambulation pattern, (2) increased freedom for hand use, (3) ability to move at a speed more closely resembling that of ambulatory people, (4) increased ability to carry or transport objects, and (5) increased potential for recreational activities.[133] The disadvantages are (1) increased risk for development of ischial-sacral pressure sores, (2) increased risk for development of hip and knee flexion contractures, and (3) risk of spinal deformity deterioration.[133]

To accentuate the advantages and diminish the disadvantages of wheelchair use, several specific items should be considered when ordering a wheelchair. Appropriate dimensions of a wheelchair seat are crucial to decreasing the risk of pressure sores and spinal deformity deterioration. The height of the seat should be set in relation to the footrests in order to provide 80 to 90 degrees of flexion at the hips and knees.[134] If the footrests are low, the person tends to slide forward in the seat and create an ischial-sacral friction or shearing force. Increased pressure on the posterior thighs from the front edge of the seat can interfere with lower extremity circulation. If the footrests are high, increased weight is shifted onto the ischial-sacral area and a gravity-assisted abduction-lateral rotation posture of the hips is facilitated. A child who has developed therapeutic ambulation skill, but demonstrates little potential for household ambulation, should have a wheelchair seat essentially level in height with the beds and chairs to which he or she will learn to transfer. This may require placement of footrests fairly high off the floor to maintain their correct relationship with the seat. On the other hand, to maintain household ambulation ability, the seat of the wheelchair should be low enough to facilitate standing transfers. For this purpose, the foot-pedals should be no less than and as close to 2 inches off the floor, while the correct relationship with seat height is maintained. The width of a wheelchair seat should allow only 1 to 2 inches between the person's lateral thighs and the edge of the seat.[134] Since long leg braces occupy considerable chair space, the seat width should be planned to accommodate them if warranted by sufficient wearing time. Both propulsion strength and endurance are compromised, as well as the work of wheelchair mobility increased, by an excessively wide seat. The depth of the wheelchair seat needs to be sufficient to prevent a gap forming at the back that traps sacral tissue causing friction and shearing forces. On the other hand, a seat that is too deep can create pressure in the popliteal area that compromises lower extremity circulation. To facilitate transfers in and out of the wheelchair, specific types of armrests and footrests, as well as variations in wheel diameter, can be provided.

Two aspects need consideration when determining the diameter of wheels for a chair. The smallest diameter wheel, 20 inches, does not rise above the chair seat and obstruct sitting transfers to the extent that larger wheels do. The smaller the wheel diameter, however, the more force the person has to generate to initiate and maintain forward movement.[134] The overall efficiency of propelling is greater with larger rimmed wheels. For this reason, larger wheels are usually thought of as helpful to people with short or weak arms. Handrims with a rubber or plastic coating to increase the ease of grasping and propelling the chair are helpful.

"Growing" chairs, which can increase in size as reupholstering is done, are generally considered cost effective for chronically involved children. These chairs generally expand from a size appropriate for an average 6- to 8-year-old to that of an average 12-year-old.[134] Consideration should be given during the ordering process to the level of maintenance required and to the use the wheelchair will receive. Without an ongoing maintenance program, this wheelchair is unlikely to survive the 4 to 6 years of active use that makes it seem a wise investment. The level of maintenance care any wheelchair receives is a primary factor determining its useful life-span and the extent to which appropriate fit can be retained.

Currently, insufficient information exists about the development of physically normal children, or those with myelodysplasia, to determine an age younger than which wheelchair mobility and transfer skill are unrealistic. The teaching of these skills, however, is frequently not initiated until the person with myelodysplasia becomes too heavy for their caregivers to lift. Clearly, there is a stage prior to this regretable situation when mobility and transfer training can and should be initiated. Once a child has developed the ability to assist with push-up and pull-up movement patterns, he or she should begin assisting with transfers on and off a prone scooter or sitting cart. Once wheelchair propulsion has been learned, the child's assistive role getting into and out of the chair needs to begin and the passive role needs to end.

Corresponding with the tendency to equate myelodysplasia with paraplegia, the shoulder depression push-up transfers used by paraplegics are generally the focus of the myelodysplasia patient's transfer training; however, the normal proportional relationship between lower extremity and trunk length characteristic of paraplegics is often not the case with this group. The normal neurologic function and capacity for strength and endurance gains in the upper body of paraplegics may not be present in the child with myelodysplasia either. The possibility that a young child may not have the central nervous system maturation required to execute these transfers also needs to be considered. For these reasons, the pull-up transfers taught more frequently to quadriplegics, using overhead loops or a trapeze, can be a more realistic starting point for transfer training of children with myelodysplasia. The child can initially practice the necessary wheelchair and body movement patterns, as well as participate in transfers by using an adult's hands as a support from which to pull upward. Ideally, an overhead trapeze can be attached to the child's bed at home so that at least one transfer is fully independent at a young age.

Because of the shortness of children's legs, particularly those with myelodysplasia, front-approach transfers can be much safer than side approach. If knee flexion contractures are not a significant problem, the child can assume a long-sitting position while facing the side of the bed from the wheelchair with the lower portion of both legs on the bed. From this position, the child can use pull-up assistance to move the hips laterally onto the bed or other surface. This transfer pattern, as well as more complex methods used by quadriplegics but modifiable for myelodysplasia patients, are thoroughly described and illustrated in other texts.[135,136]

The endurance required for functional, community-wide wheelchair mobility is often given inadequate attention in treatment. While wheelchair mobility is less energy consuming than ambulation with assistive devices, Glaser and associates[137] have found that, in general, wheelchair locomotion requires a higher maintained heart rate than ambulation by a physically normal individual. Similar studies of the cardiovascular responses of children during wheelchair locomotion have not been published. Given the size and strength of a child's upper body relative to the size and weight of a wheelchair, it seems logical that a similar, if not greater, increase in heart rate occurs. Glaser and associates[137] have identified four primary factors that influence cardiovascular responses during wheelchair propulsion. The characteristics of the wheelchair itself and the velocity at which it is propelled are two of those factors. Stability of the wheels and axle mechanism, as well as the wheel diameter, are examples of characteristics that influence the speed and efficiency with which locomotion can occur. Architectural conditions are a third factor that can increase the resistance to rolling and thereby increase energy expenditure. Increased ventilatory requirements and heart rate responses are reported to occur with propulsion across even low-pile carpet.[137] The fourth factor is the fitness level of the individual for upper extremity work. Hildebrandt and associates[138] have pointed out that average daily wheelchair use may not be of sufficient intensity or duration to have a training effect for the individual. Since average wheelchair use may not prepare a person for functional community mobility, the benefits of conditioning programs have been proposed and supported in work by Glaser et al.[139] Using apparatus that simulates wheelchair propulsion, they have demonstrated that a 5-week training program can improve cardiovascular responses of a normal subject to a heavy work load.[139] The extent to which these results can be duplicated in groups of younger and/or physically disabled subjects remains to be determined.

Similar to the problems that children with myelodysplasia encounter in learning wheelchair locomotion and transfers, their delayed development of self-care skills can be due to several interrelated factors. Obviously, the extent of spinal cord and/or brain damage is a primary factor limiting the rate of, if not overall capacity for, skill development. Parental attitudes are another major factor. Acceptance of their child's physical limitations as permanent is prerequisite to parental readiness for learning and reinforcing any of the self-care techniques. The child's attitude toward independence in dressing, bathing, and toileting is another major factor. The prospect of independence in an activity must provide more prospective, if not immediate, rewards than continued dependence.

Successful development of the ability to maneuver clothing or braces on and off the body requires certain characteristics of the braces, as well as of the person's motor skills. The lightness in weight and freedom of orthotic joint movement that facilitate ambulation and standing transfers also make the taking off and putting on of braces easier. The fewer straps and less bracing the child has to deal with, the easier the application process is. The motor skills required for development of dressing skills are the abilities to position legs, roll from side to side, sit up from a lying position, sit stably with at least one arm free, and shift weight using push-up or pull-up maneuvers.

In preparation for dressing practice, several play activities can be used to facilitate the learning process. The child can be encouraged to place rings made of various articles on the arms and legs. These rings can be made from buckled belts, knotted scarves, or colorful embroidery hoops. The more rigid the loops are, the more easily they can be maneuvered on and off an extremity. The more lax they are, however, the more closely the loops resemble clothing. Large loops of stretchable material can be manipulated from overhead to off the feet or the reverse. Initial dressing practice can be done with large stretchable garments that require the same motor patterns without the constraint of appropriately fitting clothes. This can be turned into a creative game of "dress-up" in mother's or father's clothes. Although the ages at which physically normal children accomplish independent dressing skills cannot serve as guidelines for the myelodysplasia population, the general trends of this normal sequence can. Positioning the body to help with dressing or undressing is the first independent step that occurs. After that, the ability to take off articles of clothing precedes the ability to put on the same article. The ability to open or release fasteners generally precedes the ability to secure or close them.[140]

Development of independent bathing and toileting skills is closely related to transfer skill development. Transfers between a wheelchair and bathtub or toilet represent two of the more challenging transfer situations that a child with myelodysplasia has to manage. The relatively short arms of a child, in relationship to the width of a standard bathtub, are a factor that complicates tub transfers. For this reason, as well as others previously stated, both the methods and the apparatus used by quadriplegics for tub transfers can be utilized by children with myelodysplasia. Bath transfers are made safer and more easily negotiated if a secure stool is placed at the back of the tub. This stool should be essentially level with the tub edge so that the individual can transfer onto it, then lower themselves down into the tub. A second step, providing an intermediate level, can be especially helpful in the process of getting out of the tub. Prerequisite to learning bathtub transfers, the child should be able to move up and down steps from a sitting position. Depending on the ability of the child, this up and down movement can be initially facilitated by assisting the child's push-up or pull-up efforts. For practice of a less-demanding level of this skill, scooting up and down an incline can be incorporated into play.

Transfers onto and off of a toilet do not require a specific technique of movement that is difficult to master. These transfers, however, do require apparatuses that alter the level of the toilet seat, reduce the size of the toilet opening, and provide places from which the child can securely control body movement. With some exceptions, the apparatuses used for these purposes are essentially the same as those used by adult spinal cord-injured patients. If a child is doing a standing transfer to a toilet, an elevated platform may be required to reduce the proportionate height of the toilet. For wheelchair transfers, the seat has to be elevated to the level of the wheelchair. While some commercially available seat attachments can be adjusted to the height of a child's wheelchair, many are too high. The small size of a child, plus the lack of posterior hip and thigh sensation, dictates the need for a smaller seat opening than is present in many of these seat attachments. Since the wall or back of a toilet is generally too far behind a child to provide sitting support, additional back support may be needed. Because of these specific needs, several designs for "homemade" adaptations have been published.[135]

Deficient Development of Fine Motor and Perceptual Motor Skills

Current research documents the presence of delayed or deficient development of fine and perceptual motor skills among children with myelodysplasia and hydrocephalus.[58,62,65-67] The extent to which these delays or deficiencies can be attributed to brain damage as opposed to lack of experience remains to be determined. Although the child's need for assistance from others in gaining fine and perceptual motor experiences at a relatively normal age seems apparent, the actual benefits of the intervention have not been proven. Prevention of or compensation for delays in development of these skills seems logical to expect, but the short- and long-term results of intervention programs for children with myelodysplasia and hydrocephalus are not known.

Early intervention programs for children with myelodysplasia are directed toward facilitation of fine and perceptual motor skills with as normal a rate and sequence as possible. They are also directed toward compensation for the lack of early sitting and mobility skills. While most of the goal-directed, early intervention programs that have been reported can be modified for use by children with myelodysplasia, some have been designed specifically for them. Rosenbaum and coauthors[91] have outlined a progression of play activities designed to facilitate visually directed hand function during the first year of development. Although less specific, Anderson and Spain[88] have described a progression of play that spans the preschool period. In addition to activities for facilitation of visually directed hand function, they provide play suggestions that facilitate body and tactile awareness, form and space perception, manual dexterity, number concepts, and attending or concentration ability. Nakos and Taylor[141] describe the rationale and protocol for an 8-week myelodysplasia infant treatment group. While including activities that teach parents about the facilitation of sensorimotor development, they have developed a program that also facilitates supportive interaction among the parents.

Numerous devices have been developed to assist young children to maintain a sitting position or attain mobility. Bean bag chairs can be used to support small infants in upright or to provide a sense of security to children learning to sit alone. When a child reaches the age of 6 to 8 months without the ability to maintain a sitting posture with their hands free, Menelaus[85] recommends the use of a sitting orthosis. By molding polypropylene to fit the trunk and buttocks area, a means of support is provided that frees the hands for play and can be used on the floor, in a high chair, or any place the child desires to be.

The use of prone scooters and long sitting push carts to facilitate early mobility has been described. Regardless of the type of apparatus used to aid sitting or mobility, the child has to gradually accept it and feel securely supported by it. If this is not the case, the child will not engage in the developmental play that the equipment was originally designed to facilitate.

Based on a review of the results reported from preschool programs available for children with myelodysplasia in Great Britain, Anderson and Spain[88] summarized the advantages and disadvantages of these programs. They concluded that social and emotional development was improved in terms of interaction skills and desire for independence. Motor skills improved, at least in terms of increased motivation to engage with other children in play activities requiring mobility. These factors enabled the children attending preschool programs to make a smoother transition into school settings. Anderson and Spain also concluded that these programs gave the childrens' mothers a source of support, as well as relief from responsibility for predictable time periods. The mothers also gained a more realistic perception and acceptance of their childrens' strengths and weaknesses. The disadvantages that Anderson and Spain found were the cost and difficulty of transporting the child to and from the program site. The handling of feeding and clothing articles, as well as braces or other equipment, in addition to the child, was a problem particularly for the mothers of 4- and 5-year-olds.

Although the perceptual motor problems of children with myelodysplasia and hydrocephalus have been documented by numerous studies, little information has been published about treatment and remediation methods, or their results, with this group. Gluckman and Barling[142] have reported results from use of the Frostig Program for the Development of Visual Perception during a 6-week period for 12 children with hydrocephalus and myelodysplasia. Using the Frostig Developmental Test of Visual Perception as a pre- and post-test, they found that the treatment group made gains in contrast to 12 children in an attention placebo group and 12 in a control group; however, these investigators report insufficient data for the reader to determine the significance of the nine-point average increase in all scores among the treatment group. The treatment program used in this study, as well as other less formally evaluated programs, demonstrates a problem that is yet to be resolved. The test items used to measure perceptual motor skills are very similar to the treatment or remediation activities used in many programs. When this is the case, there is considerable risk of teaching the child how to take the test more adeptly, rather than developing new skills that are transferable to functional skills, such as reading and writing.

Several researchers[61,62,71] have used portions of Ayres' Southern California Sensory Integration Test to measure perceptual motor problems among children with hydrocephalus and myelodysplasia. Minimal information, however, has been published regarding the results or methods of implementing the techniques specific to Ayres' approach to sensory integrative treatment with these children. The role that vestibular stimulation techniques might play in the treatment of hydrocephalic children with either a low tolerance for movement in space or a low threshold to the stimulus of that movement is unknown.

TREATMENT WITHIN THE PUBLIC SCHOOL SYSTEM

Approximately 15 years after the enactment of Public Law 94-142, the impact of "mainstreaming" physically disabled children into regular classroom settings is generally considered to be positive for both the students with as well as without disabilities.[143] Physically limited adolescents that have had a mainstream education experience generally achieve higher scores on tests of academic and social skills than their counterparts in special education settings.[143,144] Successful social integration of disabled children into a regular classroom clearly requires the active effort and resourcefulness of a teacher.[145] Several reports substantiate that a child's sense of social isolation can actually be increased by regular classroom experiences in which their integration into activity is not well facilitated.[146-148] Successful integration frequently requires the expertise of both special educators and occupational therapists in order to provide a program sufficient to facilitate academic as well as specific fine motor and perceptual motor development. Although a less prevalent problem, delayed development of communication skills may require the services of a speech pathologist. Because of pressure sores, urinary tract infections, fractures, and other assorted medical complications, the school absentee rate of children with myelodysplasia is high. To prevent significant disruption of the child's learning program, home- or hospital-bound teachers need to be available within the school system.

To prevent additional absenteeism, appropriate transportation to and from school needs to be arranged. Vehicles designed to accommodate wheelchairs, as well as the limitations of people ambulating with assistive devices, are needed. Whether the child uses a wheelchair or assistive devices for mobility, architectural barriers should not hinder their movement in and out of the school, between classrooms, and in and out of a bathroom. Children with myelodysplasia require bathrooms with sufficient space in which to maneuver a wheelchair, as well as stable support bars to assist with transfers. They need to have a consistently present, knowledgeable person to assist, as needed, with bowel and bladder management. In addition to assistance, they need privacy and sufficient time to attend to these self-care needs.

The extent to which a therapist can provide specific treatment of individual children varies in accordance with each school system's perception of the role of physical therapy in education. The ease with which many children fit into the school setting can be increased by individualized physical therapy directed toward increasing their transfer or locomotion skills. Improving the speed or dexterity with which toilet transfers are accomplished can simplify the child's assistive needs. The speed or quality of toileting, dressing, and self-feeding skills can be increased by individualized occupational therapy. Teaching children and their teachers how to perform transfers on and off the floor can increase a young child's ability to participate in some classroom activities. Increasing the endurance of a child in ambulation or wheelchair locomotion can alter the ability to participate in activities with physically normal children. Whether working with individual children or supervising groups of them, prevention of the side effects of prolonged wheelchair sitting can be a major concern for physical therapists to address. Pressure sores and flexion contractures need not be the price that has to be paid for mainstream educational opportunities. If daily activity periods could be planned when these children would study or play in prone lying or standing positions, many of these secondary problems could be prevented.

School placement decisions for children with myelodysplasia are usually a compromise between efforts to normalize their environments and efforts to provide special services. Ideally, these special services would be available to each child regardless of the location of their school. In reality, the funding available for the services of special education teachers, hygiene assistants, transportation assistants, physical and occupational therapists, and other related personnel has been limited. Shortages of many specialists are evident in most health and rehabilitation service centers. It seems apparent that the child whose self-care and mobility skills most closely approximate those of physically normal children has the greatest opportunity for normal social development and for educational placement based on cognitive ability and school proximity. As long as this is the case, the focus of habilitation is shifted to the preschool period, and the scope of that habilitation is widened from therapeutic ambulation to a broader perspective of functional goals.

REFERENCES

1. Freeman JM (ed): Practical Management of Meningomyelocele. University Park Press, Baltimore, 1974
2. Sharrard WJW: Congenital and developmental abnormalities of the neuraxis. p. 1076. In Sharrard WJW (ed): Paediatric Orthopaedics and Fractures. Vol. 2. 2nd Ed. Blackwell Scientific Publications, Oxford, 1979
3. Brockhelhurst G (ed): Spina Bifida for the Clinician. Clinics in Developmental Medicine, No. 57. JB Lippincott, Philadelphia, 1976
4. Stark GD, Baker GCW: The neurological involvement of the lower limbs in myelomeningocele. Dev Med Child Neurol 9:732, 1967
5. Stark GD: Spina Bifida: Problems and Management. Blackwell Scientific Publications, London, 1977
6. Laws ER: Neurosurgical management of meningomyelocele. p. 31. In Freeman JM (ed): Practical Management of Meningomyelocele. University Park Press, Baltimore, 1974
7. Stein SC, Schut L: Hydrocephalus in meningomyelocele. Child Brain 5:413, 1979
8. Gardner WJ: Etiology and pathogenesis of the development of meningomyelocele, p. 3. In McLaurin RL (ed): Myelomeningocele. Grune & Stratton. Orlando, FL, 1977
9. Padget DH: Neuroschisis and human embryonic maldevelopment: new evidence on anencephaly, spina bifida and diverse mammalian defects. J Neuropathol Exp Neurol 29:192, 1970

10. Williams B: Further thoughts on the valvular action of the Arnold-Chiari malformation. Dev Med Child Neurol, suppl. 25:105, 1971
11. Gardner WJ: Hydrodynamic mechanisms of syringomyelia: its relationship to myelocele. J Neurol Neurosurg Psychiatry 28:247, 1965
12. Leck I: Epidemiological clues to the causation of neural tube defects. p. 122. In Dobbing J (ed): Prevention of Spina Bifida and Other Neural Tube Defects. Academic Press, London, 1983
13. Shurtleff DB, Lemire R, Warkany J: Embryology, etiology and epidemiology. p. 39. In Shurtleff DB (ed): Myelodysplasia and Exstrophies: Significance, Prevention and Treatment. Grune & Stratton, Orlando, FL, 1986
14. Kaufman MN: Occlusion of the neural lumen in early mouse embryos analysed by light and electron microscopy. J Embryol Exp Morph 78:211, 1983
15. Janzer RC: Neural tube defects: experimental findings and concepts of pathogenesis. p. 21. In Voth D, Glees P (eds): Spina Bifida—Neural Tube Defects. Walter de Gruyter, New York, 1986
16. Jennings MT, Clarren SK, Kokich VG et al: Neuroanatomic examination of spina bifida aperta and the Arnold-Chiari malformation in a 130-day human fetus. J Neurol Sci 54:325, 1982
17. Carter CO, Evans K: Spina bifida and anencephalus in greater London. J Med Genet 10:209, 1973
18. Renwick JH: Hypothesis: anencephaly and spina bifida are usually preventable by avoidance of specific but unidentified substance present in certain potato tubers. Br J Prev Soc Med 26:67, 1972
19. Knox EG: Anencephalus and dietary intakes. Br J Prev Soc Med 26:219, 1972
20. Fedrick J: Anencephalus and tea drinking. Proc R Soc Med 67:356, 1974
21. Laurence KM, Campbell H, James NE: The role of improvement in the maternal diet and preconceptional folic acid supplementation in the prevention of neural tube defects. p. 85. In Dobbing J (ed): Prevention of Spina Bifida and Other Neural Tube Defects. Academic Press, London, 1983
22. Carter CO, David PA, Laurence KM: A family study of major central nervous system malformations in South Wales, J Med Genet 5:81, 1968
23. Naggan L: Anencephaly and spina bifida in Israel. Pediatrics 47:577, 1971
24. Naggan L, McMahon B: Ethnic differences in the prevalence of anencephaly and spina bifida in Boston, Mass. N Engl J Med 277:1119, 1967
25. Alter M: Anencephalus, hydrocephalus and spina bifida. Epidemiology, with special reference to a survey in Charleston, SC. Arch Neurol 7:411, 1962
26. Smithells RW, D'Arcy EE, McAllister EF: The outcome of pregnancies before and after the birth of infants with nervous system malformations. Dev Med Child Neurol, suppl. 15:6, 1968
27. Laurence KM: The recurrence risk in spina bifida cystica and anencephaly. Dev Med Child Neurol, suppl. 20:23, 1968
28. Elwood JM, Elwood JH: Epidemiology of Anencephalus and Spina Bifida. Oxford University Press, New York, 1980
29. Congenital Malformation Surveillance Report, January–December, 1979. Centers for Disease Control, Atlanta, GA, 1980
30. Windham GC, Edmonds LD: Current trends in the incidence of neural tube defects. Pediatrics 70:333, 1982
31. Brock DJH, Sutcliffe RG: Alpha-fetoprotein in the antenatal diagnosis of anencephaly and spina bifida. Lancet 2:197, 1972
32. Brock DJH, Bolton AE, Monaghan JM: Prenatal diagnosis of anencephaly through maternal serum alpha-fetoprotein measurements. Lancet 2:923, 1973

33. Bennett MJ, Blau K, Johnson RD et al: Some problems of alpha-fetoprotein screening. Lancet 2:1296, 1978
34. Marci JN, Haddow JE, Weiss RR: Screening for neural tube defects in the United States. Am J Obstet Gynecol 133:119, 1979
35. Haddow JE, Marci JN: Prenatal screening for neural tube defects. JAMA 242(6):515, 1979
36. Crandall BF, Hanson FW, Tennant F, Perdue ST: Alpha-fetoprotein levels in amniotic fluid between 11 and 15 weeks. Am J Obstet Gynecol 160:1204, 1989
37. Milunsky A, Jick SS, Bruell CL et al: Predictive values, relative risks, and overall benefits of high and low maternal serum alpha-fetoprotein screening in singleton pregnancies: new epidemiological data. Am J Obstet Gynecol 161:291, 1989
38. Cowan LS, Phelps-Sandall B, Hanson FW et al: A prenatal diagnostic center's first year experience with the California alpha-fetoprotein screening program. Am J Obstet Gynecol 160:1496, 1989
39. Michejda M, Queenan JT, McCullough D: Present status of intrauterine treatment of hydrocephalus and its future. Am J Obstet Gynecol 155:837, 1986
40. McLone DG: Technique for closure of myelomeningocele. Child Brain 6:65, 1980
41. Hall P, Lindseth R, Campbell R et al: Scoliosis and hydrocephalus in myelocele patients. J Neurosurg 50:174, 1979
42. Shurtleff D, Stuntz JT, Hayden P: Hydrocephalus. p. 139. In Shurtleff DB (ed): Myelodysplasia and Exstrophies: Significance, Prevention and Treatment. Grune & Stratton, Orlando, FL, 1986
43. Bergman EW, Freeman JM, Epstein MH: Treatment of infantile hydrocephalus with acetazolamide and furosemide: three to four years follow-up. Ann Neurol 8:227, 1980
44. Smith HP, Russell JM, Boyce WH et al: Results of urinary diversion in patients with myelomeningocele. J Neurosurg 50:773, 1979
45. Enrile BG, Crooks KK: Clean intermittent catheterization for home management in children with myelomeningocele. Clin Pediatr 19:743, 1980
46. Hanningan KF: Teaching intermittent self-catheterization to young children with myelodysplasis. Dev Med Child Neurol 21:365, 1979
47. Action Committee on Myelodysplasia, Section on Urology: Current approaches to evaluation and management of children with myelomeningocele. Pediatrics 63:663, 1979
48. Okamoto GA, Sousa J, Telzrow RW et al: Toileting skills in children with meningomyelocele: rates of learning. Arch Phys Med Rehabil 65:182, 1984
49. Shurtleff D, Mayo M: Toilet training: the Seattle experience and conclusions. p. 267. In Shurtleff DB (ed): Myelodysplasia and Exstrophies: Significance, Prevention and Treatment. Grune & Stratton, Orlando, FL, 1986
50. Drummond DS, Moreau M, Cruess RL: The results and complications of surgery for the paralytic hip and spine in myelomeningocele. J Bone Joint Surg 62B:49, 1980
51. Feiwell E: Surgery of the hip in myelomeningocele as related to adult goals. Clin Orthop 148:87, 1980
52. Menelaus MB: Progress in the management of the paralytic hip in myelomeningocele. Orthop Clin North Am 11:17, 1980
53. Lock TR, Aronson DD: Fractures in patients who have myelomeningocele. J Bone Joint Surg 71A8:1153, 1989
54. Findley TW, Agre JC, Habeck RV et al: Ambulation in adolescents with myelomeningocele: I. early childhood predictors. Arch Phys Med Rehabil 68:518, 1987

55. Allen BL, Ferguson RL: The operative treatment of myelomeningocele spinal deformity—1979. Orthop Clin North Am 10:845, 1979
56. Hall JE: Dwyer Instrumentation in anterior fusion of the spine. J Bone Joint Surg 63A:1188, 1981
57. Ward WT, Wenger DR, Roach SW: Surgical correction of myelomeningocele scoliosis: a critical appraisal of various spinal instrumentation systems. J Pediatr Orthop 9(3):262, 1989
58. Wallace SJ: The effect of upper-limb function on mobility of children with myelomeningocele. Dev Med Child Neurol, suppl. 15 29:84, 1973
59. Anderson EM, Plewis I: Impairment of a motor skill in children with spina bifida cystica and hydrocephalus. Br J Psychol 68:61, 1977
60. Sand PL, Taylor N, Hill M et al: Hand function in children with myelomeningocele. Am J Occup Ther 28:87, 1974
61. Grimm RA: Hand function and tactile perception in a sample of children with myelomeningocele. Am J Occup Ther 30:234, 1976
62. Brunt D: Characteristics of upper limb movements in a sample of meningomyelocele children. Percept Mot Skills 51:431, 1980
63. Emery JL, Lendon RG: Clinical implications of cord lesions in neurospinal dysraphism. Dev Med Child Neurol, suppl. 14 27:45, 1972
64. Variend S, Emery JL: The pathology of the central lobes of the cerebellum in children with myelomeningocele. Dev Med Child Neurol, suppl. 32:99, 1974
65. Jacobs RA, Wolfe G, Rasmuson M: Upper extremity dysfunction in children with myelomeningocele. Z Kinderchir, suppl. II 43:19, 1988
66. Mazur JM, Menelaus MB, Hudson I, Stillwell A: Hand function in patients with spina bifida cystica. J Pediatr Orthop 6:442, 1986
67. Pearson AM, Carr J, Hallwell MD: The handwriting of children with spina bifida. Z Kinderchir, suppl. II 43:40, 1988
68. Badell-Ribera A, Shulman K, Paddock N: The relationship of non-progressive hydrocephalus to intellectual functioning in children with spina bifida cystica. Pediatrics 37:787, 1966
69. Tew B, Laurence KM: The effects of hydrocephalus on intelligence, visual perception and school attainment. Dev Med Child Neurol, suppl. 17 35:129, 1975
70. Miller E, Sethi L: The effect of hydrocephalus on perception. Dev Med Child Neurol, suppl. 13 25:77, 1971
71. Gressang JD: Perceptual process of children with myelomeningocele and hydrocephalus. Am J Occup Ther 28:266, 1974
72. Mazur JM, Aylward GP, Colliver J et al: Impaired mental capabilities and hand function in myelomeningocele patients. Z Kinderchir, suppl. II 43:24, 1988
73. Lennerstrand G, Gallo JE: Neuro-ophthalmological evaluation of patients with myelomeningocele and Chiari malformations. Dev Med Child Neurol 32:415, 1990
74. Lennerstrand G, Gallo JE, Samuelsson L: Neuro-ophthalmological findings in relation to CNS lesions in patients with myelomeningocele. Dev Med Child Neurol 32:423, 1990
75. Tew B: The Cocktail Party Syndrome in children with hydrocephalus and spina bifida. Br J Disord Commun 14:89, 1979
76. Tew B, Laurence KM: The ability and attainments of spina bifida patients born in South Wales between 1956 and 1962. Dev Med Child Neurol, suppl. 14 27:124, 1972
77. Spain B: Verbal and performance ability in pre-school children with spina bifida. Dev Med Child Neurol 16:773, 1974

78. Quinton D, Rutter M: Early hospital admissions and later disturbances of behavior. Dev Med Child Neurol 18:447, 1976
79. Douglas J: Early hospital admissions and later disturbances of behavior and learning. Dev Med Child Neurol 17:426, 1975
80. Hayden PW, Davenport SLH, Campbell MM: Adolescents with myelodysplasia: impact of physical disability on emotional maturation. Pediatrics 64:53, 1979
81. Sousa JC, Gordon LH, Shurtleff DB: Assessing the development of daily living skills in patients with spina bifida. Dev Med Child Neurol, suppl. 18 37:134, 1976
82. Tzimas NA: Myelodysplasia: combined orthopedic and physiatric management, part II. In American Academy for Cerebral Palsy, 28th annual meeting: Syllabus of Instructional Courses, 1974
83. Lusskin R: The influence of errors in bracing upon deformity of the lower extremity. Arch Phys Med Rehabil 47:520, 1966
84. Dias LS: Ankle valgus in children with myelomeningocele. Dev Med Child Neurol 20:627, 1978
85. Menelaus MB: The Orthopaedic Management of Spina Bifida Cystica. 2nd Ed. Churchill Livingstone, Edinburgh, 1980
86. Frankenburg WK, Dobbs JB, Fandal A: The Revised Denver Developmental Screening Test Manual. University of Colorado Press, Denver, 1970
87. Touwen BCL: Examination of the Child With Minor Neurological Dysfunction. 2nd Ed. Clinics in Developmental Medicine, No. 71, JB Lippincott, Philadelphia, 1979
88. Anderson EM, Spain B: The Child With Spina Bifida. Methuen, London, 1977
89. Cornish SV: Development of a test of motor-planning ability. Phys Ther 60:1129, 1980
90. Kendrick KA, Hanten WP: Differentiation of learning disabled children from normal children using four coordination tasks. Phys Ther 60:784, 1980
91. Rosenbaum P, Barnitt R, Brand HL: A developmental intervention programme designed to overcome the effects of impaired movement in spina bifida infants. p. 145. In Holt K (ed): Movement and Child Development. Clinics in Developmental Medicine, No. 55. JB Lippincott, Philadelphia, 1975
92. Bayley N: Manual for the Bayley Scales of Infant Development. The Psychological Corporation, New York, 1969
93. Stillman RD: The Callier-Azusa Scale. Regional Center for Services to Deaf-Blind Children, Dallas, 1973
94. Bruininks RH: Examiners Manual for Bruininks-Oseretsky Test of Motor Proficiency. American Guidance Service, Circle Pines, MN, 1978
95. Vlach V: Some exteroceptive skin reflexes in the limbs and trunk in newborns. p. 41. In MacKeith R, Bax M (eds): Studies in Infancy. Clinics in Developmental Medicine, No. 27. Spastics International Medical Publications, Lavenham, England, 1966
96. Kopits SE: Orthopedic aspects of meningomyeloceles. p. 106. In Freeman JM (ed): Practical Management of Meningomyelocele. University Park Press, Baltimore, 1974
97. Noetzel MJ: Myelomeningocele: current concepts of management. Clin Perinatol 16:311, 1989
98. Townsend PF, Cowell HR, Steg NL: Lower extremity fractures simulating infection in myelomeningocele. Clin Orthop 144:255, 1979
99. Short DL, Schkade JK, Herring JA: Parent involvement in physical therapy: a controversial issue. J Pediatr Orthop 9:444, 1989

100. Hensinger RN: Orthopedic problems of the shoulder and neck. Pediatr Clin North Am 24:889, 1977
101. Drennan JC: Orthotic management of the myelomeningocele spine. Dev Med Child Neurol, suppl. 18 37:97, 1976
102. McKibbon B: The use of splintage in the management of paralytic dislocation of the hip in spina bifida cystica. J Bone Joint Surg 55B:163, 1973
103. Jaeger DL: Splint for infant with myelomeningocele. Phys Ther 61:913, 1981
104. Redford JB: Principles of orthotic devices. p. 1. In Redford JB (ed): Orthotics Etcetera. 3rd Ed. Williams & Wilkins, Baltimore, 1986
105. Fischer BH: Topical hyperbaric oxygen treatment of pressure sores and skin ulcers. Lancet 2:405, 1969
106. Shurtleff D: Decubitus formation and skin breakdown. p. 150. In Shurtleff DB (ed): Myelodysplasia and Exstrophies: Significance, Prevention, and Treatment. Grune & Stratton, Orlando, FL, 1986
107. Dibbell DG, McGraw JB, Edstrom LE: Providing useful and protective sensibility to the sitting area in patients with myelomeningocele. Plast Reconstr Surg 64:796, 1979
108. Krupp S, Kuhn W, Zaed GA: The use of innervated flaps for the closure of ischial pressure sores. Paraplegia 21:119, 1983
109. McFadyen GM, Stoner DL: Polyurethane foam wheelchair cushions: retention of supportive properties. Arch Phys Med Rehabil 61:234, 1970
110. Stewart SFC, Eng M, Palmieri V et al: Wheelchair cushion effect on skin temperature, heat flux and relative humidity. Arch Phys Med Rehabil 61:229, 1980
111. Carpendale MFT, Redford JB: Beds for patients. p. 518. In Redford JB (ed): Orthotics Etcetera. 3rd Ed. Williams & Wilkins, Baltimore, 1986
112. De Souza LJ, Carroll N: Ambulation of the braced myelomeningocele patient. J Bone Joint Surg 58A:1112, 1976
113. Oppenheimer S: Comparative statistics—treatment vs non-treatment. p. 41. In McLaurin RL (ed): Myelomeningocele. Grune & Stratton, Orlando, FL, 1977
114. Hoffer MM, Feiwell E, Perry R et al: Functional ambulation in patients with myelomeningocele. J Bone Joint Surg 55A:137, 1973
115. Findley TW, Agre JC, Habeck RV et al: Ambulation in adolescents with spina bifida. II: Oxygen cost of mobility. Arch Phys Med Rehabil 69:855, 1988
116. Agre JC, Findley TW, McNally MC et al: Physical activity capacity in children with myelomeningocele. Arch Phys Med Rehabil 68:372, 1987
117. Streissguth AP, Streissguth DM: Planning for the psychological needs of a young child in a double spica cast. Clin Pediatr 17:277, 1978
118. Molnar GE: Orthotic management of children. p. 352. In Redford JB (ed): Orthotics Etcetera. 3rd Ed. Williams & Wilkins, Baltimore, 1986
119. Main BJ: Effects of immobilization on the skeleton. p. 426. In Owen R, Goodfellow J, Bullough P (eds): Scientific Foundations of Orthopaedics and Traumatology. William Heinemann Medical Books Ltd., London, 1980
120. Lehmann JF: Lower limb orthotics. p. 278. In Redford JB (ed): Orthotics Etcetera. 3rd Ed. Williams & Wilkins, Baltimore, 1986
121. Fulford GE, Cairns TP: The problems associated with flail feet in children and their treatment with orthoses. J Bone Joint Surg 60B:93, 1978
122. Rose GK: Principles of splints and orthotics. p. 443. In Owen R, Goodfellow J, Bullough P (eds): Scientific Foundations of Orthopaedics and Traumatology. William Heinemann Medical Books Ltd., London, 1980

123. Smith EM, Juvinall RC: Mechanics of orthotics. p. 21. In Redford JB (ed): Orthotics Etcetera. 3rd Ed. Williams & Wilkins, Baltimore, 1986

124. Taylor N, Sand P: Verlo brace use in children with myelomeningocele and spinal cord injury. Arch Phys Med Rehabil 55:231, 1974

125. Rose GK, Henshaw JT: Swivel walkers for paraplegics: consideration and problems in their design and application. Bull Prosthet Res 10–20:62, 1973

126. Rose GK: Orthotics: Principles and Practice. William Heineman Medical Books, London, 1986

127. Rose GK, Stallard J, Sankarankutty M: Clinical evaluation of spina bifida patients using hip guidance orthosis. Dev Med Child Neurol 23:30, 1981

128. Lindseth RE, Glancy J: Polypropylene lower-extremity braces for paraplegia due to myelomeningocele. J Bone Joint Surg 56A:556, 1974

129. Nuzzo RM: Dynamic bracing: elastics for patients with cerebral palsy, muscular dystrophy and myelodysplasia. Clin Orthop 148:263, 1980

130. Taylor N, Sand PL: Verlo orthosis: experience with different developmental levels in normal children. Arch Phys Med Rehabil 56:120, 1975

131. Hester SB: Effects of behavioral modification on the standing and walking deficiencies of a profoundly retarded child: a case report. Phys Ther 61:907, 1981

132. Manella KJ, Varni JW: Behavior therapy in a gait-training program for a child with myelomeningocele. Phys Ther 61:1284, 1981

133. Kamenetz HL: Wheelchairs and other indoor vehicles for the disabled. p. 464. In Redford JB (ed): Orthotics Etcetera. 3rd Ed. Williams & Wilkins, Baltimore, 1986

134. Spiegler JH, Goldberg MJ: The wheelchair as a permanent mode of mobility: a detailed guide to prescription. Am J Phys Med 47:315, 1968

135. Ford JR, Duckworth B: Physical Management for the Quadriplegic Patient. FA Davis, Philadelphia, 1974

136. Palmer ML, Toms JE: Manual for Functional Training. FA Davis, Philadelphia, 1980

137. Glaser RM, Sawka MN, Wilde SW et al: Energy cost and cardiopulmonary responses for wheelchair locomotion and walking on tile and on carpet. Paraplegia 19:220, 1981

138. Hildebrandt G, Voigt ED, Bahn D et al: Energy costs of propelling wheelchair at various speeds: cardiac response and effect on steering accuracy. Arch Phys Med Rehabil 51:131, 1970

139. Glaser RM, Sawka MN, Durbin RJ et al: Exercise program for wheelchair activity. Am J Phys Med 60:67, 1981

140. Cohen MA, Gross PJ: The development of self-help skills. In Cohen MA, Gross PJ (eds): The Developmental Resource. Vol. 1. Grune & Stratton, Orlando, FL, 1979

141. Nakos E, Taylor S: Myelomeningocele infant mat program. p. 107. In McLaurin RL (ed): Myelomeningocele. Grune & Stratton, Orlando, FL, 1977

142. Gluckman S, Barling J: Effects of a remedial program on visual-motor perception in spina bifida children. J Genet Psychol 136:195, 1980

143. Walker DK, Palfrey JS, Handley-Derry M, Singer JD: Mainstreaming children with handicaps: implications for pediatricians. Dev Behav Pediatr 10(3):151, 1989

144. Tew BJ: Spina bifida children in ordinary schools: handicap, attainment and behavior. Z Kinderchir Suppl. II 43:46, 1988

145. Cooke T, Apolloni T, Cooke S: Normal preschool children as behavioral models for retarded peers. Except Child 43:531, 1977

146. Gresham F: Social skills training with handicapped children: a review. Rev Educ Res 51:139, 1981
147. Lord J, Varzos N, Behrman B et al: Implications of mainstream classrooms for adolescents with spina bifida. Dev Med Child Neurol 32:20, 1990
148. Borjeson MC, Lagergren J: Life conditions of adolescents with myelomeningocele. Dev Med Child Neurol 32:698, 1990

8 | Head Trauma

Jocelyn Blaskey

Of the more than 1 million children who suffer a head trauma each year, an estimated 230,000 require hospitalization. Statistics describing mortality from severe head injury vary from 6 to 59 percent.[1-12] The cause of death is seldom the primary brain damage, but rather intracranial or extracranial secondary complications of the brain damage or concomitant injuries.[13-15] Incidence is highest between the ages of 15 and 19 years, with an average male to female ratio of 2:1.[7]

The majority (70 to 98 percent) of severe head injuries result from motor vehicle accidents. These types of accidents, more prevalent in older children, often result in severe cranial injuries with focal deficits and long-lasting neurologic problems. Blunt trauma due to falls from trees, swings, or jungle gyms to grass or concrete, typical of mid-childhood, often result in skull fractures and more generalized cerebral injury. Falls and nonaccidental trauma are most frequent in children less than 1 year of age.[2-19]

PATHOLOGY

Injuries resulting from head trauma include scalp and cranium injuries, contusions, concussions, extraparenchymal or intracranial hematomas, cranial nerve injuries, and herniations caused by edema.[20-27] Head injuries can be classified according to how they are inflicted, including acceleration/deceleration injuries, crush injuries, and penetration injuries. Acceleration/deceleration injuries, the most common head injuries, result when the head hits an immobile object or a mobile object hits an immobile head.

Classification of cerebral injury into diffuse, focal, or mixed injuries considers the focal injuries (usually frontal and temporal) evident on computed tomography (CT) scan, and the diffuse axonal injury (DAI) due to shearing

213

forces apparent microscopically.[8,28–30] Gennarelli and colleagues[30] have found in monkeys that "the duration of coma, degree of post-traumatic disability and extent of DAI increased from sagittally to obliquely to laterally accelerated heads." The clinical patterns identified are consistent with those seen in human head injury. Their work supports the hypothesis that the mechanism of concussion is a "combination of stretch, shearing injury to the white matter, plus transient neuronal dysfunction"[8] resulting in dysfunction of the reticular formation rather than direct insult to the brain stem. In children and adolescents, cerebral edema may evolve after a trivial head injury and may not be associated with a hematoma, hemorrhage, or contusions as is commonly seen in adults. Cerebral blood flow studies and CT densities suggest that the brain contains more blood than usual.[17,25,26] Secondary brain damage, usually hypoxia or ischemia, can be caused by intracranial factors such as mass lesions or cerebral edema or extracranial factors such as hypoxemia or hypotension. Further discussion of mechanisms responsible for loss of consciousness and recovery are offered by Miller,[22] Shetter and Demakas,[23] Bruce and colleagues,[3,8,26] Dimitrijevic,[29] Ommaya and Gennarelli,[21,28] and Gennarelli and colleagues.[30]

MEDICAL MANAGEMENT

Acute medical management primarily prevents and treats the secondary complications of head injury to provide optimal conditions for neurologic recovery. Orthopedic intervention includes acute fracture stabilization and management of spasticity throughout the rehabilitation process.

Neurologic Evaluation

The neurologic evaluation assesses the disruption and evolution of consciousness after trauma to diagnose and thereafter manage primary and secondary traumatic brain lesions. Raphaely and colleagues,[1] Humphreys,[11] and Greenberg and colleagues[31] have discussed the significance of neurologic findings.

Documentation of level of consciousness permits ongoing assessment of progressive changes in consciousness. The Glasgow Coma Scale (GCS), devised by Teasdale and Jennett,[32] has been used internationally as an assessment of the depth and duration of impaired consciousness and coma during the acute stage. The GCS was conceived as a graded measurement of three aspects of behavior: motor responsiveness, verbal performance, and eye opening. The best response for each behavior is recorded. The sum of the grades for each response is an indication of the depth of coma ranging from 3 (deepest) to 15.[32]

Brink and associates[2,19] and Cartlidge and Shaw[4] adapted Ommaya's original classifications of five levels of consciousness[21] to evaluate depth and duration of coma and return to consciousness. At level V, no response to stimuli can be elicited. A generalized response to sensory stimuli indicates level IV.

At level III, a consistent localized response to a stimulus is evident. By level II, the child has become responsive to the environment. Level I is attained when the child is oriented to time and place, and is recording ongoing events. Brink and colleagues[2,19] designed three tables to further define behaviors appropriate to each age group in determining level of consciousness. The age groups are as follows: infants, 6 months to 2 years of age; preschool children, aged 2 to 5 years; and school-aged children, 5 years and older.

Further diagnostic tests include radiographic images of the skull and neck to identify fractures, multimodality-evoked potential studies to evaluate severity of involvement,[31,33,34] and CT scan and magnetic resonance imaging to identify focal lesions. Electroencephalogram may be used in severe cases to monitor brainwave activity.

Acute Medical Management

The goal of initial medical management is maintenance of vital functions. Because the child's reaction to cerebral damage is labile, clinical signs can change rapidly. Serial monitoring of respiratory rate, blood pressure, pulse rate and rhythm, temperature, and level of consciousness will indicate the child's change in status. Intubation and artificial ventilation control obstruction and prevent repeated episodes of hypoxia and cyanosis. Close monitoring of intracranial pressure permits appropriate management, including hyperventilation, hypertonic mannitol or dexamethasone, barbiturate therapy, or hypothermia. In prolonged coma, nasoesophageal tube feeding provides fluid and nutrient requirements. The majority of patients who have had post-traumatic seizures are treated with anticonvulsants, including phenytoin, carbamezapine, and phenobarbital.

Hypertension with systolic pressures between 160 and 180 mmHg and diastolic pressures between 100 and 140 mmHg are not uncommon. Systolic blood pressure greater than 130 mmHg and diastolic pressure greater than 100 mmHg, persisting for more than 6 weeks after injury, decreases the chance of significant neurologic recovery.[19] Return of blood pressure to normal levels coincides with neurologic improvement.[24]

Orthopedic Management

Orthopedic problems associated with traumatic head injury include spinal cord injury; brachial plexus injury; fractures and dislocations resulting from concomitant trauma to limbs and spine; and spasticity, contractures, pressure sores, ectopic ossification, scoliosis, and limb length discrepancies associated with the brain damage. Injuries are difficult to diagnose in the unconscious child.

Heterotopic ossification of soft tissues occurs in some patients with prolonged unconsciousness, typically 2 to 4 months after head injury. The most common sites are the shoulder, elbow, hip, and knee. Whether mobilization is beneficial during the acute phase is controversial. In children, ectopic bone is often spontaneously resorbed; therefore, surgical excision of bone to improve function is delayed. Recurrence of bone growth may follow surgery.[22,24]

Spasticity, a common sequela of head injury, increases during the first few months after injury, peaking at 2 to 3 months, then gradually decreases, sometimes for over 2 years.[24] Bilateral moderate to severe spasticity is most common in patients comatose for more than 4 weeks.[2] Conservative management, including passive range of motion (ROM), static stretching, serial plaster casts, dropout casts, and positional splints, attain full ROM before function returns. Early surgical management of spasticity includes release of hip contractures to prevent dislocation and phenol block to the musculocutaneous nerve and the motor branches of the median nerve for resistant elbow and finger flexor spasticity.

Later surgical management addresses scoliosis, leg length discrepancies, and residual spasticity interfering with function. Refer to Hoffer and associates[24] and Meyler and associates[35] for further discussion of acute and long-term orthopedic management.

Prognosis

Although recovery of consciousness and preinjury functional status is usually complete within 3 weeks, behavioral difficulties, shortened attention span, and irritability persist longer.[1] It is estimated that 5 to 10 percent of those hospitalized will manifest neurologic and/or psychologic sequelae 6 months or more after injury.[12,14,36] The interplay between the neurologic and psychologic sequelae, as well as the effect of the child's preinjury developmental and mental status,[3] family support and interaction, and availability of appropriate professional and nonprofessional intervention support systems, combine to determine the ultimate reintegration of the child into society.[6,7,9,10,36–39] Physical and mental improvement is evident 2, 3, and even 7 years after the injury[2,36]; however, it is generally agreed that the greatest change occurs by the first 6 to 12 months after injury.[2] Much research attempts to expand the confidence with which physicians can predict the ultimate outcome from the patient's status within the first few hours. Established outcome categories, recently reviewed by Jennett and associates[37,40] and referred to in many reports[7,10,12,31,37,41] are as follows: (1) death, (2) persistent vegetative state, (3) severe disability, (4) moderate disability, and (5) good recovery. An initial GCS ≤ 4 portends a poor outcome, which is often death.[1,10–12,41] Young and colleagues[41] and Kraus et al.[10] report outcomes equally distributed with GCSs of 5 to 7, and 95 percent good to moderate recovery with scores greater than 7. Changes in the GCS during the first 24 hours improve the precision of prediction of outcome.[41] Slow response time and difficulties with short-term memory are major residual abnormalities with initial GCSs of 5 to 8. Many detailed reviews of outcome can be found in the medical literature.[3–6,9–12,31,36,37,40,42–44]

Brink and associates[19] report that a good or moderate outcome is expected if coma does not exceed 6 weeks. Eiben and colleagues[9] reported that no patient with coma exceeding 1 month had a good outcome. Brink and others[19] reported that the frequency and severity of spasticity and ataxia increase as the length of coma increases. The incidence of spasticity and ataxia in severely head-injured children is high, approximately 65 and 50 percent, respectively, with 35 percent incidence of ataxia and spasticity combined.[2,13,31,33] A follow-up study of 53 children ≤18 years with severe closed-head injury grouped according to diffuse injury or mixed (diffuse and focal) injury found increased duration of coma and frequency of low GCS in those children with mixed injury, and presence of residual motor signs equally distributed among the groups.[42]

Psychologic sequelae, including cognitive and behavioral problems, are often present following minor injuries and may reflect diffuse injury. Assessing the outcome of a child is more complex than assessing that of an adult, as the child is not expected to just regain his or her former status, but to continue to mature developmentally and mentally, sequentially achieving "age-appropriate" milestones in all aspects of behavior. More recent studies of outcome in children attempt to measure social, emotional, psychologic, and academic abilities. Persistent deficits in learning and memory may be severe; the younger the age of onset, the more pronounced the effect on intellectual performance. The IQ score at 1 year after injury relates directly to length of coma.[2,24] Changes in personality and behavior include hyperactivity, distractibility, low tolerance for frustration, poor social judgment, lack of impulse control, and aggressiveness.[14,24,38,39] The intellectual deficits and personality changes that persist require special school placement and are difficult for the family to manage.

On long-term follow-up (6 to 133 months; mean, 34 months), children under the age of 7 years showed poorer outcome in measurements of social and school abilities than older children.[42] In all children tested using the revised Wechsler Intelligence Scale for Children, performance IQ was more affected than verbal IQ initially; both improved and equalized, but did not achieve estimated premorbid levels. Refer to Telzrow[38] and Ewing-Cobbs and Fletcher[39] for recent reviews of incidence, discussion of measurement tools, and methods of intervention in managing the significant residual behavioral and cognitive deficits.

PHYSICAL THERAPY ASSESSMENT

Assessment of the head-injured child is a continuous process. The unpredictable and varied rate of recovery and the complex mechanisms of recovery necessitate constant evaluation and modification of therapeutic intervention to appropriately enhance the recovery that is occurring. Close communication between professional team members assists each discipline to use strategies to best achieve their goals while reinforcing recovery in all aspects of performance.

A head-injured patient's loss of consciousness and diminished cognitive abilities require modification of the traditional assessment. Evoking the response appropriate to the area of assessment is a challenge to the therapist. Careful observation of the timing, force, duration, direction, and location of movement in response to controlled stimulation provides information as to the status of sensory, motor, and sensorimotor integrative aspects of movement. When evoking a response to sensory stimulation, allow for a delay for processing. After sufficient delay, the stimulus may have to be repeated a few times to evoke the desired response. Note the best response observed, as this indicates the potential of the patient. Information concerning the injury, the child's preinjury status, and rate of progress is available from a chart review and/or family interview. Physical assessment requires multiple short sessions to assure accurate judgments.

Behavioral Considerations

Decreased consciousness, maladaptive behaviors, and impaired cognition interfere with the child's ability to participate in the assessment. Techniques are modified according to the child's level of consciousness and cognitive function. A child at levels V, IV, or III, according to Ommaya's scale, is unable to follow commands; assessment, therefore, uses passive manipulation and observation of spontaneous or stimulus-induced movements. A child at level II can follow simple one-step commands; however, distractibility, limited attention span, and memory impairments may preclude following commands with more than one step, attending to a task for more than a few seconds, or attending to a stimulus at all. Elicitation of automatic activities provides purposeful motion for evaluation of motor control. A child at levels IV, III, and II may appear to change level of consciousness several times during the day. When the child is most alert, the best responses will be evoked. Fatigue may occur after 15 minutes, at which time earlier responses cannot be reproduced.

By level I, the child is oriented to self, time, and place. Although distractibility, limited attention span, and memory impairments remain, their severity has decreased sufficiently to permit use of traditional assessment tools for short testing periods. Behaviors such as aggression, lack of self-initiation, low frustration tolerance, emotional lability, or withdrawal require short sessions and a structured environment. At levels II and I, a quiet environment facilitates accurate evaluation of motor control; however, the child's ability to perform activities with the usual distractions may elucidate functional impairments limited by cognitive status.

The agitated patient presents the greatest challenge for assessment and treatment. One must remember that the child, while trying to come to grips with the environment, is also responding to cerebral irritation and internal confusion. Finding a means to calm the child facilitates assessment. In a calm environment with structured stimuli, the child may follow commands for short periods of time. Touching the child, or requesting a difficult or complex motion, may cause frustration and agitation. Purposeful movements, observed with a critical eye, provide ROM, sensation, motor control, equilibrium, and strength information. Children often demonstrate their best developmental or functional level when most agitated.

The cognitive functioning of children 12 years of age and older can be assessed using the Rancho Levels of Cognitive Functioning.[45] This scale is reversed in order compared with Brink's Scale and further defines behaviors of Brink levels II and I. Behaviors of Rancho levels I, II and III are the same as Brink levels V, IV, and III, respectively. At Rancho level IV (confused-agitated), the child is in a heightened state of activity, demonstrating bizarre and nonpurposeful behaviors relative to the environment. Assessment considerations for this child are described in the previous paragraph. At Rancho level V (confused-inappropriate), the child can follow simple commands inconsistently, shows gross attention to the environment but is very distractable, and lacks the ability to focus attention on a specific task. Memory is severely impaired so that new information cannot be learned. At level VI (confused-appropriate), the child shows goal-directed behavior, appropriate responses to the environment, can follow simple commands consistently, and can carry over relearned tasks. This child is still dependent on external cues for direction and shows little carry over of newly learned tasks. Assessment, treatment, and goal setting for a child at Rancho levels V or VI is similar to Brink level II.

At Rancho level VII (automatic-appropriate), the child appears appropriate and oriented to self and the environment, going through the daily routine automatically. Recent memory is impaired, resulting in shallow recall of activities and a decreased rate for learning new information. Judgment is impaired. At Rancho level VIII, the child can recall and integrate past and recent events and can adapt his or her responses to the environment. The child shows carry over of new learning and needs no supervision once an activity is learned. Deficits remain in abstract reasoning, tolerance to stress, and judgment in emergencies.[45] A child at Rancho level VII or VIII can cooperate with standard assessment procedures, although distractibility, fatigue, and deficits in higher level cognitive functions may require a longer testing time and more structure compared with a child without a head injury. Considerations in treatment and goal setting are the same as for Brink level I. For purposes of simplification, Brink levels I to V will be referred to in assessment, treatment, and goal setting.

Chart Review

The patient's age and preinjury developmental status provide a baseline for assessing motor ability and identifying preinjury problem areas. Preinjury behavior and cognitive abilities are apparent in school performance records and through family interview. Knowledge of favorite play activities aids in establishing a baseline as well as designing treatment activities.

The etiology of head injury and neurosurgical reports suggest the location and extent of cerebral injury. The circumstances of the injury alert the therapist to suspect concomitant injuries that may not be apparent until the patient gains consciousness. Peripheral nerve injuries and fractures may be missed during the acute stages.

The status of concomitant injuries and necessary precautions must be known before beginning the physical evaluation. Peripheral nerve injuries should be suspected if traction or external immobilization has been used.

Medical complications and present status alert the therapist to precautions necessary during assessment and treatment. During the acute stage, aggressive chest physical therapy may increase intracranial pressure. Elevation of the head 30 to 45 degrees and avoidance of neck rotation assist in preventing increased intracranial pressure. Coordination with nursing, supervision of proper positioning, and modifying chest physical therapy according to the patient's tolerance assures safety for the patient. Labile or hypertensive blood pressure may result from the head injury or medications. Muscle stretching during ROM or casting and changes in position may cause sudden increases in systolic and diastolic pressures and an associated tachycardia. Monitoring during treatment is recommended. Familiarity with nasogastric tube and tracheostomy precautions prepare the therapist for unexpected problems such as coughing out the inner cannula or regurgitation through the tube. Guidelines in some centers recommend avoidance of activities that lower the head below the stomach when the patient has a nasogastric tube in place, as the cardiac sphincter of the stomach is relaxed and open, and regurgitation and aspiration may take place.[38] Changes in position and chest physical therapy will loosen tracheal secretions, requiring suctioning. Careful review of the patient's medical record will alert the therapist as to which of these precautions may be necessary during assessment and therapy.

Level of consciousness or coma score at onset and changes during the first 24 to 48 hours are key prognosticators. The present level of consciousness, the time since the injury, and the duration of coma provide further indication of the severity of injury and the expected outcome.

A history of decerebrate or decorticate posturing alerts the therapist to expect contractures and be concerned about pressure areas. Prolonged posturing may result in unrelieved pressure, causing damage to superficial nerves, especially the ulnar or peroneal nerves. Heterotopic ossification, associated with trauma or spasticity, causes painful and limited joint ROM.

Family involvement since hospitalization gives an indication of involvement expected after discharge. A supportive and involved family facilitates rehabilitation and guarantees continuation of the process after discharge. In-hospital care only initiates the prolonged process of recovery and reintegration into society. The functional achievements must become part of the child's and family's daily routine. Goals and methods must be modified to meet the family's needs, as they will be the full-time therapists once the child leaves the hospital.

Previous therapeutic evaluation and progress reports indicate the child's progression. The child may appear totally different from the most recent assessment because neurologic improvement may occur rapidly. At times, the new environment and transition may result in an apparent decrease in level of consciousness until the child adapts to the new surroundings.

Table 8-1. Localized Response to Sensory Stimuli

Sensory Tract	Stimulus Examples	Response
Auditory	Voice	Eye opening
	Bell	Looking toward stimulus
	Hand clapping	Turning head toward/away from stimulus
Visual	Threat near eyes	Blinking
	Bright object	Focusing and tracking
	Familiar toy	
	Familiar person	
Olfactory	Ammonia	Grimace or turn away
Gustatory	Sugar	Smile
	Lemon	Grimace
Pain	Squeeze muscle belly	Pull extremity away
	Squeeze nail bed, pin prick	Look toward pain

Sensory Testing

The child's response to a specific sensory stimulus changes as level of consciousness changes. Stimuli through intact auditory, visual, olfactory, gustatory, and pain pathways evoke a response at all levels of consciousness, except level V.

A level IV child demonstrates a generalized response to any sensory input. The response is the same regardless of the type of stimulus presented. Increased respiratory rate, sweating, increased pulse rate, change in tone throughout the body, grimace, or total body movements are frequently noted.

At level III, the child's response is specific to the stimulus presented. A delay often occurs before the response, and the stimulus may need to be repeated. Examples of localized responses to selected stimuli are listed in Table 8-1.

Proprioception can be grossly assessed once the child initiates purposeful movements (level II). Specific testing is limited by cognition and the child's age. Sharp–dull and two-point discrimination testing require memory, the ability to process information, and the ability to follow complex commands.

Hypersensitivity to touch must be assessed. Total body, perioral, and oral hypersensitivity most often result from prolonged lack of stimulation and resolve nicely in response to desensitization therapy.

Range of Motion

Assessment of which factors are interfering with full ROM determines whether full range can be gained or whether the child must learn to compensate. Heterotopic ossification is often associated with a warm joint and painful range. A bony end point is noted if one can range through the child's resistance. Range may become more limited and the pain of movement through the range may interfere with functional activities. While heterotopic bone often is reabsorbed in children, short-term and potentially long-term compensation for lack of range is necessary. Hypertonus may favor prolonged habitual posturing and the potential development of soft tissue and joint capsule contractures. Positioning the patient to minimize tone aids in determining passive joint ROM. Appropriate conservative or surgical methods gain ROM to permit functional use of the extremity.

A child who is agitated, confused, or unable to follow commands may appear to resist ranging and cry as if in pain. Observing joint ROM used in spontaneous movements and functional activities confirms that full ROM is present, or further challenges the therapist to determine what is truly limiting the range.

Tone

Assessment of muscle tone, the amount of resistance to passive movement, may reveal varying degrees of increased or decreased tone. Apparent hypotonicity may result from muscle weakness, impaired sensorimotor integration, impairment in excitatory centers of postural tonic control, and, possibly, damage to reticular activating centers. Apparent hypertonicity may result from abnormalities in central programming and regulation of the motor neuron pool, as current theory proposes, or as an exaggeration of the normal tendency to revert to tonic reflex influence in difficult activities. The pattern of relative hyper- or hypotonicity reveals the balance of excitatory and inhibitory influences on the motoneurons. The child's alertness, difficulty of the task, and modified vestibular, tactile, and proprioceptive input affect the muscle tone and ability to move. Assessing the muscle tone relative to modifications in sensory input assists in program planning.

A transition from decerebrate or decorticate posturing to hypotonicity often follows neurologic recovery. Hypotonus eventually changes to hypertonus or alternating hypo- and hypertonus. Prolonged hypotonus is often associated with ataxia; however, ataxia may not be apparent until the child initiates purposeful movements.

Motor Control

Movement reflects level of consciousness, behavior, cognition, sensation, sensorimotor integration, status of supraspinal regulation, and neuromuscular status. The quality of movement is the product of the interaction of the uninvolved centers of control. Apparent deficits represent the inability of remaining centers to compensate for actual deficits caused by damage to or suppressed functioning of major motor control centers.

Initially, the quality of movement is assessed in general terms. Whether movement occurs spontaneously or only in response to stimulation reflects the level of consciousness or the presence of limb neglect as a result of sensory deficits. Level of consciousness determines whether motion is purposeful or nonpurposeful (random movement). Careful observation of spontaneous movements and manipulating position, type, and location of stimulus to encourage a selective response determines if selectivity is present. Often, selective movements and normal movement patterns replace the abnormal flexion and extension patterns as the child's level of consciousness and cognition improves and motor learning progresses; however, if moderate to severe spasticity combines with abnormal patterned motion, resolution to selective control is less likely. Assessment of movement in gravity-eliminated positions and against gravity determines the relative strength of muscle groups and assists in identifying peripheral nerve injuries. Determining good and normal strengths of individual muscles is difficult. Often a child will not maintain a joint position against resistance. Lifting body weight or weighted items and the way in which a child moves between postures and maintains postures may suggest weaknesses. Muscle endurance may be impaired from prolonged inactivity, especially if hypotonus is present. It has been argued that brain-damaged patients suffer from lack of central control over movement and not actual muscle weakness. In my experience, some children suffering severe head injuries and prolonged unconsciousness demonstrate muscle weakness and limited endurance, contributing to impaired motor control, especially of the neck and trunk. Areas of weakness then demand consideration in planning treatment.

The influence of muscle tone, sensation, and muscle strength and endurance on the selective or patterned control available determines the achievable motor control of each extremity, as well as the neck and trunk. Observation of function identifies the child's ability to use the motor control available. Deficits in sensorimotor integration (e.g., apraxia, impaired motor planning, or visual discrimination), supraspinal regulation, impaired cognition (limited attention to task and impaired memory), and decreased level of consciousness affect the functional use of motor patterns available. Observations of purposeful movement in response to a command may indicate cognitive or sensorimotor integration deficits. A classic case is the child's apparent inability to move his or her arms when asked to lift an arm as high as possible and to touch the therapist's hand or reach for a toy; however, if the therapist throws a ball, the child automatically catches it with perfect control! Whether the child is unable to attend, to initiate movement or to sequence the activity, or has sensorimotor integration deficits is difficult to determine. Team members specializing in these areas of evaluation, such as occupational therapists, often identify specific deficits and suggest intervention strategies for improvement of function or compensation for deficits.

Documenting the movement patterns observed in the developmental sequence of postures and transitions between postures assists in identifying which of the above problems impair function. The change from stereotyped patterns of movement to a greater variety of patterns of movement follows a pattern similar to normal development, but on an accelerated time line. Developmental tests have not been standardized for the head-injured population. With the complexity of deficits in each child, the validity of these tests is questionable;

however, a selection of testable items provides an index of the abilities of the child at a point in time and a baseline for comparison as recovery occurs. The validity of standardized tests in defining outcome or confirming total recovery has not been evaluated.

Testing equilibrium and righting reactions usually demonstrate delayed and exaggerated responses that resolve as level of consciousness improves. Hypertonicity interfering to prevent a protective or equilibrium response in lower-level activities portends residual impairment, although improvements occur. Ataxia or neglect interfering with protective responses may take years to resolve, necessitating compensation. Although righting and equilibrium reactions are apparent in supine, prone, and four-point positions, sitting and standing may prove too difficult or stressful, resulting in tonic reflex influences dominating motor responses; however, the quality of righting and equilibrium reactions in lower level developmental activities portends the eventual quality of these reactions in higher-level postures. It often appears that the postural response in the trunk is exaggerated, or the timing is incorrect for the extremity movement planned or when coordinating transitional movements, although the muscle synergies used are appropriate. This problem usually resolves with treatment. Consideration of the effect of lack of ROM at a key joint of the response may explain the "inappropriate" response and indicate a need to increase ROM rather than facilitate a modified response. For example, a child with limited dorsiflexion range would tend to choose a hip response rather than an ankle response when displaced posteriorly. Horak[46] describes the influence of deficits in sensory organization, motor coordination, and the musculoskeletal system on postural control.

The head-injured child may also have visual and visual–perceptual problems affecting selection of motor patterns. Shumway-Cook and Horak[47] describe a test to differentiate deficits in sensory integration interfering with balance in standing (Fig. 8-1). This test is appropriate when the child is older than 8 years, can follow simple commands, and does not have musculoskeletal problems.

Testing motor control in standing can predict the child's ability to use available control in walking. The ability to flex the hip, knee, and ankle quickly and the ability to control the hip, knee, and ankle in single-limb standing are graded on a three-point scale described by Montgomery.[48]

Cardiopulmonary Status

In the acute setting, cardiac and respiratory impairments may result from trauma to the chest, pharyngeal spasm, respiratory center depression from brain stem damage, and labile reactions to trauma. Endotracheal intubation or tracheostomy permit maintenance of an airway for provision of mechanical ventilation and suctioning.

Laboratory study results and chest radiographs assist in identifying the respiratory problem. In the acutely ill patient, mechanical devices such as arterial, central venous, and Swan-Ganz catheters, electrocardiograms, intra-

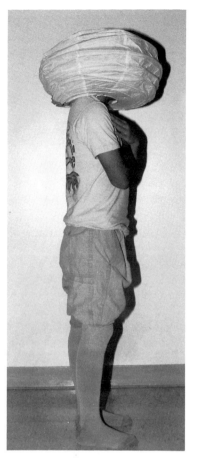

Fig. 8-1. Testing postural responses using a visual conflict globe. This is one of six testing conditions for differentiating deficits in sensory integration affecting balance.

cranial pressure transducers, and respiratory gas analyzers provide baseline data as well as indication of tolerance for treatment. Observation of breathing rate, rhythm, and pattern; chest expansion measurements; and palpation, percussion, and auscultation complete the clinical assessment.[49–51]

The child no longer needing mechanical monitors may continue demonstrating labile physiologic responses to change in position or muscle stretch. Baseline heart rate, rhythm, and blood pressure are determined at rest and in response to exercise.

Orofacial Control

Children suffering severe head injuries frequently require nasogastric tube feeding because brain stem involvement has impaired the swallow, gag, and cough reflexes. Prolonged nasogastric tube feeding often results in deprivation of oral sensation and, therefore, delay in return of normal reflex responses for swallowing and preventing aspiration. Impaired cognition may interfere with the voluntary aspects of eating, resulting in inability to monitor the amount of food in the mouth or pocketing of food instead of pushing the bolus backward. Cranial nerve deficits are often present.

Sensory assessment of the face, lips, gums, tongue, soft palate, and posterior pharyngeal wall may identify hypo- or hypersensitivity to touch. Children with a history of decorticate posturing often demonstrate abnormal reflex responses to stimulation, including the following: rooting reflex, pursing reflex, and reflex chewing followed by a reflex suck–swallow. The reflex swallow, gag, and cough are assessed in all patients. The reflex gag, normally elicited on the posterior third of the tongue, may be hypersensitive (elicited in middle to anterior third) or diminished (elicited only on soft palate or posterior pharyngeal wall). Voluntary initiation of a swallow and cough is requested if the child can follow commands. If unable to follow commands, a small amount of water placed in the side of the mouth with a straw will usually elicit a swallow. An audible swallow, multiple attempts, delayed initiation, or inadequate laryngeal excursion indicate incoordination and risk of aspiration. If a reflex cough is not elicited, active respiratory problems are present and/or the status of the swallow suggests aspiration risk; further assessment is necessary before initiating feeding. If a child has a tracheostomy, feeding the child a small amount of pureed food with blue food coloring added followed by suctioning will reveal if aspiration has occurred. A swallowing fluoroscopy may be necessary to confirm the absence of aspiration when a tracheostomy is not present.

In a review of videofluoroscopic evaluations of swallowing in 53 closed-head trauma patients, Lazarus and Logemann found delayed or absent swallow, reduced tongue control, and impaired pharyngeal peristalsis to be the most common problems.[52] Liquids were aspirated when tongue control was impaired or the swallow was delayed or absent. Most often, aspiration occurred after the swallow, when reduced pharyngeal peristalsis resulted in food left in the vallecula. These investigators suggested that because many patients did not cough following aspiration, videofluorographic assessment is an invaluable tool to identify the presence and etiology of aspiration. (If a swallowing videofluoroscopy is necessary, the therapist must consider positioning, facilitation, and inhibition techniques and the consistency of the substance swallowed for a true assessment of aspiration to be expected during therapeutic feeding. Refer to Lazarus and Logemann.[52])

Selective and voluntary control of the lips, tongue, and jaw can be observed in response to stimulation with a tooth swab, gloved finger, or tongue blade to the gums and tongue. Expected motor control for the child's age must be considered. Adequate ability to maneuver food to the sides and back of the mouth and presence of a reflex swallow, reflex gag, and reflex cough are indications for a feeding trial.

Setting Realistic Functional Goals

Ideal long-term goals include attainment of age-appropriate gross motor activities, functional abilities, and diet. Reasonable outcomes considering length of coma have been discussed. Ataxia and spasticity are the most common physical factors interfering with functional activities and, if severe, may prevent ambulation. Mental and cognitive deficits are often more disabling than physical deficits in determining overall outcome. The need for constant supervision and residual aggressive, impulsive, and destructive behavior require an involved caretaker for successful postdischarge management. Intellectual deficits, common when a severe head injury is sustained in childhood, may limit potential vocational abilities. Adolescents commonly demonstrate poor judgment and difficulty with problem solving, which seriously hinder vocational potential and financial independence.[10,22,36,38,39,45]

Considering developmental and functional abilities appropriate to the child's age, the length of time in coma, and the physical findings and cognitive status in light of the length of time from onset, a potential functional status can be estimated. To determine if the predicted status is achievable and realistic for the patient, consider preinjury development, setting after discharge, and involvement of caretakers. Family members may not be available for constant supervision, and household barriers (and monetary constraints) may prevent use of assistive devices for independence, limiting function in transfers to those requiring assistance. The availability of therapy through school or infant intervention groups permits discharge at lower levels of function with the knowledge that therapy will be continued on an outpatient basis. Unrealistic family expectations for recovery require immediate and continuing family involvement and education. If institutional placement is necessary, realistic goals and equipment are chosen as appropriate to the discharge setting, where time restraints and staffing may limit supervision and follow-through of programs.

Level of consciousness and cognitive function may limit achievement of goals expected on the basis of physical findings only. For children at levels IV and III, wheelchair positioning to prevent contractures and assist respiratory status is realistic. Bed positioning, ROM, and, possibly, a respiratory–postural drainage–vibration program may be carried out by an involved family. Feeding reflexes may permit the child to be fed a pureed or soft diet. Mobility in bed is dependent, but instructions for caretakers on body mechanics and facilitation of rolling may assist the care of the adolescent. Transfers are dependent. A lift is recommended.

A child at level II is able to follow commands and initiate purposeful activity. The child may be able to relearn automatic activities, such as rolling, coming to sit, crawling, standing, ambulation, and self-feeding, if physical deficits are minimal. The absence of judgment and problem-solving abilities requires constant supervision and, often, assistance to prevent injury to the child. Carry over of the same activity in new environments will require assistance and much repetition until the pattern is relearned in the new situation. A child with moderate to severe motor deficits has difficulty learning to compensate due to poor memory and sequencing abilities. Learning mobility with equipment may not be possible. Bed mobility and transfers may require minimal to moderate assistance.

A child reaching level I is oriented to time, place, and self, and is recording ongoing events. Independence in mobility at home, self-care, and feeding are realistic goals. Proper use of adaptive equipment can be learned. However, a child normally requires supervision in the community. This must be emphasized with caretakers because poor frustration tolerance, lack of problem solving, impaired judgment, and poor impulse control demand closer supervision than preinjury. The adolescent will also require supervision in the community, where the multitude of stimuli may be confusing and residual judgment and problem-solving deficits may make new situations difficult to manage.

PHYSICAL THERAPY

General Treatment Principles

The therapist does not cause neurologic recovery, but rather channels the spontaneous recovery that is occurring. Whether recovery is the result of diaschisis, equipotentiality, compensation, vicariation, and/or collateral regeneration and hypersensitivity remains controversial.[29,49–57] The timing, frequency, and type of therapeutic intervention to effect a given outcome has not been objectively ascertained. Valid tools to define deficits and methods of differentiating recovery based on neurophysiologic mechanisms from that resulting from learning compensatory behaviors are yet to be developed.

A systematic assessment permits determination of the major problems interfering with function, the abilities retained, and intact exteroceptive and proprioceptive systems through which adaptive behaviors can be stimulated. Treatment is an extension of the assessment process. With the complexity of deficits, uniqueness of each child, and spontaneous recovery occurring, no single method of treatment is appropriate in every situation. The patient's adaptive response to a specific intervention may change within a treatment period as well as between treatment periods. The therapist must know the adaptive response he or she is trying to evoke. The therapist must then evaluate findings and responses to this point to provide the appropriate cues. Immediate evaluation of the child's response, both subtle tone changes as well as gross movements, provides feedback as to modifications needed in the handling provided.

The normal learning process may account for apparent recovery. Carr and Shepherd[58] identified key factors in the process of relearning of movement. The goal must be identified and relevant to the child. Guiding the child through the proper sequence of movement, the therapist provides cues as needed, allowing the child to be an active participant in learning the movement through experiencing the feel of the movement. The therapist assists with the inhibition of unnecessary activity that normally occurs as the movement is refined, thus reducing the energy cost of movement. Normal postural reactions necessary to maintain balance and position against gravity permit progression from stability to controlled mobility. Guided and controlled practice, variability in practice, motivation and knowledge of results, and feedback on performance further enhance learning.[59] A learned task can be performed automatically in a variety of situations. Feedback must be specific, quantitative, and appropriate to the cognitive level of the child and to the phase of motor learning.[59] If practicing part of a motor pattern is necessary, the therapist must incorporate the single movement within the functional movement task immediately to maximize learning. When refining a learned task, practice sessions must challenge the patient to problem solve and adapt to different environments. The ability to design play activities appropriate to the child's cognitive abilities that are goal directed, provide success, encourage movement, and yet permit adequate handling by the therapist to ensure a normal sensorimotor experience is a skill developed through practice.

A coordinated team effort enhances patient learning through additional reinforcement of appropriate skills incorporated into the treatment sessions of each team member. Generally, each team member contributes to orienting at the beginning and end of each session by telling the child his or her own name, where the child is, what the child is going to do, and the therapist's name. The child's cognitive abilities and behaviors influence the therapist's approach to treatment. At levels IV and III, the child cannot actively initiate participation in the therapeutic program. Emphasis at this time is to increase the duration of attention to stimuli and decrease the response delay. Maintaining or improving ROM and stimulating equilibrium and righting reactions prepare the musculoskeletal system for the time when the child can participate. Decreasing hypersensitivity and facilitating normal reflex responses of gag, swallow, and cough prepare the child for feeding. An active respiratory program prepares the physiologic response.

At level II, the child can initiate interaction with the environment. Structuring the environment controls the sensory input and therefore assists to organize the input in evoking an appropriate response. The child may be able to perform a previously learned activity with much repetition. Providing simple verbal directions, demonstrating the command, and assisting the child through the activity provide appropriate cues and structures. However, if the child responds only verbally to verbal cues, but will roll when the command is gestured and is facilitated, these cues are then repeated without speaking. Gradually, assistance through the activity is decreased so that the therapist initiates the activity but expects the child to complete the roll. Eventually, with only a gesture or command, the child can initiate the activity with the components in the proper sequence to achieve the goal. Carry-over from session to session requires memory. Independent carry-over in a different environment is not expected until the child can solve problems; therefore, although physically able to perform an activity, the child may require assistance to repeat the same activity in a different environment. Verbal feedback of specific performance problems must be given in a way that does not confuse the child.

As the child's memory improves, the child can carry over activities to new environments and remember them from day to day. Lability and distractibility tend to decrease; however, irritability and difficulties with judgment and problem solving often persist at level I. Expecting the child to take responsibility for getting to classes on time, choosing clothes, and other age-appropriate expectations of independence are gradually encouraged. Community outings challenge the child's judgment and problem solving. Exercising safety in street crossings at busy corners and running errands to small stores or fast-food restaurants test the child's cognitive, emotional, social, and physical abilities in the community.

Inadequate Range of Motion

Management of inadequate ROM depends on the factors limiting range and the severity of the factors. Heterotopic ossification is the most difficult to manage. The child splints against passive ROM and will not move the joint through full range actively. If the pain interferes with functional activities, immobilization in plaster may relieve the pain sufficiently to permit rehabilitation to continue. The child must compensate for the limited range until the bone is reabsorbed or surgical resection is complete.

Hypertonicity, hypotonicity, or peripheral nerve injury prevent spontaneous movement of each joint through its normal ROM and encourage prolonged posturing, resulting in myostatic or capsular contracture. An ROM program incorporating positioning, myofascial stretching, joint mobilization, static stretching, casts, splints, orthoses, and/or electric stimulation is designed considering the apparent soft tissue contracture and factors affecting its development. Static stretch or serial casting may decrease soft tissue contracture over 2 to 4 weeks. Splints and positioning maintain range.

Most applicable in early management, positioning serves to maintain ROM by preventing prolonged use of abnormal postures. Bed positioning with pillows and rolls should encourage slight neck and trunk flexion, shoulder protraction, slight elbow flexion and forearm pronation, and wrist extension. Pelvic anterior tilt and slight flexion of the hip, knee, and ankle may relax lower extremity tone. Extremity positioning is alternated between flexion and extension as long as tone is relaxed. Placement in the prone position is encouraged when medically cleared. Moderate to severe tone not decreased with positioning may respond with the addition of casts and splints.

Wheelchair positioning to control tone must consider the influence of the head position on tone and the key points where control affects the tone of the rest of the body. Lateral trunk supports, a somewhat reclined wheelchair back, and H-straps or soft ties provide lateral and anterior support, preventing kyphosis and lateral lean. Upper extremities supported on a lap board or bolsters assists with lateral support and prevents forward lean of the upper trunk. A solid seat, lap belt at 45 degrees, and supported feet position the pelvis at neutral (Fig. 8-2). Hips flexed and abducted with wedged cushion and abduction bolster provide additional control of the pelvis when needed.

A stable pelvis and trunk are prerequisites for controlling head position. Maintaining slight cervical extension and capital flexion with neutral neck rotation and lateral flexion provides a normal sensorimotor experience through visual orientation and vestibular and somatic proprioceptive systems. Lateral head supports control neck rotation and lateral flexion as long as the wheelchair

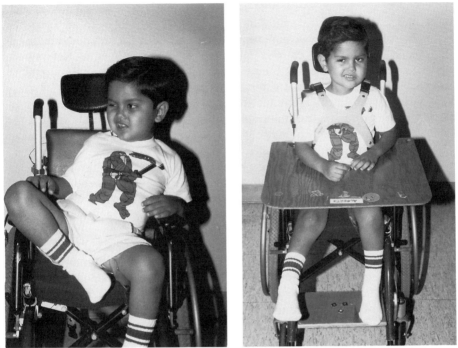

Fig. 8-2. Poor trunk control and hemiplegia often result in an asymmetric sitting posture (**A**), even with a solid seat and back insert. A butterfly chest strap, lap board, and pelvic seat belt (not seen) provide adequate anterior and lateral trunk support and eliminate the pull of the hemiplegic arm on the trunk (**B**). Midline positioning improves visual orientation and promotes equal weight-bearing on ischii and extremities.

back is well reclined. Medium density, 6-inch-thick cushions may be carved to provide appropriate cervical extension and prevent lateral flexion and rotation. Carving a cap within the foam to cover part of the forehead assists in controlling capital positioning.

Shoulder and hip ROM limitations are best managed with traditional static stretching and passive ROM methods combined with positioning to maintain the range available. An abductor bar attached to short- or long-leg casts or splints maintains hip abduction in the supine and prone positions. Depending on the child's therapy program, abductor bars and outriggers are attached permanently to present casts or splints, or are attached to plaster cups that fit on the heel of a short-leg cast, permitting removal for dressing or sidelying positioning.

Ankle and knee contractures often respond well to serial casting. Well-padded cylinder casts applied with the joint positioned just short of its maximum passive range are changed every 8 to 10 days. At each cast change, the joint is put through full range and a new cast applied at maximum available range. Generally, two to three cast changes are necessary to achieve full range. Once the desired range is achieved, a "holding cast" maintains the corrected range for 1 to 3 weeks. This cast may be bivalved and converted to an anterior–posterior splint. Gradual weaning to using splints at night, and positioning orthoses and ROM during the day, proceeds as long as range is maintained. Splinting continues until neurologic recovery results in decreased spasticity and improved motor control. Dropout casts combined with positioning for gravity-assisted ROM hasten the reduction of elbow flexion contractures and knee flexion contractures of less than 60 degrees. Dropout casts may need to be changed every 3 to 5 days as range will increase quickly. Serial casting is most often incorporated into early management to achieve functional range by the time coma has decreased, permitting the child's participation in therapy. During this time, children may demonstrate physiologic lability to pain and stretch and cannot communicate location or intensity of pain. Labile vital signs or other indications of pain necessitate changing casts to decrease stretch and/or relieve localized skin pressure.[60,61]

Tone-inhibiting casts encouraging extension of the toes, equalizing pressure on the plantar surface, and stabilizing ankle position may normalize dynamic hypertonicity when functional activities in the upright position are initiated.[62] Traditional ankle–foot orthoses or specially modified, tone-inhibiting orthoses may maintain ankle ROM and modify persistent hypertonicity during functional activities until neurologic recovery permits adequate motor control or until surgical procedures are considered at 1 to 2 years postinjury.[60]

Electric cycling of muscle groups antagonistic to spastic muscles may be incorporated with use of casts or separately to increase ROM at the knee, ankle, elbow, and wrist.[63] Cycling in a functional position, such as standing, increases joint range while assisting to reeducate normal muscular control. A child with knee flexor contractures and/or hamstring spasticity interfering with extension control in the upright position may benefit from functional electric stimulation of the quadriceps muscle in standing combined with weight shift to the involved side during stimulation. Electric stimulation of the peroneal nerve may facilitate a decrease in extensor tone and foot clearance in swing. Tolerance for electric stimulation and the effect of stimulation on spastic musculature elsewhere in the body is variable; therefore, judicious use of this modality as an adjunct to the therapeutic regimen is recommended.

Inadequate Motor Control

Ommaya describes the reintegrative phenomena displayed by patients as they slowly struggle toward full consciousness as a distorted and irregularly accelerated reproduction of ontogenetic development. The patient retraces general behavioral development as well as the neurologic pattern of his or her own growth and maturity.[21] It is fascinating to watch the recovery of young children. They often cry or refuse to progress too quickly. Tonic influences in difficult postures and reintegration of normal postural reactions are dramatic. Often, the child spontaneously progresses to the next developmental level. Facilitating normal tone, movement, and increased sensory awareness and providing a structured environment to reinforce normal postural reactions and mobility, while preventing repetition of abnormal movement, affects internalization and independent imitation of normal postural reactions and movement patterns. Whether the therapist is assisting with or permitting the learning process, enhancing access to intact control centers through amplification of previously less-developed proprioceptive access systems, or whether recovery is independent of outside intervention currently defies determination; however, maintaining the musculoskeletal status, channeling the functional use of recovery that occurs, and teaching compensation for residual deficits are minimal roles of the therapist.

Appropriate treatment strategies are suggested through evaluation of findings and observation of adaptive responses to handling, providing various types and amounts of sensory cues. Treatment evolves from appropriate integration of principles of Neurodevelopmental Treatment, Rood, Ayres, Brunnstrom, and proprioceptive neuromuscular facilitation (PNF). The child's adaptive responses provide feedback and therefore indicate modifications of intervention necessary to refine the response.

Motor control of the extremities is influenced by head and trunk control and head position. Posturing of the trunk is influenced by extremity tone and head position. Head control is influenced by trunk control. In short, the movement of any part of the body is influenced by and influences the postural control of other parts of the body; therefore, treatment planning must include consideration of the whole body (and cognitive status).

Motor control at levels III and IV is facilitated through stimulation of exteroceptors to elicit automatic responses and proprioceptors to effect tonic and postural responses. Wheelchair and bed positioning programs aim to provide appropriate proprioceptive input to encourage normalization of tone, as well as maintain range. Positioning on the tilt table and supported sitting on a mat provide varying somatic proprioceptive, vestibular, and visual input. Assisted rolling and coming to sit facilitate righting and equilibrium reactions to somatic proprioceptive and vestibular input. Handling encourages appropriate adaptive responses while inhibiting abnormal tonic influences.

As the child reaches level II, play activities encourage purposeful goal-directed responses initiated by the child. The therapist assists the child with inhibition of abnormal postures and movement and facilitation of the greatest possible variety of innate and potentially normal motor patterns. Head control, head and trunk righting, extremity control for support and mobility, rotation, and equilibrium reactions are considered in choosing activities and treatment techniques. Tactile stimulation and techniques of proprioceptive neuromuscular facilitation, such as use of resistance and rhythmic stabilization, as well as tapping, approximation, and weight-bearing, provide increased sensory input in the presence of apparent or real weakness of muscles after decreasing abnormal tone or hypotonicity.[64] Withdrawing assistance and varying activities are key to the child's learning and internalizing the movements for functional tasks.

Play activities are designed with combinations of postural demands of head and trunk and gross and fine motor demands of extremities. Progression of treatment includes decreasing the amount of postural assistance provided through handling or increasing the difficulty of movement expected. Providing sufficient handling for postural control while using an activity to facilitate or challenge postural control may require two people (Fig. 8-3). The therapist handling the child receives constant feedback as to the child's postural response. The therapist then directs the assistant or designs the play to encourage mobility, which challenges the postural control to the point just short of where the child reverts to abnormal responses. If the task is too difficult, the therapist providing stability will feel a decrease in postural tone or a reversion to primitive tonic reflexes to provide the tone needed. Dynamic modification of handling will guarantee successful completion of the task and a normal sensorimotor experience.

Goldberger[65] suggests that spontaneous recovery from cerebellar ataxia is dependent on peripheral feedback and is not dependent on training or enhanced by training. Inaccuracy in timing and movement is compensated for by greater accuracy in position (mediated in part through the cerebral cortex). Initial ataxia is replaced by tremor as the oscillation amplitude decreases, frequency increases, and rhythm becomes more regular. The dorsal roots, dorsal columns, pre- and postcentral cortical gyrus, and pyramidal tract are implicated in compensating for cerebellar dyskinesia resulting from dentate-interpositus lesions.[65]

Ataxia becomes apparent once the child initiates purposeful movements. The oscillations decrease in amplitude as each developmental level is mastered; however, progression to a less stable posture or demanding a fine motor activity with the hand at a distance away from the body exacerbates the oscillations. The child stabilizes against a firm object, with upper extremities against the body or a table when performing fine motor activities. When moving from one position to another, the child will maintain as many points of contact with a steady surface as possible. Postural stability, rotation within the body axis, and equilibrium reactions are facilitated through proprioceptive input. Studies on long-term follow-up of resolution of ataxia and long-term interference with ambulation as an adult are not available.

Nelson,[66] in reviewing neuro-otologic aspects of head injury, presented evidence of cervical vertigo produced in animal studies and apparent in clinical experience without a pathophysiologic explanation. Ataxia can be produced in rabbits, monkeys, and humans by local anesthetic injected into the neck muscles. Humans report a sense of falling or tilting. Nystagmus cannot be demonstrated. Unilateral injection results in a clinical picture of ipsilateral ataxia, past pointing, and hypotonia. A cervical collar relieves the ataxia. Clinical symptoms arise 12 hours to 1 day after a whiplash injury and may persist for weeks or months, even when near-normal neck ROM is attained.

The comatose head-injured patient demonstrates vestibulo-ocular reflex impairment to head-turning or caloric irrigation of the ears. As the patient regains consciousness, a strong direction-fixed nystagmus, suggestive of a uni-

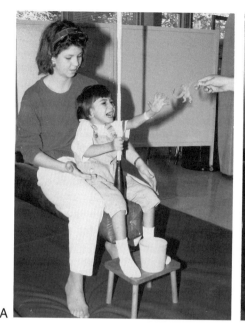

A

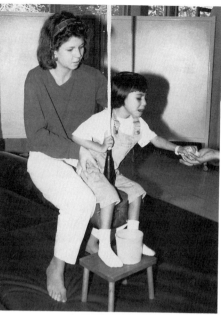

B

Fig. 8-3. The physical and occupational therapists co-treated A.J., who was fearful of movement and had poor head and trunk control and difficulty with sustained grip. She reached for the toy by extending her head and flexing her shoulder **(A)**. With approximation at her pelvis, she could lean forward and grasp the bean bag in front of her **(B)**. Reaching diagonally, A.J. needed assistance with the weight shift and trunk rotation **(C)**. Holding the rope on the suspended bolster encouraged sustained grasp and gave her a sense of security and control of her trunk in space.

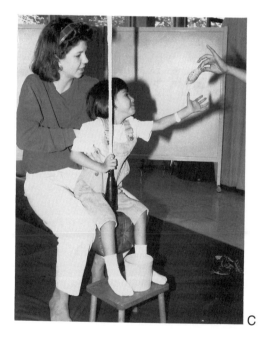

C

lateral vestibular lesion, is demonstrated. Nystagmus and vertigo largely sub-side over a 2- to 3-week period because of central compensatory mechanisms. Ambulatory patients complain of ataxia, in the absence of paresis or cerebellar tremors, with a tendency to list toward one side or difficulty changing directions when sudden head turns are required. Residual ataxia is apparent for up to several weeks, and symptomatic treatment is suggested.[66]

Generally, as cognition and level of consciousness improve, motor control improves. Refinement of sensorimotor integration and, therefore, motor control in upright postures often occur spontaneously in preschool children or are enhanced by intervention through school therapy units. Once the children are mobile, they are in constant motion, thereby naturally refining and adapting present motor patterns to perform more difficult activities. Treatment should be designed considering muscle strength and endurance and physiologic responses to exercise to decrease the demand of functional activities. Auditory rhythm[67] and dance therapy[68] provide further enhancement of postural control.

Neuromuscular electric stimulation may assist in increasing sensory input for muscle reeducation in a child with low tone or limb neglect. Lower extremity stimulation during standing and ambulation are generally preceded by a period of increasing tolerance to stimulation and strength and endurance of muscle contraction. Specific muscle strengthening may also be a goal of electric stimulation.[63]

Pick-up walkers with front wheels provide balance assistance for household mobility. Troughs can be added when upper extremity control is impaired. The addition of weight (lead BBs in the walker legs) enhances walker stability for ataxic children. Helmets are generally recommended for all ambulatory children lacking protective balance reactions sufficient for safety. Ankle–foot orthoses, besides controlling hypertonicity, may provide additional tibial stability for children with weak plantar flexors. An adjustable ankle joint orthosis allows modifications as ankle strength and control improve. Beveling the heel of the shoe or allowing limited plantar flexion motion at the ankle decreases the demand on the quadriceps muscle during loading. Bathroom equipment may include strategically placed grab bars to assist balance during transfers. A towel or nonskid stickers on the floor of the tub may assist with safety in sitting and transfers; bath loungers may be necessary if balance reactions in sitting are poor.

Reintegration of the child into the school setting requires ongoing coordination with teachers and school therapists. Sensorimotor integration deficits not apparent initially may manifest later when the child appears clumsy in certain playground activities. Observing the child performing the activity and determining the motor and sensorimotor integration skills necessary for smooth completion of the task permit identification of the residual deficits. Baum and Hall reported a significant relationship between dressing ability scores and three constructional praxis scores and concluded that a portion of the patient's inability to dress was perceptual rather than motor in nature.[69] Activities to encourage development of missing skills and suggestions for modifying activities to compensate for deficits permit continued motor control improvement while promoting self-esteem through peer interaction.

Inefficient Cardiopulmonary System

In the acutely ill patient, chest physical therapy assists in preventing the complications of atelectasis and pneumonia. Positioning, bronchial drainage, and manual techniques of percussion and vibration assist in mobilizing secretions, increasing airflow to the dependent lung.[51,58] Becker and colleagues[70] report reduced values for vital capacity, inspiratory capacity, total lung capacity, and forced expiratory volume at 1 second in young adult head-injured patients when compared with normal individuals. Less efficient circulatory and ventilatory responses to exercise among the head-injured group were identified. Becker et al. suggest that these inefficiencies may be inherent in brain stem disturbances, resulting in deficient automatic motor performances, which contribute to the development of secondary deconditioning.

Inadequate Orofacial Control

The major problems interfering with feeding are cognition, hypo- and/or hypersensitivity to stimulation, level of consciousness, and poor head and trunk control. Although voluntary initiation and modification of orofacial motor control is lacking, most children, even at levels III and IV, demonstrate the rhythmic transient or phasic jaw closing and opening reflexes, the tonic opening reflex, and the repeating tongue-movement reflex followed by reflex swallow described by Campbell.[71] These rhythmic oral motor patterns follow a yawn, oral stimulation, and, at times, noxious tactile stimulation as a generalized response to stimulation. Although the rooting and pursing reflexes may be elicited, generally these do not interfere with feeding and tend to be inhibited after three or four repetitions of stimulation.

Perioral and intraoral hypersensitivity resulting in a tonic bite and a gag will interfere with jaw opening to get food into the mouth and the swallow reflex, respectively. Techniques of desensitization, such as firm pressure on the lips, firm stroking of the gums, and firm stroking and pressure with a toothette or tongue blade intraorally and on the tongue, inhibit these responses. Densensitization may be necessary preceding each feeding session.

Hyposensitivity, often seen with prolonged nasogastric tube feeding, will modify the rhythmic oral motor patterns such that the rhythmic tongue movement may cease before the bolus reaches the pharynx, the reflex swallow may be delayed, and laryngeal excursion may be incomplete. Considering that a central pattern generator may exist in the brain stem reticular formation,[71] sensitization techniques such as quick stroking periorally and intraorally prior to feeding, which also tends to increase the alertness of the patient, may be affecting the rhythmic motor reflexes through affecting the general excitatory status of the reticular activating system. A thermogustatory bolus, such as lemon ice, and use of chilled utensils may facilitate awareness and completion of swallow.

At level III and, occasionally, level II, the brief alert periods and short attention span of the patient are most limiting to actual feeding because the motor reflexes are elicited for only short periods of time. Generally, the amount of time the child is alert is insufficient to maintain nutritional status through oral feeding. The lack of fine motor control necessary to swallow liquids without aspiration (possibly due to hyposensitivity) precludes safe and sufficient oral liquid intake.

Head and trunk control affect orofacial control in three ways. The alignment of the structures of the oropharynx and larynx affect the speed and ease of the flow of liquids and food and, therefore, the needed motor control to facilitate or control the food. The strength and endurance of neck and trunk musculature, as well as oral musculature, affect the energy cost of this simple activity and the length of time the child can sustain it. The status of the central nervous system, which accounts for hypertonicity or hypotonicity of the musculature, may influence the central control mechanism if one accepts the hypothesis that the central pattern generator can be influenced by voluntary commands from higher centers, by sensory information from the oral cavity and from the muscles, and by the state of the central nervous system.[71]

Techniques of facilitation and inhibition, such as positioning of head, trunk, and extremities; manual jaw and lip control; and quick stretch, ice, and resistive exercises to lips, larynx, orofacial, and neck musculature, appear to improve motor control in response to sensory input. Silverman and Elfant[72] suggest treatments for specific deficits noted. Whether voluntary control, increased muscular strength and endurance, a change in acuity or threshold of peripheral sensory endings, or the neurophysiologic changes of the state of the central nervous system account for improved motor control, few children lack sufficient recovery for oral feeding.

Initiation of feeding may occur earlier than one might expect. Winstein[73] lists six indications for initiation of feeding: (1) adequate cognition, (2) adequate intraoral manipulation, (3) adequate laryngeal elevation observed with reflex swallow after administration of a small amount of water, (4) presence of gag or weak posterior pharyngeal wall motion, (5) no active respiratory problem, and (6) no evidence of aspiration. (Confirm with a swallowing videofluoroscopy as indicated—*see Orofacial Control.*)

When initiating a feeding trial, head and trunk positioning and handling techniques will modify the motor control. The consistency of food and viscosity of liquids are modified according to the motor control and endurance of the musculature. Pureed foods over the middle part of the tongue will elicit the repeating tongue-movement reflex, which leads to a swallow. Soft foods of a thicker consistency require greater endurance of intraoral musculature. Ground foods provide a greater variety of sensory input and require a greater variety of tongue control to gather the pieces into a bolus, but they often stimulate this activity and may be handled better than soft foods. A regular diet requires tongue lateralization and control of jaw motion for chewing. Progression of diet follows assessment of motor control and muscular endurance and must take into consideration age expectations. Considerations in choice of foods include hypersensitivity to taste, often present initially, cultural preferences (even a taco can be pureed in a blender), and the tendency of dairy products to increase secretions.

Liquids are the most difficult to swallow as they may pass quickly through the oropharyngeal passages and provide little sensory stimulation to elicit adequate motor control. Thickening liquids with gelatin or cereal may increase the viscosity sufficiently to permit adequate motor control. Proper hydration often requires continued nasogastric tube feedings. The increased sensory stimulation of carbonated beverages or very cold beverages may facilitate adequate motor control to prevent aspiration. (The advisability of hydration through carbonated beverages must be discussed with the physician, but do not be surprised to find Johnny easily downing a Coke during a visit with Mom and Dad and yet aspirating on milk for dinner.) Once a child can complete a meal in 30 minutes without aspiration, family members and/or nursing staff are instructed on proper positioning and simple facilitation techniques. Progressing the child to completing three meals a day orally may initially require supplemental feedings through a nasogastric tube.

Cognition and behavior often interfere with self-feeding even after adequate orofacial motor control and endurance are achieved. A short attention span and absent memory result in distractibility and confusion. The child may forget to swallow and be attending to other stimuli, but when reminded to swallow and redirected to the eating activity, can complete a meal. The confused child does not know that you drink from a cup and may put it on his or her head. The child may continually stuff food into the mouth, apparently forgetting that food has just been put into the mouth, and also forgetting to swallow. (A more highly textured diet or thermogustatory bolus may facilitate swallowing completion.) Supervision and structure initiated by the therapist may be carried through by the family or nurses to remind the child to swallow after each bite, not allow scooping more food from the plate before swallowing, and to structure him or her not to use the spoon when "eating" the milk or try to drink from the plate. If initiation and sequencing are a problem, appropriate assistance and supervision are provided. If upper extremity motor control does not preclude self-feeding, once a child reaches level II, initiating purposeful activities, necessary supervision, and assistance to permit successful self-feeding are preferred over passive feeding of the patient. Although one meal may take an hour to complete, self-feeding for at least one or, preferably, two meals is encouraged.

PARENT/CLIENT EDUCATION

Education of the parents during the acute and in-hospital rehabilitation phases of recovery involves the whole team. By the time of discharge, the parents must have accepted the role of primary therapist for all aspects of the child's behavior. The parents must implement the child's reintegration into society, the ultimate goal of rehabilitation. They must recognize the child's abilities and understand his or her disabilities, structuring the day and activities to meet the child's needs and eventually to nurture independence while continuing their own lives and caring for other family members.

Education of the family during the acute stage includes comprehension of the significance of the trauma and the prognosis expected. The inability of the neurosurgeon to accurately predict outcome 100 percent of the time adds to the confusion. The stages of grieving the family experiences often preclude actual hearing and understanding of explanations.

As the level of consciousness improves, hope is nurtured. Unrealistic expectations of recovery may interfere with therapeutic intervention and family education. Following evaluation of the child by each team member, a conference is held for team members and the child's parents. Each team member identifies his or her role in rehabilitation, the abilities and problems the child has at present, and the expected abilities at discharge from the hospital. Team members must explain the child's problems and reasons for expected discharge abilities (which are less than normal function) so that the family can begin to understand problems that will remain and become involved in the rehabilitation program.

Family educational programs involving several families, mediated by a social worker or psychologist, provide education and interaction with the child's therapists as well as supportive therapy from other families experiencing similar feelings and problems. Short slide presentations and discussions by each team member convey the role of that discipline in the child's rehabilitation, demonstrate the usual progression of improvement and therapeutic activities the child will experience, and define terms commonly used to identify cognitive problems and behaviors.

Although most families of young children have working parents, they are encouraged to spend an occasional day attending the child's therapy sessions. Nursing staff provide most of the ongoing education when the parents visit in the evenings. Assistance and supervision in play, self-care, and transfers are encouraged early in preparation for home therapeutic passes.

Home therapeutic passes usually begin when the child is eating, although training parents in nasogastric tube or gastric tube feeding permits earlier passes. Assistance and supervision in play, feeding, self-care, and mobility are practiced at home and updated weekly. Structural barriers and safety hazards are identified and solutions explored immediately to facilitate the discharge process.

As discharge approaches and adaptive equipment needs are identified, the family participates in choosing adaptive equipment and determining acceptable methods of mobility to assure carry over. By the time of discharge, the family understands the child's needs and is able to assist and progress his or her activities.

Follow-up as an outpatient is usually through clinic visits. Evaluation of neurologic recovery and improvement in play, socialization, speech, feeding, and mobility provides team members with information for further intervention and appropriate referrals to outside agencies or staff team members. As the child matures into an adult, needs change and residual problems cause effects in different ways. Continued follow-up assures family and child education to facilitate reintegration into society. Referral to appropriate community resources, such as special schools, school therapy units, vocational training centers, driver's training centers, health professionals, the National Head Injury Foundation (333 Turnpike Road, Southborough, MA 01772; telephone: 508/485-9950), and other nonprofit organizations, assists in meeting the needs of the family and client.

OTHER MANAGEMENT

The members of the rehabilitation team include a pediatrician, psychologist, social worker, nurses, occupational therapist, and speech therapist, with consultation by orthopedic surgeons, neurologists, and neurosurgeons. The roles of health team members vary according to the center, the team members available, and the strengths of the staff. I will briefly highlight the management characteristic of each professional at our center.

The speech pathologist assesses and treats the cognitive and language deficits. At levels IV and III, treatment is focused on facilitating responses and establishing a means of communication, beginning with indicating "yes" and "no" with a head nod or gesture. Increasing attention, concentration, visual discrimination, sequencing, categorization, memory, and orientation to time, self, and place are emphasized at level II. At level I, therapeutic activities encourage the development of skills in analysis and synthesis, judgment, problem solving, reasoning, and abstract thinking. The higher cognitive functions of decision making, judgment, and problem solving are usually not expected to recover by discharge and require constant supervision to assure the child's safety. Observation of performance in actual community situations is used to assess the child's ability and to identify deficits.

Specific speech production problems, linguistic function, auditory and visual reception and retention, hearing language formulation, and expression are tested. If deficits impair speech intelligibility, assistive communication modes such as word/picture boards are explored. Relearning of reading, spelling, and writing skills is initiated in the rehabilitation hospital and continued in the school setting.

Social workers, psychologists, speech pathologists, and psychiatrists may provide family counseling to deal with residual hyperactivity, lack of impulse control, low tolerance for frustration, aggressiveness, and poor social judgment. Psychologic testing identifies significant slowing of response, reduction in performance IQ compared with the preinjury state, and difficulty with auditory and visual perception, all of which markedly limit school performance. Only 30 percent in a series of 300 severely head-injured children had normal intelligence; however, 64 percent could benefit from an educational program.[24] Psychological testing prior to discharge assists with school placement.

Social worker intervention with families varies with the child's level of consciousness. Assessment of the family support system facilitates assisting family adjustment. Through individual and group mediums, initial intervention assists the family to cope with the devastating disruption to their lifestyle and the issue of life or death. Education on the rehabilitation process and the family's coping strategies attempts to shift them to coping day to day rather than trying to prepare for the long term. As the child recovers, the family responds on an emotional roller coaster of highs (as the child lives, wakes up, and progresses) and lows (as progress hits plateaus and residual physical, cognitive, and psychologic deficits, and behavioral changes are compared with preinjury identity). The social worker assists families to deal with their feelings, anxieties, frustrations, and depression in considering the child's reentry to home and the resultant threat to their lifestyle and marriage. As discharge approaches, families are informed of financial, school, mental health, regional center, and voluntary agency resources. The social worker and psychologist also assist other team members in coping with the family's and child's behaviors. Outpatient intervention assists the family and child in dealing with the child's inappropriate social behavior, social isolation, peer rejection, and low self-esteem to assist reintegration into society.

A nurse specializing in assisting the return to school coordinates the necessary testing and referrals to smooth the transition. As a liaison to the community, the nurse confers with the team members to identify proper school placement where appropriate therapy and educational needs can be met.

Occupational therapists and physical therapists work closely together. The occupational therapist emphasizes fine motor, self-care, and perceptual skills. Age-appropriate socialization and play skills are encouraged within the child's physical abilities. Social and play development, perceptual motor development, and daily living skills at home and in the community are impaired after a head injury. Activities and intervention to develop these skills to age-appropriate levels are continued in outpatient follow-up and therapy at school. Disabilities in these areas contribute to peer rejection, isolation, and poor self-esteem.

Ongoing evaluation and intervention by psychologists, speech pathologists, and physical and occupational therapists assist the child in successful reintegration into academia. Current research is aimed at identification of subtle deficits and appropriate management strategies to prevent the impressive social and academic problems often seen.[10,36,38,39,74] It has been said that people who suffer head injuries all too often "passed rehabilitation but failed real life."[38]

Case Study: J.J.

J.J. was 18 months old when he suffered a basilar skull fracture to the foramen magnum with brain stem contusion in an automobile versus pedestrian accident. Computed tomography scan demonstrated hemorrhage and edema in the cerebellar area. His GCS (initially 3–4) improved to 7–8 within 24 hours. The third day postinjury, his course was complicated by an infarct of the right middle cerebral artery.

By 9 days postinjury, J.J. demonstrated spontaneous movement of his right side and a generalized response to stimulation (level IV). At 3 weeks, he could eat half a jar of baby food when fed, turned when his name was called, and withdrew from pain (level III).

At 4 weeks postinjury, he was transferred to a rehabilitation hospital. Family interview revealed normal development premorbidly and an intact, supportive family. Communication disorders staff reported that he had phonation, but no communication (level III). He focused on a bright object and withdrew from a noxious stimulus. The occupational therapist reported the absence of self-care and play, no spontaneous movement of the left upper extremity, and increased tone in left shoulder, wrist, and finger flexors and forearm pronators. The physical therapist reported poor head and trunk control: he could not roll, maintain his head or trunk upright in sitting, or demonstrate balance reactions to tilting. In supine, he postured with his head rotated toward the right. His legs demonstrated spontaneous flexion pattern bilaterally with more frequent movement of the right. Spasticity was present in his plantar flexors; ankle dorsiflexion range of motion was limited to zero degrees bilaterally. J.J. appeared hypersensitive to touch, crying and squirming when touched or held. Tactile sensation was generally intact. Proprioception, presence of ataxia, or sensorimotor deficits could not be assessed because his movements were not purposeful. He demonstrated good oral control of food, with a functional swallow and gag. Initially, he demonstrated incoordination when drinking liquids, but this resolved within 2 days. Paresis of cranial nerves VI and VII was evident on the left.

Discharge goals were established with age-appropriate levels in fine motor, gross motor, adaptive and social skills, and residual deficits in left extremity motor control. Treatment emphasized improving head and trunk control by facilitating postural responses in supine, positioning in midline, increasing movement and awareness of the left side, decreasing hypersensitivity, and decreasing the delay and increasing the amount of time he could attend to stimulation. A reclined wheelchair back, wedged seat, head and trunk supports, and a lapboard provided adequate support for midline positioning.

By 5 weeks postinjury, J.J. was at level II, participating in play, feeding himself, and recognizing familiar people. Postural responses could be elicited in his head and trunk in supported sitting. By 6 weeks postinjury, he was beginning level I, initiating interaction with his environment. His restlessness had resolved. He could feed himself crackers and use a spoon and a cup. He could roll to the left, and maintain his head upright in supported sitting for short periods of time. Prone over a wedge, supporting on extended elbows, he could maintain neck extension for 30 seconds, but, supported on hands and knees, he could not lift his head. Supported on a tilt table, he could control his head and upper trunk.

By 11 weeks postinjury, J.J. could play when prone on elbows; in tailor sitting, he could play catch and cross midline challenging his equilibrium within a limited range. Receptive language was at the appropriate age level, while expressive language was mildly to moderately delayed.

By 18 weeks postinjury, his trunk control was adequate to get to sitting from supine, maintain sidesitting, scoot in sitting, and don his socks independently, although protective reactions were delayed and nonfunctional to the left and backward. He was assisted in pulling to stand and standing. A psychologist began to work with the family on coping with J.J.'s low frustration tolerance, agitation, and impulsivity.

Within a week, he could pull to stand with his right upper extremity and attempted to cruise. A mild hearing loss was diagnosed.

At 5 months postinjury, he was discharged home with intervention from physical and occupational therapists twice a week, a speech therapist three times a week, and a home-based infant program for the deaf and hard-of-hearing twice a week. Testing with the Gesell developmental test showed age-appropriate personal/social skills and minimally age-appropriate cognitive/adaptive and fine motor skills.

Equilibrium and protective responses were delayed and inadequate in his left lower extremity for independent standing. Tactile sensation on the left was impaired. He was discharged with a wheelchair, short-leg braces for stance stability, and a ring walker for upright mobility. On his clinic return in 1 month, he was maneuvering the ring walker well.

At 1 year postinjury, J.J. could ambulate with the left short-leg brace, but short attention span, distractibility, and left-sided neglect made him unsafe. His vocabulary had increased and he was putting two words together.

By 2.5 years postinjury, he could ambulate independently without his short-leg brace, although he demonstrated a collapsing tibia during stance and occasional toe drag during swing. Clonus remained present in his left plantar flexors and left lower extremity equilibrium reactions were delayed.

Case Study: A.W.

A.W. was 6 years old when she suffered a skull fracture, right femur fracture, and cerebral concussion in a motor vehicle versus pedestrian accident while crossing the street on her bicycle. Her GCS (initially 3) improved to 5 within 24 hours. Three days postinjury, she was at level III; she withdrew from painful stimulation. Two weeks postinjury, she was at level II; she could follow simple commands and was tolerating water and pureed food by mouth.

Five weeks postinjury, a cast brace was fitted to control her right femur fracture and she was transferred to a rehabilitation hospital. She was at level I, indicating yes and no by nodding her head and her age by holding up her fingers. Team evaluation found that her premorbid development was normal;

A.W. was living with her father, brother, and stepmother. Physical findings included paresis of the right facial nerve. Range of motion was normal and sensation was intact. Ataxia was evident in both upper extremities and her left lower extremity. She used her left upper extremity as her dominant arm, with impaired fine motor control and moderate ataxia. Her right upper extremity was used inconsistently as a gross assist. She demonstrated apraxia and neglect of the right upper extremity and had fair-plus strength with increased tone in her biceps, wrist, and finger flexor muscles.

A.W.'s neck and trunk strength was fair-plus, with ataxia apparent. Head-righting responses were present; equilibrium responses in sitting were delayed and exaggerated. Her left leg had good strength with minimal ataxia. Apraxia was apparent when trying to perform gross motor actions. She was assisted in rolling and coming to sit, but could sit independently with upper extremity support. She was unable to creep, crawl, kneel, or ambulate. She was assisted in self-feeding, hygiene, and grooming because of apraxia, ataxia, and cognitive impairment. She demonstrated moderately delayed cognitive and language deficits and severely reduced speech production, speaking in four to five-word sentences at a rate of one syllable per second. She was easily distracted by visual and auditory stimuli and had a severely impaired attention span.

Team goals for discharge were for A.W. to be an independent, household ambulator with equipment, independent in self-care with residual delay in play and school readiness skills, and a limited community communicator. Her program included a cognitive reorganization and language/speech program and therapeutic activity to improve motor control and function with appropriate equipment. Her family attended family evening classes to learn about brain injury and typical residual problems, as well as for group support. She had weekend passes within 3 weeks so that her family could carry over care at home in preparation for discharge.

Within a week, motor control had improved so that A.W. could roll and get to sitting independently. She could sit without hand support for 60 seconds; her neck muscles fatigued in 40 seconds when prone on elbows. She had less neglect of her right upper extremity and occasionally used it as her dominant hand. Weighted cuffs and stabilizing with her forearms improved her control for table activities; however, visual perceptual deficits were noted at this time. Her physical therapy included use of blow bottles to improve breath control, PNF activities to improve trunk control in rolling and sitting, and tilt table to begin weight-bearing.

By 2 months postinjury, apraxia and motor control had improved so that A.W. could feed herself with a regular spoon with her right arm and was age-appropriate in play. She was minimally assisted in dressing and hygiene due to ataxia. She could maintain her balance sitting astride a bolster for 5 minutes, but needed assistance to reach to the floor and recover; she was assisted in getting to hands and knees and maintaining that position. She could control her breath to produce a soft puff, hard puff, and sustained output for three seconds. Her receptive and expressive language skills and auditory sequencing were 1 year behind age level. Within the next 2 weeks, she could independently reach to the floor and recover in sitting with no hand support and began ambulating in the parallel bars with assistance.

At 12 weeks postinjury, the right fracture brace was removed. Knee flexion ROM was limited to 80 degrees. A.W.'s right lower extremity had fair-plus strength, except that plantar flexors were poor. She had minimal patterning and impaired proprioception.

By 3 months postinjury, A.W. was demonstrating more spontaneous emotional responses. Her receptive and expressive language skills were at age level and she was age-appropriate in personal/social skills and play activities. She could sustain exhalation for 5 seconds, during which she would speak 7 to 10 syllables. Her residual deficits at discharge included monopitch and slowed speech due to reduced breath control. She required cuing to complete her self-care, dressing, and feeding because of residual distractibility and decreased attention span, although physically she could perform the tasks independently. Residual ataxia, weakness in her lower extremities, and delayed balance reactions dictated the need for assistance in getting to standing and transferring. Double adjustable ankle–foot orthoses greatly improved her stance stability. She ambulated with standby assistance using a walker with front wheels for 30 meters at 19 percent of normal velocity. Her distractibility and poor judgment interfered with safety in walking, bathing, and toileting. She was discharged home with a wheelchair, grab bars, walker with front wheels, double adjustable ankle joint ankle–foot orthoses, and a helmet. She received speech and physical therapy three times a week in a school setting for the orthopedically handicapped.

At 7 months postinjury, A.W.'s ataxia had diminished significantly so that she ambulated at home with only her ankle–foot orthoses. In the community, she required assistance on stairs and uneven surfaces because of residual ataxia and impaired balance responses of the right lower extremity. She had a wide-based gait, had difficulty catching and kicking a ball, and was unable to run, jump, balance on one leg, or hop. Hyperactive reflexes were still present in her right extremities.

At 1 year postinjury, A.W. ambulated at school independently using the ankle–foot orthoses and at home without them. Mild ataxia and muscle weakness (fair-plus plantar flexors and hip abductors) remained. Speech therapy continued at school.

By 1.5 years postinjury (7.5 years old), A.W. had good strength throughout both lower extremities and could run and jump, but she could not hop or tandem walk. Mild ataxia was noted. Her speech rate and prosody remained somewhat diminished. She was transferred to a special education program in a regular school setting. Her school work was between first- and second-grade level.

REFERENCES

1. Raphaely RC, Swedlow DB, Downes JJ et al: Management of severe pediatric head trauma. Pediatr Clin North Am 27:715, 1980
2. Brink JD, Garrett AL, Hale WR et al: Recovery of motor and intellectual functions in children sustaining severe head injuries. Dev Med Child Neurol 12:565, 1972

3. Bruce DA, Schut L, Bruno LA et al: Outcome following severe head injuries in children. J Neurosurg 48:679, 1978
4. Cartlidge NEF, Shaw DA: Head Injury. p. 213. In Walton Sir JN (ed): Major Problems in Neurology. Vol. 10. WB Saunders, Philadelphia, 1981
5. Mayer T, Walker ML, Johnson DG et al: Causes of morbidity and mortality in severe pediatric trauma. JAMA 245:719, 1981
6. Gilchrist E, Wilkinson M: Some factors determining prognosis in young people with severe head injuries. Arch Neurol 36:355, 1979
7. Goldstein FC, Levin HS: Epidemiology of pediatric closed head injury: incidence, clinical characteristics and risk factors. J Learning Dis 20:518, 1987
8. Bruce DA: Head injuries in the pediatric population. Curr Probl Pediatr 10:67, 1990
9. Eiben CF, Anderson TP, Lockman L, et al: Functional outcome of closed head injury in children and young adults. Arch Phys Med Rehabil 65:168, 1984
10. Kraus JF, Fife D, Conroy C: Pediatric brain injuries: the nature, clinical course and early outcomes in a defined United States population. Pediatrics 79:501, 1987
11. Humphreys RP: Outcome of severe head injury in children. Concepts Pediatr Neurosurg 3:191, 1983
12. Wagstyll J, et al: Early prediction of outcome following head injury in children. J Pediatr Surg 22:127, 1987
13. Jennett B: Head injuries in children. Dev Med Child Neurol 14:137, 1972
14. Ommaya AK: Head injuries: aspects and problems. Med Ann DC 32:18, 1963
15. Carlsson C-A, von Essen C, Löfgren J: Factors affecting the clinical course of patients with severe head injuries. J Neurosurg 29:242, 1968
16. St. James-Roberts J: Neurological plasticity, recovery from brain insult, and child development. Adv Child Dev Behav 14:253, 1979
17. Hardman JM: The pathology of traumatic brain injuries. Adv Neurol 22:15, 1979
18. Bruce DA, Schut L: The value of CAT scanning following pediatric head injury. Clin Pediatr (Phila) 19:719, 1980
19. Brink JD, Imbus C, Woo-Sam J: Physical recovery after severe closed head trauma in children and adolescents. J Pediatr 97:721, 1980
20. Morley TP: Some considerations of head injury. Postgrad Med 22:53, 1957
21. Ommaya AK: Trauma to the nervous system. Ann R Coll Surg Engl 39:317, 1966
22. Miller JD: Pathophysiology of human head injury. p. 507. In Becker DP, Gudeman SK (eds): Textbook of Head Injury. WB Saunders, Philadelphia, 1989
23. Shetter AG, Demakas JJ: The pathophysiology of concussion: a review. Adv Neurol 22:5, 1979
24. Hoffer M, Brink J, Marsh JS et al: Head injuries. In Lovell WW, Winter RB (eds): Pediatric Orthopaedics. JB Lippincott, Philadelphia, 1990
25. Clifton GL, McCormick WF, Grossman RG: Neuropathology of early and late deaths after head injury. Neurosurgery 8:309, 1981
26. Bruce DA, Alavi A, Bilaniuk L et al: Diffuse cerebral swelling following head injuries in children: the syndrome of "malignant brain edema." J Neurosurg 54:170, 1981
27. Miller JD, Butterworth JF, Grudeman SK et al: Further experience in the management of severe head injury. J Neurosurg 54:289, 1981
28. Ommaya AK, Gennarelli TA: Cerebral concussion and traumatic unconsciousness. Brain 97:633, 1974
29. Dimitrijevic MR: Restorative neurology of head injury. J Neurotrauma 6:25, 1989
30. Gennarelli TA, Thibalt LE, Adams JH et al: Diffuse axonal injury and traumatic coma in the primate. Ann Neurol 12:564, 1982
31. Greenberg RP, Newlon PG, Hyatt MS et al: Prognostic implications of early mul-

timodality evoked potentials in severely head-injured patients: a prospective study. J Neurosurg 55:227, 1981

32. Teasdale G, Jennett B: Assessment of coma and impaired consciousness. Lancet 2:81, 1974

33. Tubokawa T: Assessment of brainstem damage by the auditory brainstem response in acute severe head injury. J Neurol Neurosurg Psychiatry 43:1005, 1980

34. Chiappa KH, Gladstone KJ, Young RR: Brain stem auditory evoked responses. Arch Neurol 36:81, 1979

35. Meyler WJ, Bakker H, Kok JJ et al: The effect of dantrolene sodium in relation to blood levels in spastic patients after prolonged administration. J Neurol Neurosurg Psychiatry 44:334, 1981

36. Klonoff H, Low MD, Clark C: Head injuries in children: a prospective five year follow-up. J Neurol Neurosurg Psychiatry 40:1211, 1977

37. Jennett B, Snoek J, Bond MR et al: Disability after severe head injury: observations on the use of Glasgow Outcome Scale. J Neurol Neurosurg Psychiatry 44:285, 1981

38. Telzrow CF: Management of academic and educational problems in head injury. J Learn Dis 20:536, 1987

39. Ewing-Cobbs L, Fletcher JM: Neuropsychological assessment of head injury in children. J Learning Dis 20:526, 1987

40. Jennett B, Bond M: Assessment of outcome after severe brain damage: a practical scale. Lancet 1:480, 1975

41. Young B, Rapp RP, Norton JA et al: Early prediction of outcome in head-injured patients. J Neurosurg 54:300, 1981

42. Filley CM, Cranberg LD, Alexander MP et al: Neurobehavioral outcome after closed head injury in childhood and adolescence. Arch Neurol 44:194, 1987

43. Mayer T, Walker ML, Shasha I et al: Effect of multiple trauma on outcome of pediatric patients with neurologic injuries. Child Brain 8:189, 1981

44. Mayer T, Matlak ME, Johnson DG, Walker ML: The modified injury severity scale in pediatric multiple trauma patients. J Pediatr Surg 15:719, 1980

45. Malkmus D: Integrating cognitive strategies into the physical therapy setting. Phys Ther 63:1952, 1983

46. Horak FB: Clinical measurement of postural control in adults. Phys Ther 67:1881, 1987

47. Shumway-Cook A, Horak FB: Assessing the influence of sensory interaction on balance: suggestion from the field. Phys Ther 66:1548, 1986

48. Montgomery J: Assessment and treatment of locomotor deficits in stroke. In Duncan P, Badke MB (eds): Stroke Rehabilitation: The Recovery of Motor Control. Year Book Medical Publishers, Chicago, 1987

49. Kigin CM: Chest physical therapy for the postoperative or traumatic injury patient. Phys Ther 61:1724, 1981

50. Ciesla N, Klemic N, Imle PC: Chest physical therapy to the patient with multiple trauma. Phys Ther 61:202, 1981

51. Hammon WE, Martin RJ: Chest physical therapy for acute atelectasis. Phys Ther 61:217, 1981

52. Lazarus C, Logemann JA: Swallowing disorders in closed head trauma patients. Rehabilitation 68:79, 1987

53. Robinson RO: Equal recovery in child and adult brain? Dev Med Child Neurol 23:379, 1981

54. Bishop DVM: Plasticity and specificity of language localization in the developing brain. Dev Med Child Neurol 23:251, 1981

55. Robinson RO: Plasticity and specificity of language localization in the developing brain. Dev Med Child Neurol 23:387, 1981
56. Goldman PM: Plasticity of function in the CNS. In Stein DG, Rosen JJ, Butters N (eds): Plasticity and Recovery of Function in the CNS. Academic Press, San Diego, 1974
57. Geschwind N: Late changes in the nervous system: an overview. In Stein DG, Rosen JJ, Butters N (eds): Plasticity and Recovery of Function in the CNS. Academic Press, San Diego, 1974
58. Carr JH, Shepherd RB: Physiotherapy in Disorders of the Brain. Heinemann, London, 1980
59. Riolo-Quinn L: Motor learning considerations in treating brain injured patients. Neurol Rep 14:12, 1990
60. Winstein C, Thompson S, Briggs D et al: Treatment techniques of gaining motor control. In Professional Staff Association of Rancho Los Amigos Hospital: Rehabilitation of the Head Injured Adult. Comprehensive Physical Management, Downey, CA, 1979
61. Hoffer MM, Garrett A, Brink JD et al: The orthopedic management of the brain-injured children. J Bone Joint Surg 53A:567, 1971
62. Zachazewski JE, Eberle ED, Jefferies M: Effect of tone-inhibiting casts and orthoses on gait. Phys Ther 62:453, 1982
63. Benton LA, Baker LL, Bowman BR et al: General uses of electrical stimulation. In Professional Staff Associates of Rancho Los Amigos Hospital. Functional Electrical Stimulation Workshop, Downey, CA, 1979
64. Bobath K, Bobath B: The facilitation of normal postural reactions and movements in the treatment of cerebral palsy. Physiotherapy 50:246, 1964
65. Goldberger ME: Recovery of movements after CNS lesions in monkeys. p. 235. In Stein DG, Rosen JJ, Butters N (eds): Plasticity and Recovery of Function in the CNS. Academic Press, San Diego, 1974
66. Nelson JR: Neuro-otologic aspects of head injury. Adv Neurol 22:107, 1979
67. Safranek MG, Koshland GF, Raymond G: Effect of auditory rhythm on muscle activity. Phys Ther 62:161, 1982
68. Couper JL: Dance therapy: effects on motor performance of children with learning disabilities. Phys Ther 61:23, 1981
69. Baum B, Hall KM: Relationship between constructional praxis and dressing in the head-injured adult. Am J Occup Ther 35:438, 1981
70. Becker E, Bar-Or O, Mendelson L et al: Pulmonary functions and responses to exercise of patients following craniocerebral injury. Scand J Rehabil Med 10:47, 1978
71. Campbell SK: Neural control of oral somatic motor function. Phys Ther 61:16, 1981
72. Silverman EH, Elfant IL: Dysphagia: an evaluation and treatment program for the adult. Am J Occup Ther 33:382, 1979
73. Winstein C: Evaluation and management of swallowing dysfunction. In Professional Staff Associates of Rancho Los Amigos Hospital: Rehabilitation of the Head Injured Adult. Comprehensive Physical Management, Downey, CA, 1979
74. Oddy M, Humphrey M: Social recovery during the year following severe head injury. J Neurol Neurosurg Psychiatry 43:798, 1980

9 | Children with Severe and Profound Retardation

Karen Yundt Lunnen

There is increasing recognition that retarded individuals are more like us than they are different; that they need, just as we all do, love, joy, activity, a chance to grow and progress, and a chance, wherever possible, to become independent.[1]

Senator Hubert H. Humphrey

The most widely accepted definition of mental retardation is that adopted by the American Association on Mental Retardation (AAMR): ". . . significantly subaverage intellectual functioning existing concurrently with deficits in adaptive behavior and manifested during the developmental period."[2] (The developmental period had been interpreted as being from birth until the 18th birthday, but is now thought to begin at conception.) Put another way, retardation is the result of conditions that prevent, reduce, or delay the development of effective ways of interacting with the environment. "Mental retardation is the number one health problem affecting children today."[3]

CLASSIFICATION OF MENTAL RETARDATION

There is considerable controversy about the classification of individuals with mental retardation, the validity of the intelligence quotient (IQ), and the effects of labeling. IQ testing is an adequate measurement of cognitive ability (short-term memory, reasoning, etc), but it is more difficult to objectively measure the influence of achievement, motivation, and personality/temperament.

251

Table 9-1. Intellectual Classification Based on Standardized Test Scores[2] and Percentage of All Retarded Persons in Each Category[1]

Level of Retardation	Approximate Percentage of All Retarded Persons	Quotient Range	
		Cattell or Stanford-Binet	Wechsler
Mild	89	52–68	55–69
Moderate	7	36–51	40–54
Severe	3	20–35	25–39
Profound	1	0–19	0–24

Despite its difficulties, however, "classification of exceptional children is essential to get services to them."[4] The definition adopted by the AAMR at least dictated that classification be based on intelligence *and* adaptive behavior, thus expanding the concept of mental retardation to include more than just intellectual functioning.

Intellectual classification is based on a quotient determined by standardized testing (usually Stanford-Binet, Cattell, or Wechsler Scales). Those scoring below 70 are classified as mentally retarded, with subgroupings of increasing severity established at increments of standard deviation units below the normative mean of 100 (one standard deviation being 15 or 16 points, depending on the test). Table 9-1 presents the usual classification system and also gives the approximate percentage of all retarded persons in each category.

The AAMR has provided general guidelines for the adaptive behavior classification, and many adaptive behavior rating scales have been published. The appropriateness of any behavior, of course, varies with age. Table 9-2 presents a summary of an adaptive behavior classification for individuals who are severely and profoundly retarded based on the AAMRs expanded definition of mental retardation.

A variety of behaviors are considered to be reflective of intelligence: "the ability to learn and profit from experience . . . the ability to reason . . . the ability to adapt to changing conditions . . . and the will to succeed."[5] It is important to keep in mind that each of these areas will be affected when intelligence is impaired.

ETIOLOGY AND PATHOLOGY OF MENTAL RETARDATION

Known, discrete causes of mental retardation are found in only a small percentage of cases, although significantly more of the children with IQ levels less than 50 have an identifiable etiology than those with higher IQ levels.

Table 9-2. Adaptive Behavior Classification (Severe and Profound)[a]

Severe: Such persons require continuing and close supervision, but may perform self-help and simple work tasks under supervision (dependent).
Profound: Such persons require continuing and close supervision for survival, but some may be able to perform simple self-help tasks. Often have associated handicaps.

[a] Summarized from the expanded definition of mental retardation of the AAMR.[2]

Treatment strategies are seldom dependent on etiology, and etiology is notably absent from the AAMR definition of mental retardation, but it can be important in the prevention of future cases.

Over 200 conditions are known to cause retardation. In general, these conditions include genetic defects in the developing embryo, environmental deprivation in early childhood, or disease/damage to the central nervous system (CNS; including metabolic and nutritional disorders, physical insult, hypoxia, infections, and intoxications).[3] It is believed that greater than 50 percent of the known causes of mental retardation are preventable, and prevention is a major theme of the President's Committee on Mental Retardation.[3]

In a study of children with severe mental retardation, Gustavson and associates[6] reported that mean gestational age and birth weights were lower than in average newborns. They also determined that at this level of mental retardation, the insult occurred prenatally in 69 percent, perinatally in 8 percent, postnatally in 1 percent, and at an unknown age in 22 percent.

Intelligence is a polygenic phenomenon; in other words, at least 10 pairs of genes, and probably more, determine intelligence. With severe and profound levels of retardation, there are almost always diffuse brain abnormalities and neurologic insult. Serious physical handicaps and deficits in physical growth (stunting of skeletal development) frequently accompany mental retardation, with the frequency and severity roughly proportional to the degree of IQ deficit.[7] One study reported autopsies conducted on 1,410 individuals with severe or profound retardation over a 14-year period and found that 97.5 percent had neurologic damage.[8]

Conley[9] states that almost 95 percent of individuals with IQ levels less than 30 and almost 78 percent of those individuals with IQ levels between 30 and 55 suffer from at least one major physically handicapping condition. Among the severely and profoundly retarded, the handicaps are proportionately more common and more severe. Capute and associates[10] examined the major presenting symptoms of children at a nonresidential facility who were mentally retarded and found them to be (1) overall slowness, (2) motor disability, (3) language disorder, and (4) behavioral disturbances. Correspondingly, those who were profoundly mentally retarded had mortality rates 50 percent higher than those with severe mental retardation.[11]

There are many theories and considerable controversy about the development of individuals who are retarded compared with those with normal intelligence.[12] Weisz and Zigler developed one of the more popular theories, the "similar sequence hypothesis" based on Piagetian concepts.[13] The hypothesis holds that "during development retarded and nonretarded persons traverse the same stages in precisely the same order and differ only in the rate of development and in the ultimate ceiling they attain." Some theorists believe that the hypothesis is valid only for those persons who are not retarded or have cultural–familial retardation, thus, in essence, proposing a different sequence of cognitive development for individuals who are severely or profoundly retarded and who may have brain damage or genetic impairment. Weisz and Zigler, however, drew evidence from three longitudinal and 28 cross-sectional studies of developmental phenomena described by Piaget and found that the evidence supported their hypothesis with respect to every subject group, with the "possible exception of individuals with pronounced electroencephalogram abnormalities."

Children who are severely and profoundly retarded reach an ultimate mental age of less than 6 years and the profoundly retarded never progress out of Piaget's sensorimotor period. These children will always need supervision and, because of associated handicaps, they seldom achieve independence in activities of daily living.

SOCIAL POLICIES AND PROGRAMS

Public awareness, political support, and legal action are important for progress in the management of mental retardation. A historic perspective on these issues is necessary to understand the direction of current programs for the mentally retarded. Several informative publications are the *President's Committee on Mental Retardation: A Historical Review* (1966 to 1985),[14] Rosen's *The History of Mental Retardation* (Volumes I and II),[15] and Scheerenberger's *A History of Mental Retardation*.[16] President Kennedy's appointment in 1961 of a panel of experts to make recommendations for national action to combat mental retardation was the beginning of new social and political awareness that resulted in a dramatic surge in activity related to treatment, research, education, and legal action.

The so-called normalization movement of the 1970s was a concerted attempt to end the segregation of mentally retarded individuals in large state institutions and had its roots in political, social, and legal activities. Special education programs were among the recommendations of President Kennedy's panel in 1963. However, more dramatic in its impact and the legal direction it provided was Public Law 94-142, "The Education for All Handicapped Children Act of 1975,"[17] which guaranteed the availability of special education programming to handicapped children and youth who require it. The basic tenets of this law were expanded to cover the younger age groups (0 to 5 years) via Public Law 99-457, "Education of the Handicapped Act Amendments of 1986," which is in the process of implementation at the state level.[18] Congressional intent to streamline services to the developmentally disabled is detailed in the "Developmental Disabilities Assistance and Bill of Rights Act" of 1984,[19] and broad guarantees of access are guaranteed in the "Americans With Disabilities Act of 1990."[20]

There are many groups, both governmental and nongovernmental, that have a significant impact on the population of mentally retarded citizens in the United States. Several deserve mention as they can provide valuable resources for professionals:

Association for Retarded Citizens (National Headquarters, PO Box 6109, Arlington, TX 76011), the largest national voluntary health organization, comprised of over 300,000 parents, educators, and professionals (organized in 1950). Influential as a political lobby group for public policy issues. (Telephone: (817) 640-0204)

American Association on Mental Retardation, previously the American Association on Mental Deficiency (1719 Kalorama Rd NW, Washington, DC 20009), a multidisciplinary organization of professional practitioners and researchers. Responsible for the publication of the research journal, *American Journal of Mental Deficiency*; the *AAMR Monograph Series*; and the *Manual on Terminology and Classification in Mental Retardation*. (Telephone: (202) 387-1968)

Council for Exceptional Children (1920 Association Dr, Reston, VA 22091), comprised of approximately 70,000 teachers. Has made significant contributions to the education of the mentally retarded. (Telephone: (703) 620-3660)

President's Committee on Mental Retardation (US Department of Health and Human Services, Washington, DC 20201), established by executive order in May 1966 with a mandated function of providing assistance and advice concerning mental retardation to the President. Annual reports and other publications are available to the public. (Telephone: (202) 245-7634)

MEDICAL MANAGEMENT

Neurobiologic factors are the primary cause of severe and profound retardation and it is logical that medical problems would be concurrent. If one uses a functional definition of health, it is often hard to diagnose poor health among the severely handicapped and difficult to judge whether a specific treatment will improve the quality of life for these individuals. Severe medical complications accompanying mental retardation are a major concern in planning residential environments and other services.[21]

Dental Care

Prophylactic care and management of dental problems is seldom mentioned in the literature but is a critical component of comprehensive medical care and one frought with difficulties. Few dentists specialize in pediatrics, and even fewer specialize in the special problems of the mentally retarded. Third-party payers like Medicaid reimburse approximately one-eighth to one-third of the regular fee charged in the average dental office, so a growing number of dentists refuse to even accept Medicaid patients.[22] Sedation or total anesthesia is often necessary to perform even routine work and reimbursement is minimal or non-existent. Lack of incentives and countless roadblocks impede the provision of adequate dental care to individuals who are mentally retarded.

Orthopedic Surgery

Orthopedic intervention with the child who is multiply handicapped must be "long range continuum care" rather than "episodic" because of the complexity of the problems and the necessity of considering a multitude of contributing factors.[23] Three phases of orthopedic treatment are prevention, control/support, and correction. Fraser and colleagues[23] review these various treatment phases for spinal curvatures and upper and lower extremity deformities. Another comprehensive resource on the subject of orthopedic surgery in the mentally retarded is *Orthopedic Clinics of North America* (Vol. 12, 1981). The question arises whether the potential benefits of orthopedic surgery are worth the risks. Hoffer and Bullock[24] estimate that the length of hospital stay for the severely mentally retarded is two to four times longer than normal, and the rehabilitation period is complicated by the patient's inability to comprehend what has occurred or to cooperate maximally.

Pettitt[25] listed what she believed to be the legitimate reasons for considering surgery for the severely mentally retarded: (1) alleviation of pain, (2) improvement of posture for wheelchair mobilization, and (3) increased ease of nursing care. Lindsey and Drennan[26] would add to that list the achievement or maintenance of ambulation.

Drug Therapy

"One of the most heavily medicated segments of our society is the mentally retarded people who live in public institutions or community residence facilities."[27] The use of medication to moderate or alter behavior, to control seizure activity, and to manage a wide variety of concurrent medical problems is often a necessity in this population, but considerable controversy exists.

One topic that has received much attention in the past few years is psychopathology in mentally retarded children and youth. "Without exception, studies on prevalence of psychopathology in mentally retarded persons have shown rates much higher than the general population."[28] Some studies indicate that as many as 50 percent of the children who are severely and profoundly retarded can be viewed as emotionally disturbed. One approach to treatment of psychopathology is the use of neuroleptic drugs, which control behavior by general sedation and tranquilization. There are many side effects, including tardive dyskinesia.

Medications used to control seizure activity (anticonvulsants or antiepilectics) are another common type of drug therapy used with this population. In a study by Richardson and colleagues,[29] almost half of the individuals with an IQ of less than 50 had experienced one or more seizures by the age of 22, most occurring during the first year of life. Anticonvulsants are powerful central nervous system depressants whose side effects can include paresthesias, drowsiness, anorexia, nausea, dizziness, ataxia, tremors, nystagmus, diplopia, lethargy, irritability, and nervousness.[30] Because so many of these side effects can interfere with psychomotor development, knowledge about drug use is an important part of obtaining a medical history. A problem that is common but frequently neglected is nutrient–drug interactions. For example, seizure medications can interfere with the absorption of folic acid, other B vitamins, and vitamin D.

Nutrition

Altering diet or using nutritional supplements to affect the actual intellectual functioning or behaviors of the mentally retarded is an area of continuing controversy. Critics maintain that the results have been exaggerated and the treatments turned into a profitable market directed at families who are clutching at any offering of hope. Proponents speak to the relatively harmless side effects of a basic approach they believe is proven effective. Harrell and associates[31] maintain that nutritional supplements can improve both the IQ scores and functioning of some severely mentally retarded children. They conducted a partially double-blind experiment with 16 retarded children (initial IQ levels ranging from 17 to 70) who were given nutritional supplements or placebos over an 8-month period. Those children receiving supplements had statistically significant increases in their IQ scores when compared with those on placebos. The researchers had particular success with Down syndrome and believe that their results support the hypothesis that mental retardation is in part a genotrophic disease.

Hitchings[32] reported several case studies in which the basic diet was changed to one high in protein and low in carbohydrates and supplemented with megadoses of vitamins and minerals. His clinical impression was that this treatment approach is beneficial for children with autism, schizophrenia, brain damage, and the learning disabilities that may arise as a result of these disorders.

A good basic review of the literature on the advocacy of additive-free diets for hyperkinetic children (popularized by Feingold) is presented by Mailman and Lewis,[33] who are skeptical about the benefits. They stated that there was no significant difference noted in well-controlled studies. Along similar lines, Pollitt[34] reported no effects of sugar on either normal children or children with attention-deficit disorders except possibly in preschool children.

Good basic nutrition is important for mentally retarded children, however, and can be a problem area because of associated problems with feeding.

PHYSICAL THERAPY ASSESSMENT

Physical therapy assessment of the child who is multiply handicapped and severely or profoundly retarded must be comprehensive and as objective as possible. Flexibility in assessment must be maintained in order to recognize and appropriately adapt to behavioral problems, unique or absent communication, and limited capacity to cooperate. Several approaches to assessment of the child with neurologic impairment are covered in other chapters and are applicable to this population. In this section we will review assessment tools that are particularly useful for the severely and profoundly retarded populations and discuss characteristic problem areas that must be considered when conducting a definitive assessment. For organizational purposes, various aspects of the assessment are discussed separately, but these various functions cannot, and should not, be isolated.

Background Information

It is essential to obtain a general knowledge base by reviewing available records and talking with family members, teachers, and other important individuals who interact with the child. These children are an emotional strain on the best of families. What is the structure of the basic family unit and what attitudes are displayed by various members? Multiple problems often make them eligible for a variety of services and programs. What agencies are involved? In what programs is the child participating? For what services and financial support systems is the child eligible?

What medical care has the child received, and by whom? Is there a history of seizures and, if so, what type? Are the seizures controlled with medication or is the child on any other type of medication? Have side effects from these medications been observed? Is there evidence of recurrent problems as one reviews the medical history? For example, recurrent pneumonia is a red flag to carefully assess oral motor function and feeding behaviors. Has there been surgical intervention for physical deformities or other problems? Have hearing and vision been evaluated, and with what result? What equipment is available for the child's use and how is it being used?

Obtaining accurate and complete information in areas such as these provides the basis for planning a comprehensive assessment.

Communication

It would seem, at times, that the specialty skill one needs most in pediatrics is the ability to establish sufficient rapport to gain the cooperation of the child in performing activities and allowing handling or positioning. Carenza[35] compiled a book of strategies successful in gaining the cooperation of children for medical examination and cleverly entitled it *Pediatricks*. Because expressive and receptive communication skills are often absent or delayed, and behavioral problems are common among the severely and profoundly mentally retarded, it is important to obtain information about the child in these areas prior to testing. Are there characteristic behaviors, reinforcement schedules, or communication aids developed for the child that should be used to facilitate cooperation? The reliability and validity of the assessment may depend on how effectively behaviors are managed and communication established.

Encouraging imitation is one of the "tricks" sometimes used to gain co-operation from children, but it is fairly well-documented that individuals with severe retardation lack spontaneous imitative behavior, although they can be trained to copy the behavior of others.[36] This may be directly attributable to diminished intelligence, to sensory deficits, or to some experiential concomitant of retardation, such as institutionalization[37]; it also may be the result of per-ceptual inconsistency and the subsequent difficulty of distinguishing self from the outside world.[38]

Language problems in the mentally retarded are four times as common as in the general population, and the frequency and severity are generally inversely proportional to IQ.[10] Difficulties with language may be caused by the cognitive deficits or by associated neurophysiologic problems.

Piaget[39] believed that cognitive structures necessary for development of meaningful expressive language are not present until an individual is functioning at stage 6 of the sensorimotor period, and many individuals with profound retardation function below this level. Piaget based this belief on the premise that no mental images are formed during stages 1 through 5 of sensorimotor imitation. Research by Kahn,[40] who compared the language abilities of pro-foundly retarded persons with their sensorimotor level of function (as tested with the Uzgiris-Hunt Ordinal Scales of Psychological Development) supported Piaget's hypothesis.

Many nonverbal children have been instructed in alternative modes of communication. Nonspeech communication modes used with the mentally re-tarded include mime, manual sign language, Blissymbolics, or a variety of communication boards.[40] Basic familiarity with these systems is strongly rec-ommended for anyone working with children with severe or profound retar-dation.[41,42]

Assessment Instruments

One of the outcomes of legislation in behalf of the mentally retarded pop-ulation (specifically Public Law 94-142) is that it provided legal direction and guidelines for the assessment of handicapped children. It is mandated that testing be "multifactored" and that tests and other evaluation procedures used in a multifactored evaluation must "have been validated for the specific purpose for which they are used."[17] The intent of this section is to assure more com-prehensive and valid assessment of the multiply handicapped, severely or pro-foundly retarded population, for whom previous testing, if it was done at all, was a hodgepodge of modified instruments originally designed for a less se-verely involved group, resulting in marked discrepancies.[42]

Several resources are available that provide annotated listings of assess-ment programs for the multihandicapped child.[43-45] Some of the tests designed specifically for the severely or profoundly retarded population are listed below:

1. *Adaptive Behavior Curriculum: Prescriptive Behavior Analyses for Moderately, Severely and Profoundly Handicapped Students* (Popovich and Laham, 1982): a curriculum of 3,500 behavioral objectives, designed primarily for use by teachers (Paul H Brooks Publishing Co., PO Box 10624, Baltimore, MD 21204).

2. *AAMD Adaptive Behavior Scales* (Nihara et al., 1975): provides information on adaptive behavior functioning in 12 essential categories of daily living (Pro-Ed, 8700 Shoal Creek Blvd, Austin, TX 78758).

3. *Balthazar Scales of Adaptive Behavior* (Balthazar, 1976): appropriate for assessing ambulatory severely or profoundly retarded individuals aged 5 to 57 years. Scales on functional independence and social (coping) behaviors (Research Press Company, 2612 North Mattis Ave, Champaign, IL 61820).

4. *Bayley Scales of Infant Development* (Bayley, 1969): useful for young children who are severely or profoundly retarded. Naglieri[46] has extrapolated the developmental indices below 50 for the lower functioning group. For additional reference, Haskett and Bell[47] discuss the descriptive and theoretic utility of the Bayley Mental Scale for the severely and profoundly retarded (The Psychological Corporation, 757 Third Ave, New York, NY 10017).

5. *Behavior Rating Inventory for the Retarded* (Sparrow and Cicchetti, 1978): assesses skills in areas of communication, self-help, and physical and social behavior (Child Study Center, Department of Psychology, 333 Cedar St, New Haven, CT 06511).

6. *Camelot Behavioral Checklist* (Foster, 1974): checklist of 339 behavioral objectives arranged in age-expectancy order, all ages (Camelot Behavioral Systems, PO Box 3447, Lawrence, KS 66044).

7. *Gestural Approach to Thought and Expression, An Index of Non-verbal Communication and Its Critical Prerequisites* (Langley, 1968): data regarding the child's communication system, collected in a variety of natural settings, from birth to 36 months (Box 158, Child Study Center, Peabody College for Teachers, Nashville, TN 37203).

8. *Prescriptive Behavioral Checklist for the Severely and Profoundly Retarded* (Popovich, 1977): checklist ratings on motor development, eye-hand coordination, and physical eating problems (University Park Press, Baltimore, MD 21202).

9. *Programmatic Guide to Assessing Severely/Profoundly Retarded* (Crebo and Heifetz, 1981): provides information in self-help, communication, gross motor, sensory discrimination, preacademics, and prereading (Experimental Educational Unit, WJ-10, Child Development and Mental Retardation Center, University of Washington, Seattle, WA 98195).

10. *TMR Performance Profile for the Severely and Moderately Retarded*: scales in the areas of social behavior, self-care, communication, basic knowledge, practical skills, and body usage for severely multihandicapped children (Educational Performance Associates, 563 Westview Ave, Ridgefield, NJ 07657).

11. *Vulpe Assessment Battery* (Vulpe, 1969): performance analysis and developmental assessment in basic senses and functions, gross and fine motor

behaviors, language behavior, cognitive processes, organizational behaviors, activities of daily living, and assessment of the environment (National Institute on Mental Retardation, Ontario, Canada).

Motor Development

Many of the published assessments for the severely and profoundly retarded include a motor performance checklist, which is essentially a yes/no format for accomplishment of the basic motor milestones. What the physical therapist can and must contribute to completion of that checklist is a description of motor behaviors and deductive reasoning as to the causes of delays. The physical therapist's role is analysis of the contribution to deficient sensorimotor performance being made by behavior, motivation, cognition, perception, strength, muscle tone, contractures, joint limitation, or reflexes.

Reports in the literature vary about the extent of motor deficit in mentally retarded persons. The variability seems to exist, however, because of inconsistencies in what is meant by the term *mental retardation*. It is important to determine the level(s) of retardation being discussed (i.e., mild, moderate) or specific excluded subgroups (e.g., those with neurologic dysfunction). In general, research indicates delays in sensorimotor development among the mentally retarded—the extent of the delay roughly paralleling the extent of intellectual impairment.[48,49]

Reflex Development

A comprehensive reflex assessment is essential because the often extensive brain damage may be manifested in the persistence of primitive reflexes that interfere with normal development and predispose to asymmetries in muscle tone, sometimes leading to serious deformity.[50] Recognition of a child's inability to suppress the effect of primitive reflexes on motor behavior can be the key to making appropriate recommendations about positioning, handling, the use of adaptive equipment, and general treatment.

Muscle Tone

The tonus of muscles must be carefully evaluated and some judgments made as to the interference of abnormal tone with functional abilities and how this contributes to musculoskeletal deformity. Because primitive reflexes can greatly influence tone and movement,[51] assessment should be based on observation and handling of the child in a variety of positions and postures. Hypotonia is a common characteristic of the severely mentally retarded population when cerebral palsy (CP) and other defined neuromusculoskeletal problems are excluded.

Muscle Strength and Function

It is very difficult to test muscle strength with any objectivity in the severely and profoundly retarded. One must extrapolate muscle capabilities from observation of general motor activity and posture.

Joint Range of Motion and Muscle Length

The functional mobility of each joint should be carefully assessed as well as the length of key muscle groups. Awareness of problems in these areas can prevent serious deformity later.

Samilson[50] investigated the incidence of hip subluxation or dislocation among individuals who were severely involved, neurologically immature, or developmentally retarded and found it to be about 28 percent. The mean age when hip problems were discovered was 7 years; 62 percent of those with hip problems were quadriplegic total bed-care patients. Postures that predisposed to dislocation were hip flexion, adduction, and medial rotation; scoliosis; and pelvic obliquity, with rotation and inclination.

Lindsey and Drennan[26] conducted a study of institutionalized mentally retarded persons, which excluded CP and other recognizable neuromuscular disorders. Hypotonia, ligamentous laxity, and delayed motor milestones were general characteristics in this population. From a total of 1,600 mentally retarded patients, they found 48 (24 with Down syndrome) who had either isolated major foot problems or a combination of significant foot and knee disorders. The use of appropriate foot orthoses to permit proper weight-bearing alignment until skeletal and ligamentous maturity has been achieved is recommended.[52]

In their study, Lindsey and Drennan[26] found that knee problems were uniformly associated with antecedent foot problems. The most common problem was genu valgum, associated with varying degrees of joint laxity and sometimes with chronic patellar dislocation, but normally no interference with function. The most common functional knee deformity was flexion contracture, which can be attributed to the prolonged part-time use of a wheelchair and the stance adaptation of a crouch gait.

Posture

Sherrill[53] defines posture as "good body alignment and proper body mechanics" and stresses that posture evaluation should be based on dynamic postures (e.g., walking, sitting, stair climbing, and lifting and carrying objects) rather than a single static stance. Table 9-3 summarizes her findings from a posture assessment done on 69 persons with severe mental retardation, using the New York Posture Rating Chart.

A pictorial description of positions that predispose to posture problems is provided by Kendall and Kendall[54] and is helpful in evaluating the severely

Table 9-3. Percentage of Severely Mentally Retarded Persons Having Each Posture as Measured by the New York Posture Rating Chart

Posture	Normal	Mild	Moderate/Severe
Head tilt	88.41	10.14	1.45
Shoulder obliquity	59.42	39.13	1.45
Scoliosis	59.42	36.23	4.35
Hip obliquity	62.32	33.33	4.35
Ankle valgus	28.99	59.42	11.59
Protrusion of abdomen	20.29	46.52	23.19
Lordosis	31.88	56.52	11.60
Kyphosis	57.97	40.58	1.45
Forward head	27.53	62.32	10.15

(Adapted from Sherrill,[53] with permission.)

and profoundly retarded who may be "locked in" to positions as a result of abnormal tone and primitive reflex posturing.

Samilson[50] provides a comprehensive review of the incidence, etiology, and management of problems in the spine among the mentally retarded. He found that the incidence of scoliosis in ambulatory patients with CP was 7 percent and in total bed-care patients, 39 percent. Of 232 scoliosis patients, 193 were spastic quadriplegics, 68 percent had fixed pelvic obliquity, and 81 percent demonstrated deformity of one or both hips that ranged from soft tissue contracture to dislocation.

Under what conditions surgery is indicated for scoliosis is often a difficult decision. Rinsky[55] believes that the most common indications for spinal fusion in neurogenic curves of patients who are retarded include the following:

1. pelvic obliquity interfering with sitting tolerance with impending ischial breakdown,
2. collapsing curves requiring use of the upper extremity to maintain sitting balance,
3. pain (usually rib impingement against the iliac crest),
4. interference with respiration,
5. progressive curves when use of a brace is not feasible, and
6. interference with the ability of others to care for the patient.

Even with the above problems, Rinsky does not believe that the profoundly retarded, multiply handicapped child would realize enough benefit from the surgery to warrant the risks involved.

Kyphotic deformities in the mentally retarded may be secondary to tight hamstrings (with absence of the normal lumbar lordosis) or to an increased lumbar lordosis (with hip flexion contractures).[50] Surgical release of shortened thigh muscles is recommended as a consideration for correction.

Excessive lumbar lordosis, like kyphosis and scoliosis, may be functional or structural. Tight hip flexors, weak hip extensors, and weak abdominals are commonly associated problems.

Sensory Processes and Integration

Because the brain damage in children with severe or profound retardation is often diffuse, sensory losses are common. Ellis[56] states that ". . . up to half the multiply handicapped population need[s] optical corrections and most . . . will benefit from such correction." It has long been known that individuals with Down syndrome are particularly susceptible to hearing loss, but research also indicates an increased frequency of exudative otitis media among mentally handicapped people in general.[56]

Sensory integrative dysfunction in the mentally retarded population is the subject of increasing attention in the literature, and it is implicated as a major causative factor in everything from learning disorders and self-abusive behavior to abnormal and delayed motor development. Ayres[57] has written one of the primary references on the topic of sensory integration. An excellent resource for physical and occupational therapists, which condenses the applicable theories of Ayres, is an article by Montgomery[58] on the assessment and treatment of the child with mental retardation. Although general principles are discussed, the emphasis is on sensory integration with specific assessment and treatment strategies for visual, auditory, tactile, olfactory-gustatory, proprioceptive-kinesthetic, and vestibular functions.

Ambulation

Ambulation is an extremely complex task requiring the interaction of multiple levels of the CNS. A good summary of the biomechanical, neuromuscular, and kinesiologic components required for ambulation is given by Wilson[59] in a chapter entitled "Developing Ambulation Skills" and by Wilson and Parks[60] in an article entitled "Promoting Ambulation in the Severely Retarded Child."

It is difficult to predict the ambulatory potential of children who are mentally retarded. Illingworth[61] predicts that children with mental retardation but without CP may walk with an IQ less than 20 and will walk with an IQ above 20. Of those with an IQ less than 40 who do learn to walk, the onset will be delayed in approximately one-third.[10]

Because it is generally accepted that the lower the IQ, the less the probability of developing ambulation, the results of two studies investigating the ambulatory capabilities of mentally retarded children with and without CP are somewhat confusing. In a study of individuals with IQ levels less than 50, Donoghue and associates[62] found that only 10 percent of those with CP walked, while 79 percent of those without CP walked. One would expect lower percentages in a study by Shapiro and colleagues[63] that focused on children with IQ levels of less than 25. Their results, however, indicated that 11 percent of those children with CP walked (at a median age of 63.5 months), and 92 percent of those without CP walked (at a median age of 20 months).

Molnar[64] conducted a prospective longitudinal study with 53 infants and young children having mental retardation primarily in the mild to moderate range and delayed motor development without evidence of neuromuscular disability. She found that primitive reflexes did not seem to persist beyond the expected age, but that postural adjustment reactions were significantly delayed. Once specific postural reactions appeared, the attainment of the appropriate motor milestone followed within 1 to 4 weeks.

If one looks at the population of mentally retarded individuals who do not have identified neuromuscular problems, some characteristic gait patterns are evident. Lindsey and Drennan[26] refer to the "Chaplinesque" gait of the mentally retarded. The hips are in moderate lateral rotation, the knees are in flexion and valgus, the tibias are in lateral rotation, and the feet are placed with the medial longitudinal arch as the presenting aspect of the foot accompanied by marked valgus of the heel and forefoot pronation.

Many children with mental retardation walk in a crouched posture, which can lead to fixed flexion deformities of the hips and knees. One reason for the development of this type of gait pattern is the delay in motor maturation and balance.[26] Some children will initially stand with a normal posture of full extension at the hips and knees, but develop a crouched posture as they approach adolescence. An interesting postulate for this, proposed by Lindsey and Drennan,[26] is that children have a "predetermined functional height." Once they reach that functional height, they compensate for continued skeletal growth by assuming a crouched posture, which enables them to maintain their head position at a constant distance from the floor. It would seem to be an attempt to maintain consistency in specific types of sensory feedback. It is also common to see children with mental retardation walk with a wide base of support and arms held in a high guard posture. Grady and Gilfoyle[65] theorize that the child is using the basic pivot prone posture in an upright position to facilitate extensor tone.

Toe walking is a typical isolated finding in populations that are severely and profoundly retarded. There are generally three possible reasons for toe walking: hypertonicity in the gastrocnemius-soleus muscle group increased by assumption of the upright posture, behavioral aberrancy (i.e., "it feels good" for whatever reason), or in the absence of CP or spasticity, a problem of sensory dysfunction. Montgomery and Gauger[66] theorize that the latter group of children are generally hypotonic and hyperflexible and demonstrate vestibular dysfunction exacerbated by tactile defensiveness. Weight-bearing on the toes triggers persistent influence of the positive support reaction (seen normally in infancy) and gives them additional extensor tone. This type of toe walking must be differentiated from that seen in individuals with spasticity in the gastrocnemius-soleus muscle group. Whereas surgical release and bracing or inhibitive casting may be indicated in the spastic child, it would not benefit the child with primarily sensory dysfunction.

Orthotics or casts can be very effectively used to inhibit abnormal tone and to promote optimal foot position.[52,67] If the foot is not well positioned, all structures above are abnormally aligned. If a child has orthotics or casts, they should be carefully checked to assure appropriate fit and the child should be observed ambulating with and without them.

Several other aspects of gait should receive attention as part of an observational assessment of gait. Are the arms held high, as in the early walker, for increased balance and stability? Is there overflow of muscle tone when upright (evidenced possibly by tight elbow flexion with retraction of the scapulae and subsequent interference with normal use of the arms for balance)? Is there reciprocal, coordinated movement of the arms with the legs?

Where is the focal point of the eyes? Children with poor equilibrium may keep their eyes on the floor as they walk, rather than looking straight ahead.[68] Is the head maintained in midline? Tilting of the head to one side or the other may indicate sensory dysfunction, poor integration of primitive reflexes, or asymmetric muscle tone. Are the hips relatively stable? Is there a good heel–toe pattern? The common foot problems of the mentally retarded child often result in flat feet and concomitant inability to establish a good heel–toe gait. What type of shoes are usually worn? Is there a difference in the gait with and without shoes?

Although the physical therapist's assessment of gait will emphasize the problematic physical components, it is often true that cognitive and affective factors are the most important determinants of the functional use of walking. Some aspects of intelligence not measured by tests are the awareness of a goal, the will to succeed, and the motivation to perform a skill as a means to an end. It is often difficult to make a motor task like ambulation meaningful to a child who is severely or profoundly retarded and therefore reinforce its execution sufficiently that it will occur spontaneously. The following case study illustrates this point.

Case Study: Angie

Angie is an 8-year-old student with an unspecified genetic disorder who has relatively low muscle tone and profound mental retardation. Her motor development has progressed through a relatively normal sequence but at an extremely slow rate, primarily because of the difficulty in making motor tasks meaningful. For about 24 months she has been able to creep reciprocally on hands and knees and will do so occasionally, usually to interact at some level with the peers in her classroom. Wilson and Parks[60] summarize the necessary components for ambulation in a severely retarded child, which include balance, physical strength, the ability to perceive sensory stimuli, a sense of awareness and body image, motivation to progress, a feeling of security, and a sense of autonomy. Angie seems to have most of these components, but lacks motivation. She can kneel and pull to stand at a table or bookcase with a physical prompt but not true assistance. She seems motorically capable of stance and assisted ambulation, but tends to lean into whatever support is given, twisting around to grin at the therapist.

Angie may never be a functional ambulator in the sense that she would accompany her class on a walk or come to the table for lunch when called;

however, even if she could ambulate short distances with supervision/ reinforcement within the classroom or home, it would make her care much easier, especially as she grows in physical stature. Her physical therapy program combines behavior modification, positively reinforcing incremental stages of the walking process, with neuromuscular facilitation.

The therapist stands behind Angie, facilitating the motor components of ambulation. Initially, this required a true weight shift and rotation of the pelvis to encourage swing phase with the free leg. It was necessary to frequently change points of control (for example, alternating quick side-to-side pelvic prompts with shift to shoulder as needed) to avoid her leaning into available support or fixing posturally. Gradually, the physical prompts have been decreased, the distance lengthened, and the reinforcement phased out. Ambulation is assisted by having her push a cart with an appropriate-height handle, which offers minimal support, is motivating in itself, and creates a more positive image than the traditional walker. The teacher and therapist designed the initial program but, once established, the parents and support staff in the classroom were instructed so that there could be frequent repetition and consistent reinforcement throughout the day. The long-term goal is for Angie to walk 20 feet with only verbal encouragement. At this time, the formal program will be terminated and ambulation will become part of her routine by having her walk to regular, pleasurable events in her day (e.g., lunch).

Oral Motor Function

The development of normal oral motor patterns for feeding, respiration, phonation, speech, and language is a complex process influenced by reflexes, muscle tone, positioning, sensory integration, and behavior. It is one of the most important areas in evaluation of the severely handicapped population because problems are so common. Aspiration of food was found to be the direct cause of 3.5 percent of deaths of profoundly retarded individuals (the seventh leading cause).[69] Pneumonia, frequently the result of a chemical reaction to the aspiration of food in the profoundly retarded, accounts for 30 to 50 percent of the deaths in this population.[70] Malnutrition is another serious health-related problem. Diet is often deficient in calories, iron, vitamins, and minerals.

Behaviors like drooling or messy eating, over which the child has no control, may be aversive to caretakers and may affect social interaction, possibly resulting in isolation. Feeding, which should be a pleasurable experience for the child and a time of positive interaction, becomes instead a tension-filled experience. The lack of speech as a result of oral motor dysfunction can prevent meaningful communication and affect the type of interaction in which the child is engaged. A feeding scale is part of a comprehensive assessment of caregiver–child interaction developed as part of the Nursing Child Assessment Scale Training.[71]

Much has been written on the assessment and treatment of oral motor problems. One of the most comprehensive resources, which includes a variety of reproducible recordkeeping forms, is *Pre-Feeding Skills: A Comprehensive Resource for Feeding Development*.[72] Detailed information on oral motor assessment cannot be included in this chapter, but the following guidelines may be useful as a basis for organizing the approach to this important area of development.

I. General. An assessment should begin by observing the child and caregiver in a typical feeding situation and attending to positioning; the use of special equipment (e.g., chairs, spoons, cups, plates); the type, texture, and temperature of food; the sequence of presenting food; and the quality of social interaction that occurs. Information should also be obtained about the child's basic diet to ensure that there is adequate intake of calories and nutrients. Dietary supplements may be indicated.

II. Oral reflexes (refer to chapter on oral reflexes in *Pre-Feeding Skills: A Comprehensive Resource for Feeding Development*[72]).

III. Muscle tone and sensitivity of oral structures (cheeks, lips, and tongue).

IV. Feeding behaviors. Knowledge of the normal developmental sequence is essential to determine the difference between normal, delayed, and abnormal patterns. Regardless of other variations in position, the child's head should be in midline, stabilized if necessary, during this part of the assessment.

   A. Sucking
     1. Smooth, rapid initiation?
     2. Rhythmic pattern?
     3. Good coordination with breathing and swallowing?
     4. Effect of positioning (e.g., flexion may improve the child's oral motor function)

   B. Food from a spoon (try various textures and tastes)
     1. Mouth quiet until food presented?
     2. Graded mouth opening to receive spoon?
     3. Good lip closure around spoon?
     4. Food cleaned from spoon with upper lip?
     5. Stable position of head maintained?
     6. Effective mobility of tongue and jaw?
     7. Swallow and breathing coordinated?

   C. Drinking from a cup
     1. Jaw excursion graded?
     2. Jaw sufficiently stabilized to allow normal placement of cup?
     3. Lip closure adequate?
     4. Coordination of drinking, breathing, and swallowing?

   D. Biting and chewing
     1. Jaw movement: early up and down "munching" or more mature rotary movement?
     2. Tongue moving laterally to keep food between teeth?
     3. Lips closed adequately?

    E. Self-feeding
V. Associated behaviors
    A. Frequent gagging or choking?
    B. Vomiting (when and how often?)
    C. Drooling
    D. Attitude toward feeding: relaxed? tight? interactive?
    E. Expression of food preferences: texture? avoidance? flavor?

Respiratory Function

Respiratory problems are common in the child with multiple handicaps and can interfere with phonation, feeding, and general good health. A single cause of respiratory problems is uncommon. The problems frequently result from a combination of (1) improper positioning, which can cause deformities of the rib cage, pooling of secretions in dependent areas of the lung, and poor chest excursion; (2) weakness, incoordination, or spasticity of the respiratory muscles, resulting in an ineffective, weak cough and poor chest excursion; (3) incoordination of oral motor and respiratory movements with frequent aspiration; (4) increased saliva production and ineffective means of clearing the saliva so that it tends to collect in the throat; (5) increased incidence of allergies causing respiratory symptoms (milk products are often implicated); and (6) lack of exercise and overall poor cardiovascular and respiratory fitness.[73]

In a study by Bjure and Berg[74] of the dynamic and static lung volumes of school-aged children with CP, it was found that their total lung capacity averaged 85 percent of the predicted normal values. "Noisy" respirations are a frequent finding. Most often this is the result of secretions or saliva in the upper airways gurgling as inspired and expired air tries to pass through. The only way to differentiate upper airway congestion from the more serious lobar congestion (pneumonia) is to auscultate the chest. Experience allows one to distinguish true rales, rhonchi, and wheezes from transmitted sounds originating in the upper airways.

Careful observation of the child's respiration in various positions can be diagnostic of many problems and provides the key to effective remediation. The normal infant primarily uses the diaphragm for breathing, so that one sees significant rise and fall of the abdomen. As the child gains the upright position there is a gradual transition to thoracic breathing, the normal adult pattern. Normal rate per minute for a newborn is 35 to 50, decreasing to approximately 30 for a 2-year-old and 16 for a normal adult. The ability to breathe through the nose is important, as the obligatory mouth breather will have problems coordinating respiration and feeding, and a tendency to aspirate food. As mentioned earlier, aspiration and aspiration pneumonia are significant causes of death among the mentally retarded.

Activities of Daily Living

Individuals who are severely and profoundly retarded are unable to be independently functioning members of society, but many will be capable of independence in at least some of the activities of daily living and their independence should be encouraged by all possible means. They will be proud of their accomplishments and their family or primary caretakers will be relieved of some of the many time-consuming aspects of basic care. The appropriate use of adaptive equipment and behavior modification can be very helpful in developing skills for daily living. Langley[75] emphasizes the importance of a child's developing a sense of contingency awareness and a sense that they can effect some control over their environment. She reviews the research on the use of microswitches and microcomputers to circumvent learned helplessness and "foster learning and skill acquisition in severely impaired children." It is important that the child "perceive that the activity is meaningful and related to function in order for the toy to promote continued practice."

Adaptive Equipment Needs

Assessment of the child's function with the various pieces of equipment designated for his or her use as well as a projection of potential benefit from other types of adaptive equipment is critical. Especially for the child who is multihandicapped and nonambulatory, the proper use of adaptive equipment can be one of the most important aspects of a therapeutic program. Presperin states that "seating and positioning can have a direct correlation with the prevention of pressure sores, orthopedic deformities, and muscle contractures as well as with qualitative improvement of respiration, digestion, heart rate, and functional skills."[76]

The process of selecting appropriate equipment requires consideration of the following areas: (1) availability, (2) cost, (3) source of funding, (4) portability, (5) stability, (6) ease of adjustment, (7) ease of modifications, and (8) construction, materials, and aesthetics.[77]

Skills in correctly identifying equipment needs, locating resources for financial support, and obtaining the right piece of equipment (whether it is purchased or made) are some of the most important within the specialty area of pediatrics. Several published resources are available that provide general guidelines for positioning and some creative ideas for the construction of homemade equipment.[76–84] In recognition of the complexity of the task of identifying optimal seating for severely involved children, there are now commercially made simulators available.[76]

A child should have a variety of positioning alternatives available that are comfortable, that enable him or her to interact maximally with the environment, and that provide the support necessary for the activity intended, but still stimulate independent mastery of the necessary postural stabilization. The following areas should be assessed:

1. **Floor positions.** Several alternatives should be available for positioning on the floor or mat.

Prone: the child may benefit from a properly sized bolster or wedge. Size selection and positioning on the equipment will depend on the developmental readiness of the child for head control, forearm support, or extended arm support.

Sidelying: commercially made sidelyers are available, but the appropriate use of bolsters and pillows may be sufficient.

Sitting: a seating arrangement at floor level may help the child to participate in group activities.

2. **Seating.** Several different seating arrangements may be necessary for the multihandicapped child. For instance, a severely involved child with athetosis may need a chair that provides maximum support (head, trunk, and legs) for eating or for fine motor activities. At other times during the day, a chair with less support will allow the child to practice the necessary cocontraction of postural muscles for head and trunk control. Attention should be given to optimal seating for the following activities:

Feeding: a chair that supports the head in midline and helps to normalize muscle tone can be critical in allowing safe, effective feeding behaviors.

Fine motor skills: In the hypertonic child, a seat that provides secure flexion at hips and knees and wide abduction at the hips may normalize tone and enable significant increase in the functional use of the arms and hands.

Interactive play: sufficient support to allow the child's focus to be on interaction rather than stability.

Transportation: with seat belt laws now in effect in many states, the federal government has started officially approving adaptive seating that meets rigorous safety testing. Only this type of approved seating should be used and all directions as to its safe use should be adhered to. When needed, tie downs should be ordered for safe transport on public school buses or vans.

3. **Mobility.** If possible, some form of mobility is desirable for independence and exploration. Possibilities include tricycles, Irish mails, scooter boards, walkers, or wheelchairs, all adequately adapted and fitted for effective use.

4. **Supported weight-bearing.** Options for supported weight-bearing include a prone or supine board, with multiple adjustments available for standing or kneeling with optimal alignment; a standing box, which provides more behavioral than physical control; or a standing frame, which promotes fully upright stance with foot, knee, and pelvic support.

Finally, the physical or occupational therapist must evaluate procedures for toileting, bathing, and dressing, and identify the presence of architectural barriers preventing access to opportunities for recreation, education, and medical care.

Behavior

The behavior of children who are mentally retarded and behavioral approaches to management have received considerable attention in the literature. Webster's defines behavior as, first, "the manner of conducting oneself," and, second, "anything that an organism does involving action and response to stimulation."[85]

The behavior manifested at any particular time has its origins in an intricate matrix of physiologic and environmental systems. Hutt and Gibby[86] devoted several chapters in their book, *The Mentally Retarded Child: Development, Training, and Education*, to discussion of social, emotional, and psychological development, comparing and contrasting normal and mentally retarded children and factors in their environment that influence personality and may contribute to maladaptive behavior. Behavior is the substrate of a child's response system and must therefore be assessed and taken into consideration when determining potential and establishing a treatment program. Deviant behavior can be more of a deterrent to the success of a treatment program than deficient intelligence.

Stereotypic behaviors among the retarded can interfere with functional behaviors and can be harmful to the individual. Stereotyped mannerisms of children who are mentally retarded vary with the environmental setting and the nature of ongoing activities, and the frequency of stereotyped behavior appears to be inversely related to the potential for alternative activity. This is true for infants as well as older persons. MacLean and Baumeister[87] found that several stereotypes are dependent on a particular physical positioning of the child, which suggests that stereotypic movements are related to motor development.

PHYSICAL THERAPY

The markedly reduced capacity of the child with severe or profound retardation to cooperate at a cognitive level with treatment objectives will definitely limit the ultimate level of achievement. Short-term goals may be achieved in minute increments and at a frustratingly slow pace. As one would expect, studies that have investigated the effectiveness of various treatment regimens have found relatively better results with children functioning at higher cognitive levels. For example, Scherzer and colleagues[88] investigated physical therapy as a determinant of change in the infant with CP and found definite changes in motor, social, and management areas, "particularly among children expected to show higher intelligence."

Sommerfeld and colleagues[89] conducted a pilot study with 19 severely mentally impaired CP students ranging in age from 3 to 22 years. The study compared the following types of physical therapy management over a 5-month period: (1) direct physical therapy treatment, (2) supervised physical therapy management, and (3) no physical therapy provision. Their study showed no significant differences in the development of mature developmental reflexes, improvement of gross motor skills, or increase of passive joint motion between the three groups. Although the sample size was small and the length of time (5 months) relatively short, the results point out the importance of using reliable measures to assess treatment outcomes and the need for more research in this area to help clarify priorities for physical therapy intervention.

This is not meant to discourage those who work with children with severe or profound retardation, but there are several important concepts that must be kept in mind when establishing a treatment program with realistic and obtainable goals. Mentally retarded individuals characteristically have a short attention span and require extensive repetition for learning. They seldom copy the behaviors of others unless trained to do so,[90] so one cannot rely on imitation as a means of instruction. Curiosity, motivation, and the will to achieve are all behaviors that correspond roughly with level of intelligence and are likely to be absent or very limited in the individual with severe and profound retardation.

Goals of the treatment program should be based on the development of appropriate adaptive behaviors and should be formulated in cooperation with the child, parents, teachers, aides, and others regularly involved with the individual. Awareness of and adherence to any already planned programs for communication or behavior modification are necessary.

Isolated therapy sessions of relatively short duration will be minimally effective without the cooperation of those primarily responsible for the child's care and education. Because learning is often at a very basic level and consistency of approach is critical, highly specialized treatment regimens may not be appropriate. Emphasis should be placed on activities that can be performed by all levels of personnel and easily incorporated into various aspects of the daily routine so that frequent repetition can be accomplished with relative ease. Westervelt and Luiselli[91] found, while trying to establish standing and walking behaviors in a profoundly retarded, institutionalized 11-year-old, that they were unsuccessful until the independent efforts of the clinician were relinquished and the attendant staff was taught how to work on target behaviors.

Professionals will commonly assume a transdisciplinary rather than interdisciplinary team approach[92] depending, of course, on the training and experience of the team members and the type of setting. Published curricula for the severely and profoundly retarded, which are usually multidisciplinary in design, are available and can be helpful as a focus for a team of professionals in an educational or institutional setting.

- Fraser BA, Hensinger RN: *Managing Physical Handicaps: A Practical Guide for Parents, Care Providers and Educators.* Paul H Brooks Publishing, Baltimore, 1983
- Shanley E (ed): *Mental Handicaps—A Handbook of Care.* Churchill Livingstone, Edinburgh, 1986
- Jegard S, Anderson L, Glazer C, Zaleski WA: *A Comprehensive Program for Multihandicapped Children.* Alvin Buckwold Centre, Saskatchewan, Canada, 1980

- Jaeger L: *Home Program Instruction Sheets for Infants and Young Children.* 3rd Ed. Therapy Spill Builders, Tucson, 1987
- Kissinger EM: *A Sequential Curriculum for the Severely and Profoundly Mentally Retarded/Multihandicapped.* Charles C Thomas, Springfield, IL, 1981
- Popovich D, Laham SL (eds): *The Adaptive Behavior Curriculum.* Vol. 2. Paul H Brooks Publishing, Baltimore, 1982
- Popovich D: *Effective Educational and Behavioral Programming for Severely and Profoundly Handicapped Students.* Paul H Brooks Publishing, Baltimore, 1981
- Falvey MA: *Community-Based Curriculum Strategies for Students with Severe Handicaps.* Paul H Brooks Publishing, Baltimore, 1985
- Galka G, Fraser B: *Gross Motor Management of Severely Impaired Students.* Vol. 2. *Curriculum Model.* University Park Press, Baltimore, 1980

Positive reinforcement for appropriate behavior and the integration of treatment objectives with pleasurable experiences are important for children at any level of cognitive development. Kielhofner and Miyake[93] describe "play" itself as a learning and survival behavior and conducted an exploratory study on the therapeutic use of games with a group of adults with moderate or severe retardation. The clients who participated showed improvement in motor behavior, cognitive abilities, affect, attention, self-confidence, and social interaction.

Motor Activity

The use of motor activity to enhance the learning process of individuals who are mentally retarded has been popularized by many publications. According to Godfrey and Kephart,[94] learning is "dependent upon motor activities and the ability to control motor responses." Chaney and Kephart believe that the "efficiency of the higher thought processes can be no better than the basic motor abilities upon which they are based."[95] Kephart has developed a comprehensive theoretic framework for the evaluation of "slow learners" and a program of remediation based on the use of various types of motor activities.[96]

Although Cratty and Martin[97] are proponents of the facilitation of motor activity for a variety of reasons, they question Kephart's major hypothesis, that movement is the basis of intellect. Cratty stresses that the child must be able to think about the movement he or she is doing and be involved in a way that encourages the process of decision making.[98] He suggests the use of perceptual motor activities presented in a specified sequential fashion to enhance the educational process of children with mental retardation.[99]

The basic theories of Kephart and Cratty help us to understand the importance of the interaction between reflex, motor, and sensory systems and the learning that occurs from the direct and immediate feedback resulting from a motor act on the environment. However, the specific programs they suggest require a level of cognitive development beyond that of the severely and profoundly retarded.

Approaches to Treatment

Some current theorists are dividing approaches to physical therapy into two different models based on interpretations of how the CNS operates and responds: the facilitation model and the motor control model.[100]

1. *Facilitation model.* As summarized by Ostrosky,[100] five basic assumptions underly this model: (1) "the brain controls movements, not muscles"; (2) ". . . a patient's movement patterns can be altered by applying specific patterns of sensory stimulation, especially through proprioceptive afferent pathways"; (3) ". . . the CNS is hierarchically organized" and therefore, "abnormal movement patterns and tone disorders are assumed to result from a lack of inhibitory control by the higher centers"; (4) ". . . recovery from brain damage follows a predictable sequence that parallels the development of normal motor behavior from infancy"; and (5) ". . . all motor phenomena associated with brain damage have a neurophysiological basis."

2. *Motor control model.* The motor control model assumes that "every movement is a response to a motor problem presented to the CNS" and it looks to a more circular, distributed control system composed of four areas: the cerebellar dentate nucleus, the cerebral motor cortex, the cerebellar interposed nucleus, and the muscle. Under this model, when "higher" CNS damage occurs, "other neural structures can continue to operate the motor system in some capacity." Carr and Shepherd[101] are two of the major clinical proponents of this model. They encourage therapists to select meaningful, functional goals that are task specific and difficult, but obtainable, and to clearly communicate these goals to the patient; therapist-guided active movements are minimized, a problem-solving approach is established so that carry over is maximized, and the patient is encouraged to practice both overtly and mentally.[100,101]

The motor control model places much greater emphasis on the importance of cognitive participation by the patient and, if the model gains acceptance, there is an implicit challenge for therapists to objectively demonstrate the benefit of their intervention with populations that cannot participate well on a cognitive level.

The neurophysiologic approaches most commonly used in the treatment of the pediatric patient are based on the facilitation model. These include the neurodevelopmental, sensorimotor, and sensory integrative techniques of the Bobaths, Rood and Stockmeyer, and Ayres which are described in subsequent text. As stated by Montgomery, these approaches seem particularly appropriate for the child with mental retardation because all of these approaches emphasize functions that are relatively automatic for the individual (i.e., based on normal reflex and sensorimotor development) and therefore demand learning at a sub-cortical level.[58] Also falling under the facilitation model is neuromuscular reflex therapy, a controversial treatment approach first described by Fay and popularized by Doman-Delacato (described in subsequent text).

Neurodevelopmental Therapy

Neurodevelopmental therapy (NDT) was developed by Karl and Berta Bobath[102] as an approach to the management of the sensorimotor disorders seen in patients with CP. By definition, CP is a non-progressive lesion affecting the immature brain and "interfering with the normal process of neurodevelopment."[102] The Bobaths' treatment approach is applicable to that relatively large segment of the severely and profoundly retarded population in whom there is involvement of the portion of the brain that integrates and controls sensorimotor activity.

The Bobaths theorized that in upper motor neuron lesions producing CP, tonic and spinal reflexes are released from the normal integrative and control functions of the brain. Movement is uncoordinated and tends to occur in primitive, synergistic patterns. Sensory and perceptual deficits are common and affect the feedback mechanism, which, when functioning normally, enables refinement of movement activity. An underlying premise is that the primary deficit in CP is a derangement in the normal postural reflex mechanism.[103]

The aim of NDT is to normalize postural tone and improve the quality and control of movement, following the normal developmental sequence as closely as possible. This is accomplished by using reflex-inhibiting patterns with manual control at key points (e.g., shoulder girdle or pelvis) to normalize postural tone. With tone normalized, active automatic reactions are facilitated to develop elements of the normal postural reflex mechanism. The handling techniques used in NDT are designed to elicit active, automatic movements from the child, and therefore do not require that the child cooperate at a cognitive level. As the Bobaths stated, "it is this aspect of the approach which has made this [NDT] treatment so eminently adaptable to the needs of the mentally subnormal and uncooperative child."[102]

Sensorimotor Therapy

Stockmeyer[104,105] has described in the literature an interpretation of Rood's approach to the treatment of neuromuscular dysfunction. It is an approach that "seeks to activate the movement and postural responses of the patient in the same automatic manner as they occur in the normal, without need for conscious attention to the response itself."[104] Reliance on automatic reactions makes Rood's approach, like the Bobath's, applicable to the child with severe or profound retardation.

Several premises form the basis for Rood's approach to treatment.[104,105]

First, motor and sensory functions are inseparable. Stimuli, carefully chosen to activate, facilitate, or inhibit motor responses, are an important part of the treatment program. The effect of various stimuli on not only somatic, but also on autonomic and psychic function is an ongoing consideration. Second, there are two major sequences in motor development that are distinctly different and yet inextricably interrelated: skeletal functions and vital functions. Third, skeletal function can be separated into four sequential levels of control: mobility (shortening and lengthening of the agonist with its antagonists), stability (co-contraction of agonists and antagonists), mobility superimposed on stability in a weight-bearing position (proximal part moving on fixed distal part), and mobility superimposed on stability in a non–weight-bearing position (free distal part moving on a proximal part that is dynamically holding). Fourth, children normally traverse a specific skeletal function sequence (also termed *ontogenetic motor patterns*). This sequence is the guideline Rood proposed for the assessment and subsequent treatment of neuromuscular dysfunction.

Sensory Integrative Therapy

The basis for Ayres' use of sensory integrative therapy is rooted in the Piagetian theory that concrete action precedes and makes possible the use of the intellect and that sensorimotor experiences are the foundations of mental development.[106] Stated another way, intelligence may be viewed as a progressive transformation of motor patterns into thought patterns. The results of an interesting longitudinal study with normal infants and infants with Down syndrome conducted by Bradley-Johnson and associates[107] provide support for Piaget's basic theory. They found that children's performance on the Stanford-Binet at age 3½ years was significantly correlated with the length of time spent on the exploration of novel objects at age 6 months.

Ayres[57] developed a comprehensive theoretic basis for sensory integrative therapy and a rationale for its use with brain-damaged children. She informally defined sensory integration as the ability to organize sensory information for functional use in producing an adaptive response and believed that this ability is the essence of perception. A motor act is a typical response to a perception, and the sensory feedback gained from the motor act enables the child to evaluate the accuracy of the perception and the effectiveness of the response (Fig. 9-1). Ayres believed that a strong relationship exists among cognitive function, motor development, and reflex integration, but that the child first experiences the environment through information conveyed by afferent pathways. Inability to accurately receive or organize sensory input causes dysfunction in the whole process of learning via sensorimotor experience. Sensory integrative therapy is not directed toward the mastery of specific tasks or skills, but toward improving the brain's capacity to perceive, to remember, and to plan motor activity. Montgomery and Richter[68] published a handbook for physical and occupational therapists based on the principles of sensorimotor integration and other neurophysiologically based intervention techniques.

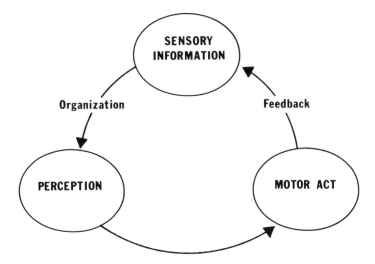

Fig. 9-1. Sensory integration. Diagrammatic representation of the basic process.

Trainable mentally retarded children (IQ levels less than 50) were the subjects of Montgomery and Richter's[108] study, which compared the effectiveness of three different motor programs on neuromotor development. On a test battery that assessed gross, fine, and perceptual motor skills and reflex integration, the children receiving sensory integrative therapy showed the greatest gains, followed by those who participated in a developmental physical education program and, finally, those in an adaptive physical education and arts and crafts program. The investigators concluded that neuromotor development may be enhanced more effectively by activities that facilitate improved postural responses than by practice of specific motor skills.

Several studies have investigated the effectiveness of sensory integrative therapy with the severely and profoundly retarded. A pilot study by Norton[109] indicated improved motor skills in profoundly mentally retarded preschoolers after participating in a program of sensory stimulation. A study by Clark and associates[110] collaborated the findings of Webb[111] that a sensory integration program elicited increases in eye contact and vocalization and promoted postural adaptation in adults with profound retardation.

Controlled vestibular stimulation is one of the most popular types of sensory stimulation. In a review article, Ottenbacher[112] relates that "controlled vestibular stimulation has had positive effects on arousal level, visual exploratory behavior, motor development and reflex integration." Ottenbacher and colleagues[113] used a group of 38 severely and profoundly retarded, nonambulatory, developmentally delayed children to compare the results of sensorimotor therapy alone or sensorimotor therapy combined with controlled vestibular stimulation. They found that the group receiving the combined therapies "made significantly greater gains on measures of reflex integration and gross and fine motor development." Magrun and colleagues[114] used vestibular stimulation prior to a monitored free play situation to increase the spontaneous use of verbal language in trainable mentally retarded children. Effects were generally positive and better results were obtained with younger children who were more severely language disabled.

Two theories have wide currency regarding the basis for the self-injurious behavior (SIB) often seen in the severely and profoundly retarded. One theory postulates that SIB is learned and therefore is most effectively treated with contingency-based management techniques (i.e., behavior modification). The other theory suggests that SIB is a type of self-stimulation and should be ameliorated by treatment with various forms of sensory and environmental enrichment. Bright and associates[115] assumed sensory deprivation was at least a partial cause of the SIB of a profoundly retarded adult, and they were successful in reducing the frequency of the behavior using sensory integrative techniques. Evans[116] was able to reduce the hyperactive behavior of three profoundly retarded adolescents by increasing the visual and auditory stimulation in their environment.

Neuromuscular Reflex Therapy

Fay's approach, known more commonly as patterning, is based on the concept that primitive movements resulting from reflexes, spinal automatisms, and tonic responses to stimuli are possible without a highly developed cerebral cortex.[117] Doman et al. and Delacato expanded Fay's basic patterning procedures and developed a popular method of treatment that they claim can benefit children with neuromuscular disorders, learning disabilities, behavioral disturbances, and mental retardation.[118,119]

Delacato[118] categorized a developmental progression based on the belief that the ontogenetic development of normal humans recapitulates the phylogenetic process. The progression starts with truncal movements of the newborn, which correspond to the swimming movements of the fish and represent a medullary level of function, proceeds through homolateral crawling, cross-pattern creeping, and crude walking, and ends with cross-pattern walking, which is considered to be a distinctly human form of locomotion and is identified with mature cerebral function and the establishment of hemispheric dominance. Important to the theory is the premise that each of the levels is stage dependent and that adequate organization at any subsequent level is dependent on mastery of the coordination requisite for the antecedent stages.

Basic to the treatment method is the application of a variety of sensory and motor experiences directed toward facilitation of "neurologic organization."[118] The patterning aspect of the regimen involves three to five adults passively manipulating the child's arms, legs, and head in a rhythmic pattern, according to a meticulously ordered sequence. Other aspects of the regimen include visual, tactile, and auditory stimulation, a breathing technique designed to increase the amount of carbon dioxide inhaled, expressive activities, gravity and antigravity activities (e.g., rolling, somersaulting, and inverted hanging), and a plan of restriction and facilitation of selected experiences to foster the establishment of left hemispheric dominance.[118,119] If fully implemented, the program demands many hours of treatment each day; it must be done 7 days a week and it usually necessitates involving friends as well as family members in a demanding schedule.

The patterning treatment has remained relatively popular for severely and profoundly handicapped children because it does not require any cognitive level of participation by the child, is prescribed for use at home (after a period of training), and has been credited with miraculous cures in the popular press. Criticism has centered around the lack of scientific evidence to support the results claimed for the treatment regimen and the tremendous emotional, psychological and financial burden it places on families.[120,121] In 1981, Zigler[122] published an article, "A Plea to End the Use of the Patterning Treatment for Retarded Children." He regrets the appeal this type of program holds for parents who are seeking a "last hope" and who are then faced with the emotional burden of failing to see results from a program whose success was presented to them as strongly dependent on their perseverance.

The American Physical Therapy Association (APTA) has joined with other professional groups (including the American Academy of Pediatrics) in expressing concern about the efficacy of the Doman-Delacato techniques. In APTA's view, "the available research indicates: that claims as to the benefits of the Doman-Delacato method remain largely unproven; that considerable doubt exists concerning its efficacy; and that there is reason for concern that parents and children may be ill-served by its use."[123]

Behavior Modification

Consideration of treatment of the mentally retarded is impossible without discussion of behavior modification. The basic principles of behavior modification as described by Skinner[124] are simple. A target behavior is selected, and the specific responses that are desired are selected and defined. Correctly completed responses are immediately reinforced. By continued specific reinforcement and by successive and more generalized reinforcement procedures, the learning sequence is established, leading to accomplishment of the target behavior. In establishing a behavior modification program, one must (1) specify target behaviors in an objective and measurable manner, often breaking down a desired behavior into many small increments; (2) determine the method of measuring changes; (3) choose appropriate reinforcers; (4) specify the conditions (contingencies) under which the desired behavior will be rewarded; (5) establish a plan that provides for consistent reinforcement and frequent "success"; (6) monitor the effectiveness of the contingencies; and (7) modify as indicated. Clinical researchers have used it to shape a variety of gross motor behaviors, including reduction of time in reverse tailor sitting,[125] development of standing and walking,[91,126–131] raising an arm to pull a ring,[132] reduction of drooling,[133] and cessation of crawling.[134] Behavior modification has also been used to reduce or eliminate SIB[135–137] and stereotypic behavior.[138] Alberto and Troutman have written a good basic text on the effective application of behavior modification techniques.[139]

The use of automated learning devices is based on the principles of behavior modification—a concrete action immediately reinforced by a pleasurable consequence—and can be very effectively applied with a population that is severely handicapped.[140,141] A switch, either purchased or homemade,[141,142] is interfaced between the power source (usually batteries) of the selected reinforcer so that the switch must be activated before the reinforcer will "perform." The switches can be generally categorized into one of two types: a mechanical switch that requires a basic manipulation like light pressure or grasp to complete a circuit, or a mercury switch that is activated by its position relative to gravity and can be placed on an individual in such a way as to be activated by a specific position of that body part in space. The reinforcer activated by the switch can be any battery-operated (or, with an adapter, electrically powered) device: a toy, small fan, vibrating pillow, light, tape recorder, etc. Researchers have used automated learning devices to train a wide range of behaviors, including head posture,[142–145] range of motion (ROM);[146,147] finger praxis,[148] and prehension,[149] and to eliminate stereotypic behavior and SIB in individuals with CP and mental retardation.

Sometimes, nonpurposeful repetitive behaviors are so frequent that it is very difficult to elicit purposeful behaviors. In such a situation, the physical therapist may be involved in a team effort to design and implement a plan to decrease the frequency of nonpurposeful behaviors prior to work on meaningful motor behaviors. A case example illustrates a situation of this type.

Case Study: Annie

Annie is an 8-year-old girl with Down syndrome and a profound level of mental retardation. She is ambulatory (despite unstable hip joints), but nonverbal, and dependent in all aspects of daily living. She demonstrates a variety of stereotypic behaviors that, although not self-injurious, do interfere with her effective interaction with her environment. She makes infrequent eye contact or social engagement and seldom shows meaningful manipulation of an object, tending to be off in a world of her own with a set of self-stimulatory behaviors (SSBs). The team working with her decided that implementation of other aspects of a program was pointless until there was a decrease in the frequency of stereotypic behaviors. The four most frequent behaviors were listed, and three were found to involve the hands: mouthing, hand flapping, and scratching the palms.

Many theorists believe that stereotypic behaviors are used by an individual to compensate for a lack of adequate stimulation or to act as a filter because of too much environmental stimulation.[150] With this in mind, Annie's environment is kept as homeostatic as possible.

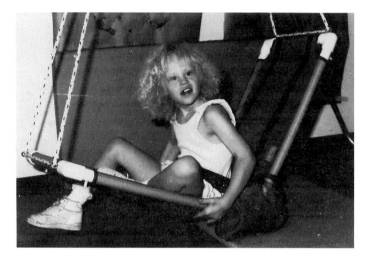

Fig. 9-2.   Case study: Annie. Means of vestibular stimulation—suspended hammock.

Based on reports in the literature of a reduction of SSB with sensory integrative techniques,[151,152] especially vestibular stimulation, a trial of this was initiated. As a baseline, the Southern California Test of Postrotary Nystagmus[153] was administered. Annie had no nystagmus and no clinical signs of change after spinning, except that she obviously enjoyed it.

For 20 minutes twice a day, she was strapped into a hammock suspended from an overhead frame. She was close enough to a mat on the floor that she could easily drop a leg and mobilize the hammock in a rotary or linear direction (Fig. 9-2). She kept herself moving almost continuously, seemed happy, and significantly reduced her SSB when she was thus engaged. The problem was that there seemed to be no carryover; once out of the hammock, the frequency of SSB returned quickly to the baseline rate. It seemed that this type of vestibular stimulation simply substituted for other stereotypic behaviors and still allowed no meaningful interaction with her environment.

Annie also enjoyed vestibular stimulation provided over a large inflatable therapy ball (bouncing in a sitting position, segmental rolling on top of the ball, and rocking back and forth in a prone position over the ball *toward* the therapist). This type of therapist-directed stimulation resulted in increased eye contact and increased vocalization.

Over the course of a year, with input from all team members (including the parents), a review of the literature, and various trial and error programs, a treatment plan was developed that incorporated a combination of techniques and proved effective in reducing SSB, increasing eye contact, increasing vocalization, and maximizing Annie's potential for interacting meaningfully with the objects and people in her environment.

When Annie engaged in one of the three targeted stereotypic behaviors, she was told "no" and then was prompted to use her hands in a purposeful

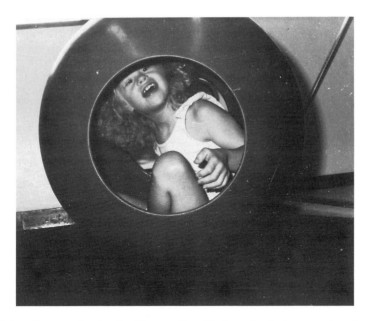

Fig. 9-3. Case study: Annie. Means of vestibular stimulation—enclosed sphere.

activity with social praise, coupled with an edible reinforcer initially, for the latter. Behaviorists term this approach the *differential reinforcement of other behaviors*. At times, when it was difficult to pay close attention to Annie, she was seated on an adaptive tricycle that was more comfortable for her to use with both hands on the handlebars, or she was given toys attached to her lap tray (so she would not throw them), an automated learning device that requires bilateral manipulation to activate,[154] or the means to provide vestibular stimulation for herself, including sitting in a large plastic half sphere or bubble, swinging in the suspended hammock described earlier, or rocking in a large red sphere open at each end and big enough to climb into (Figs. 9-3 and 9-4). "Play" time on the big therapy ball was scheduled each day for midmorning and incorporated some of the activities recommended by the speech therapist.

Other Treatment Priorities

In addition to the facilitation of neuromotor development and behavior modification, the prevention of deformity, the prevention of respiratory complications, and the treatment of oral motor problems must be made priorities in a comprehensive management program.

Prevention of Deformity

The more common types of deformity and the forces that tend to cause deformity in the mentally retarded were summarized in the section on assessment. To prevent deformity and the subsequent loss of function, an effective

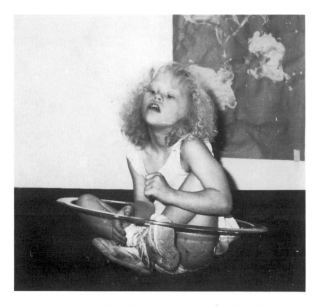

Fig. 9-4.   Case study: Annie. Means of vestibular stimulation—half sphere.

program must be developed that includes suggestions for handling and positioning, exercise, and the appropriate use of adaptive equipment. Two case examples illustrate these points.

Case Study: Christopher

Christopher is a 3-year-old boy who has a spastic quadriplegic type of CP, with profound retardation, impaired vision, and a seizure disorder. Extensor tone predominates in the lower extremities with a posturing of adduction, medial rotation and extension of the hips, extension of the knees, and plantar flexion of the feet. Other prominent patterns are strong retraction of the scapulae and shoulder girdle; flexion of the elbows, wrists, and fingers; and pronation of the forearms. Primitive reflexes are not integrated, with particular influence on postural tone from persistence of the crossed extension, tonic labyrinthine, positive support, and asymmetric tonic neck reflexes (Fig. 9-5). Oral motor function is markedly abnormal. Mouth opening is associated with neck extension, and there is profuse drooling. Chest excursion is minimal and he almost always has upper airway congestion.

A priority for Christopher was a well-fitted chair to be used for feeding and other activities (Fig. 9-6). To reduce the extensor tone in his legs, the chair selected has foot rests that promote full contact of the soles of his feet (to avoid

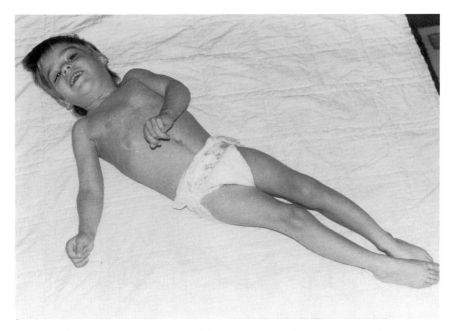

Fig. 9-5.   Case study: Christopher. Abnormal posture in supine.

stimulating a positive support reaction), an abduction wedge with sufficient depth to generalize the contact with the hip adductors and help to keep his hips back in the chair, a seat that is tilted back at a slight angle to promote hip flexion of slightly more than 90 degrees, and basic trunk and head supports for midline positioning. Tie downs on the van enable Christopher to be safely transported to developmental day care in his chair.

   The supine position is avoided because of the influence of the tonic labyrinthine reflex. Sidelying with hips and knees well flexed is a good position to use to work on hand function (e.g., a pressure switch activating a cassette recorder) or for general positioning, because it provides stabilization in midline and inhibits the tonic labyrinthine reflex (Fig. 9-7). The prone position, supported under the chest with a bolster or wedge with the shoulders forward for elbow propping and the knees flexed, helps to stimulate head and upper trunk control, to inhibit retraction of the shoulder girdle, and to provide some weight-bearing through the shoulder.

   A prone stander promotes lower extremity weight-bearing with its associated benefits (Fig. 9-8), and a suspended hammock allows vestibular stimulation in a relaxed position of flexion. A beanbag chair is used for comfortable semi-upright sitting at floor level. Carrying suggestions include straddling the adult's hip or fully flexed at hips and knees and facing away from the adult. Support is used as minimally as possible to stimulate independent head and trunk control.

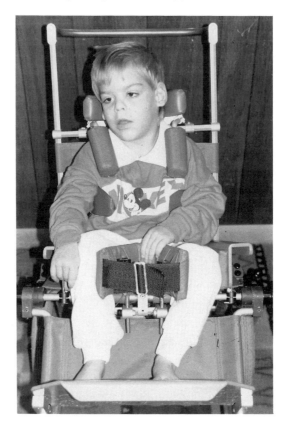

Fig. 9-6. Case study: Christopher. Well positioned in adaptive seating.

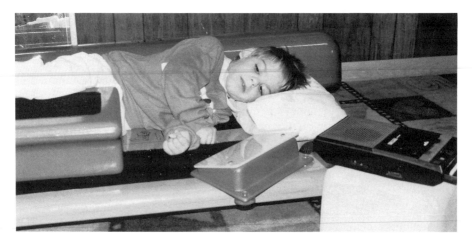

Fig. 9-7. Case study: Christopher. In sidelying, relaxed enough to activate a pressure switch attached to a cassette tape player.

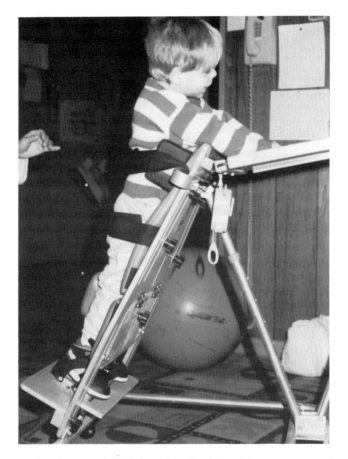

Fig. 9-8. Case study: Christopher. Positioned in a prone stander.

Case Study: Tony

Tony is a 17-year-old student with a nonspecified genetic disorder characterized by hypothyroidism, absence of sweat glands (causing hypersensitivity to heat and susceptibility to skin breakdown), partial blindness, musculoskeletal abnormalities, and profound mental retardation. General hypotonicity and ligamentous laxity are present. Tony has no means of communication and is upset by movement and handling. He demonstrates distress with a throaty scream and self-inflicted blows to his head. He is ambulatory with assistance (required primarily because of his blindness). Figure 9-9 illustrates his severe kyphoscoliosis and the deformities of his feet.

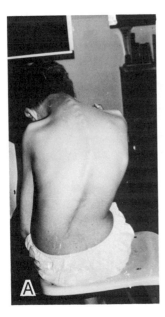

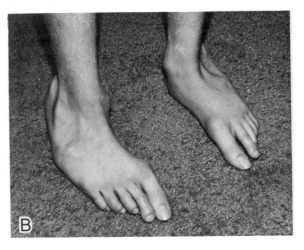

Fig. 9-9. Case study: Tony. **(A)** Severe kyphoscoliosis in unsupported sitting. **(B)** Bony collapse of the feet.

Ideally, Tony should have received orthopedic care (surgery and/or bracing) at an early age to prevent deformities, but he was discharged from orthopedic follow-up at the age of 3 years because of his "lack of potential." His parents, intelligent and caring people, were faced with a difficult decision for managing his kyphoscoliosis. It had progressed too far for electrical stimulation to be a viable alternative. The fear of skin breakdown eliminated the choice of surgery followed by full body casting or bracing. Surgery followed by 6 to 9 months of skeletal traction was an option. However, the closest medical center that could perform the surgery was 6 hours from home, and Tony's parents were apprehensive about his emotional response to separation from them, as well as the discomfort and strangeness of the immobilization. They decided that the benefits of surgery did not outweigh the risk of severe emotional trauma. Because the arches of the feet were thought to have collapsed maximally, with further progression unlikely, surgery and/or bracing were presented as alternatives for the future should his continued ability to ambulate become jeopardized or the feet cause pain or discomfort.

The "rightness" or "wrongness" of the orthopedic physician's decision not to follow Tony at an early age and the parent's decision not to allow spinal surgery are moot at this point. Therapists are frequently presented with such "regrettable" situations. In this case, a realistic explanation of the purpose of exercise and positioning was given to the classroom teacher and the parents. They were made aware that exercise and positioning were not likely to affect the progression of the scoliosis, but were encouraged to follow a basic program to prevent soft tissue contractures, maintain flexibility in the trunk, and minimize impingement of the rotated thorax and twisted spine on the lungs and other vital organs.

Several suggestions for positioning were made: (1) avoid sitting on the floor; (2) use a chair with a firm back and a table or lap board of an appropriate height to allow arm support; (3) lie prone over a large wedge with arms forward to minimize the kyphosis, stimulate use of the extensor muscles of the neck and upper trunk, and reduce the scoliosis by the mild traction effect of gravity pulling against fixed shoulders; and (4) lie on either side with appropriate support.

Instruction was given to the caregivers in basic exercise to stretch the soft tissues in the feet, legs, and trunk, which are at risk of shortening because of the persistent deforming forces. Handling suggestions included activities to stimulate Tony's ability to support himself in the prone and four-point positions. A program of appropriately graded stimulation to decrease Tony's sensitivity to touch and a program of sensory stimulation and behavior modification to eliminate his self-abusive behavior were also included.

Prevention of Respiratory Problems

Frequent change of position in the severely handicapped child is probably the single most important measure for preventing respiratory problems. Proper positioning helps to prevent rib cage deformity and pooling of secretions and facilitates improved chest excursion. For feeding, the child should be positioned with the trunk at a minimum of a 45-degree angle (seated at 90 degrees is preferable), with the head balanced in a neutral position between flexion and extension. If the neck is allowed to extend in what has been termed the *bird feeding position*, the glottis is not able to close effectively over the trachea and there is essentially an open channel for the aspiration of food into the lungs.

Inverted positioning is of value in promoting the drainage of secretions from the airways. Traditional postural drainage, however, with specific positioning to drain various lung segments, accompanied by percussion and vibration to those areas, is not indicated for upper airway congestion. Theoretically, the effect of postural drainage is to remove secretions, such as are produced in a lobar pneumonia, from the alveoli of specific lung segments. Its use for less serious upper airway congestion is not harmful, but neither is it likely to be particularly beneficial.

Treatment of Oral Motor Problems

Following a careful assessment of oral motor problems, remediation of the problem areas can be accomplished following the guidelines provided by Morris and Klein[72] or others. Consistency is particularly important in an oral motor program. Rarely can a therapist be available for all, or even most, of a child's feeding sessions, so that provisions for carryover to other mealtime situations are essential. It may be that the therapist will choose not to instruct others in specialized techniques like jaw control, but, if possible, consistency in the position the child is in, the utensils used, and the type, texture, and temperature of foods offered should be provided.

It is important for therapists to support families or other primary caregivers in what can be initially a frustrating experience. Somehow, eating seems to be such a basic function that we just expect children to eat well. In the face of a sloppy, slow eater who may have poor nutrition and choke frequently, this unmet expectation may lead to serious feelings of personal inadequacy or non-acceptance of the child on the part of a parent. Patience is essential. Feeding is such a habitual process that any change will at first seem to worsen rather than improve the situation and it takes time, sometimes as much as an hour and a half, to complete a meal when a new program is initiated.

Mealtime should be a relaxed time, a sometimes rare opportunity for one-to-one interaction. In a book entitled *Mealtimes for Severely and Profoundly Handicapped Persons: New Concepts and Attitudes*, more than 50 professionals, as well as parents, volunteers, and handicapped persons themselves, describe and interpret the value of mealtimes.[155] Creative situations and meal-time atmospheres are described that can be the strata for positive interaction, development, and education.

PARENT AND STAFF EDUCATION

The parents of children with severe or profound retardation should be an important focus and an integral part of the team approach to management. It is interesting to note that cultural familial factors are the leading cause of mild retardation, but the majority of parents of severely and profoundly retarded individuals are normal and have characteristics of the general population in terms of education, social status, etc.[156]

Parents of children with severe or profound retardation are faced with tremendous emotional strains, the need to make critical decisions (sometimes from birth), and the responsibility for a person who will, all of his or her life, require supervision and have special needs. Prior to the normalization movement of the 1970s, parents had basically two alternatives: to send their children away to large state or private institutions (often a choice encouraged by professionals because of a general hopeless outlook) or to keep them at home with virtually no support and no services. Fortunately, alternatives are being created that bridge the large gap between home care and institutionalization. These alternatives include group homes, foster home care, home care with day school, home care with respite care (either community-based or in an institution), and short-term institutionalization for the purpose of intensive training or respite for the family.

Enactment of Public Laws 94-142 and 99-457 guaranteed privileges that other parents take for granted: assistance with the education and social development of their offspring and a break from the 24 hour-a-day responsibility for their supervision and care. The law also mandated that parents be included in the formulation of appropriate goals and programs for their children.

Denhoff[157] states that one of the major benefits of infant stimulation or enrichment programs is that they enable infants who are severely handicapped to stay at home. "A good (infant enrichment) program not only instructs and supports parents in carrying out a therapeutic regimen at home, but also helps them to cope with irregularities of feeding, sleeping, crying, and other problems which lessen the chances of survival of the family."

The passage of laws does not guarantee that the rights of individuals with mental retardation will be supported in philosophy and practice. Parents need to know what the rights of their children are and how to become effective advocates in their behalf. They need opportunities to meet other parents of children with handicaps and assistance in developing support groups. The concept of community-based programs is an important one for parents, but ideas can be a long way from reality. Too many families do not have access to group homes, respite care, or other support services in their community. Although, in general, public awareness and concern for individuals with mental retardation have improved, parents still often feel isolated and guilty. The persistence of architectural barriers in public facilities is a too-frequent reminder that society is not yet concerned enough. Many of the programs and much of the research effort that benefits individuals with mental retardation is funded through government sources. With severe cuts in state and federal budgets, it is more important than ever that citizens in every community become advocates for the mentally retarded and help support the children and their families.

Professionals must resist the tendency to make prejudgments about what is appropriate for the severely handicapped and to give parents "stock" answers.[158] The ability to listen and to consider compassionately not only the financial but the emotional economy of each family is vital. Parents must be encouraged to voice their own needs and concerns, guided to an understanding of their child's many problems, assisted in finding constructive ways to interact with and "teach" their child, and supported in their efforts to work in the child's behalf.

Educational materials specifically addressed to parents have been published by a wide variety of public organizations and private citizens. Bibliographies listing publications of interest to parents are available from The Association for the Severely Handicapped and the Association for Retarded Citizens. Both of these associations provide excellent support to parents and effective advocacy for their children with handicaps. More is needed.

With the development of new types of programs—new facilities as well as traditional institutional settings—paraprofessionals with a variety of job descriptions are providing care for the profoundly and severely retarded. These workers need to receive instruction in how to develop effective patient management skills, so that the mentally retarded can benefit from their consistency. Recommending specific measurable objectives for the staff to work on will facilitate cooperation and consistency in program implementation and provide the reward of seeing positive growth in the children under their care.[159]

Another group that needs guidance in how to understand and support the mentally retarded are the normal children, who, as a result of mainstreaming, are interacting with their mentally retarded peers in school on a regular basis. Successful attempts at shaping positive attitudes have been achieved with group discussion, role playing, and the use of audiovisuals.[160-163] "The Kids On the Block, Inc."[164] is a commercially available program that includes puppets with a variety of problems, including mental retardation and CP. The puppets with problems interact with normal peers in prescribed scripts, appropriate for a range of ages, but targeted for fourth graders. A special book review section in an issue of *Physical and Occupational Therapy in Pediatrics* provides information about numerous children's books written to help provide information and promote acceptance/understanding of children with handicapping conditions, including mental retardation.[165]

CONCLUSION

Individuals who are severely and profoundly retarded are people with needs and rights, like all of us. Caring for and about them adequately simply demands a little extra insight, creativity, resourcefulness, and patience.

"Cortical function can be curtailed in a great variety of patterns, but barring the totally comatose state, there are always residual perceptions and expressions. These latter elements can be reached, usually in stimulation and training programs, and the expression of such established function is the core of 'fulfillment' at any level. Gratification of this need for fulfillment will add grace to what can otherwise be a dismal atmosphere."[162]

REFERENCES

1. Humphrey H: Quoted in: The Problem of Mental Retardation. President's Commission on Mental Retardation. US Department of Health and Human Services (79-21021), Washington, DC, 1977
2. Grossman HJ (ed): Classification in Mental Retardation. American Association on Mental Deficiency, Washington, DC, 1983
3. President's Committee on Mental Retardation: Report to the President—MR 79. Mental Retardation: Prevention Strategies that Work. Department of Health and Human Services, Office of Human Development Services, Washington, DC, 1980
4. Hobbs N (ed): Issues in the Classification of Children. Vols. 1 and 2. Jossey-Bass, San Francisco, 1975
5. Baroff GS: Mental Retardation: Nature, Cause, and Management. 2nd Ed. Hemisphere Publishing Corporation, New York, 1986
6. Gustavson KH, Holmgren RJ, Son Blomquist HK: Severe mental retardation in children in a northern Swedish county. J Ment Defic Res 21:161, 1977
7. Bruincks RH: Physical and motor development of retarded persons. p. 209. In Ellis N (ed): International Review of Research in Mental Retardation. Vol. 7. Academic Press, New York, 1974
8. Malamud N: Neuropathology. p. 429. In Stevens HA, Heber R (eds): Mental Retardation: A Review of Research. University of Chicago Press, Chicago, 1964

9. Conley RW: The Economics of Mental Retardation. John Hopkins University Press, Baltimore, 1973
10. Capute AJ, Shapiro BK, Palmer FB: Spectrum of developmental disabilities: continuum of motor dysfunction. Orthop Clin North Am 12:3, 1981
11. Eyman RK, Miller C: Introduction: A demographic overview of severe and profound mental retardation. In Meyers CE (ed): Quality of Life in Severely and Profoundly Mentally Retarded People: Research Foundations for Improvement. American Association for Mental Retardation, Washington, DC, 1978
12. Zigler E, Balla D: Mental Retardation: The Developmental Difference Controversy. Lawrence Erlbaum Associates, Hillsdale, NJ, 1982
13. Weisz JR, Zigler E: Cognitive development in retarded and nonretarded persons: Piagetian tests of the similar sequence hypothesis. Psychol Bull 86:831, 1979
14. President's Committee on Mental Retardation: A Historical Review, 1966–1985. US Department of Health and Human Services, Office of Human Development Services, Washington, DC, 1986
15. Rosen M (ed): The History of Mental Retardation. Vols. 1 and II. University Park Press, Baltimore, 1976
16. Scheerenberger RC: A History of Mental Retardation. Paul H Brookes Publishing Co, Baltimore, 1983
17. Public Law 94-142: "The Education for All Handicapped Children Act of 1975": Signed, November 29, 1975. US Congress, Washington, DC
18. Public Law 99-457: "Education of the Handicapped Act Amendments of 1986": Signed, October 8, 1986. US Congress, Washington, DC
19. Public Law 98-457: "Developmental Disabilities Assistance and Bill of Rights Act": Signed, October 19, 1984, US Congress, Washington, DC
20. Public Law 101-336: "Americans With Disabilities Act of 1990": Signed, July 26, 1990. US Congress, Washington, DC
21. President's Committee on Mental Retardation: A Presidential Forum—Citizens with Mental Retardation and Community Integration. Forum Proceedings, Department of Health and Human Services, Office of Human Development Services, Washington, DC, 1989
22. Anderson AL: Dental care for persons with mental retardation. p. 187. In President's Committee on Mental Retardation: A Presidential Forum—Citizens with Mental Retardation and Community Integration. Forum Proceedings, Department of Health and Human Services, Office of Human Development Services, Washington, DC, 1989
23. Fraser BA, Hensinger RN, Phelps JA: A Professional's Guide—Physical Management of Multiple Handicaps. Paul H Brookes Publishing Co., Baltimore, 1987
24. Hoffer MM, Bullock M: The functional and social significance of orthopedic rehabilitation of mentally retarded patients with cerebral palsy. Orthop Clin North Am 12:185, 1981
25. Pettitt B: Surgery of the lower extremity in cerebral palsy: considerations and approaches. Arch Phys Med Rehabil 57:443, 1976
26. Lindsey RW, Drennan JC: Management of foot and knee deformities in the mentally retarded. Orthop Clin North Am 12:107, 1981
27. Gadow KD, Poling AG: Pharmacotherapy and Mental Retardation. College Hill Press, Boston, 1988
28. Matson JL, Frame CL: Psychopathology among mentally retarded children and adolescents. p. 13. In Kazdin AE (series ed): Clinical Psychology and Psychiatry Series. Vol. 6. SAGE Publications, Beverly Hills, 1986

29. Richardson SA, Koller H, Matz M: Seizures and epilepsy in a mentally retarded population. Appl Res Ment Retard 1:123, 1981

30. Gever LN (Clinical Pharmacy ED): Nursing 81 Drug Handbook. Intermed Communications. Horsham, PA, 1981

31. Harrell RF, Capp RH, Davis DR et al: Can nutritional supplements help mentally retarded children: an exploratory study. Proc Natl Acad Sci USA 78:574, 1981

32. Hitchings WD: Megavitamins and diet. p. 92. In Feingold B, Bank C (eds): Developmental Disabilities of Early Childhood. Charles C Thomas, Springfield, IL, 1978

33. Mailman RB, Lewis MH: Food additives and developmental disorders: the case of erythrosin (FD and C red #3) or guilty until proven innocent? Appl Res Ment Retard 2:297, 1981

34. Pollitt E: Developmental impact of nutrition. p. 33. In Bray NW (ed): International Review of Research in Mental Retardation. Vol. 15, Academic Press, New York, 1988

35. Carenza EC: Pediatricks. Van Nostrand Reinhold, New York, 1974

36. McCuller WR, Salzburg CL: The functional analysis of imitation. p. 285. In Ellis NR (ed): International Review of Research in Mental Retardation. Vol. 11. Academic Press, New York, 1982

37. Altman R, Ralkington LW, Cleland CC: Relative effectiveness of modeling and verbal instruction on severe retardates' gross motor performance. Psychol Rep 31:695, 1972

38. Ritvo ER, Ornitz EM, La Franchi S: Frequency of repetitive behaviors in early infantile autism and its variants. Arch Gen Psychiatry 19:341, 1968

39. Piaget F: The Origins of Intelligence in Children. Norton, New York, 1963

40. Kahn JV: Relationship of Piaget's sensorimotor period to language acquisition of profoundly retarded children. Am J Ment Defic 79:640, 1975

41. Silverman FH: Communication for the Speechless. Prentice-Hall, Englewood Cliffs, NJ, 1980

42. Gould J: The use of the Vineland Social Maturity Scale, the Merrill-Palmer Scale of Mental Tests (non-verbal items) and the Reynell Developmental Language Scales with children in contact with the services for severe mental retardation. J Ment Defic Res 21:213, 1977

43. Langley MB: Assessment of the Multihandicapped, Visually Impaired Child. Stoelting, Chicago, 1980

44. Murray JN (ed): Developing Assessment Programs for the Multi-handicapped Child. Charles C Thomas, Springfield, IL, 1980

45. Mulliken RK, Buckley JJ: Assessment of Multihandicapped and Developmentally Disabled Children. Aspen Systems, Rockville, MD, 1986

46. Naglieri JA: Extrapolated developmental indices for the Bayley Scales of Infant Development. Am J Ment Defic 85:548, 1981

47. Haskett HJ, Bell J: Profound developmental retardation: descriptive and theoretical utility of the Bayley Mental Scale. p. 327. In Myers CE (ed): Quality of Life in Severely and Profoundly Retarded People: Research Foundations for Improvement. AAMR, Washington, DC, 1978

48. Hardman ML, Drew CJ: The physically handicapped retarded individual: a review. Ment Retard 15:43, 1971

49. Francis RJ, Rarick GL: Motor characteristics of the mentally retarded. Am J Ment Defic 63:792, 1959

50. Samilson RL: Orthopedic surgery of the hips and spine in retarded cerebral palsy patients. Orthop Clin North Am 12:83, 1981

51. Fiorentino MR: A Basis for Sensorimotor Development: Normal and Abnormal. Charles C Thomas, Springfield, IL, 1981
52. Cusick BD: Progressive Casting and Splinting: For Lower Extremity Deformities in Children With Neuromotor Dysfunction. Therapy Skill Builders, Tucson, AZ, 1990
53. Sherrill C: Posture training as a means of normalization. Ment Retard 18:135, 1980
54. Kendall HO, Kendall FP: Developing and maintaining good posture. Phys Ther 48:319, 1968
55. Rinsky LA: Perspectives on surgery for scoliosis in mentally retarded patients. Orthop Clin North Am 12:113, 1981
56. Ellis D (ed): Sensory Impairments in Mentally Handicapped People. College-Hill Press, San Diego, 1986
57. Ayres AJ: Sensory Integration and Learning Disorders. Western Psychological Services, Los Angeles, 1976
58. Montgomery PC: Assessment and treatment of the child with mental retardation: guidelines for the public school therapist. Phys Ther 61:1265, 1981
59. Wilson JM: Developing ambulation skills. p. 83. In Connelly B, Montgomery P (eds): Therapeutic Exercise in Developmental Disabilities. Chattanooga Corporation, Chattanooga, TN, 1987
60. Wilson V, Parks R: Promoting ambulation in the severely retarded child. Ment Retard 8:17, 1970
61. Illingworth RS: The Development of the Infant and Young Child. 5th Ed. Churchill Livingstone, London, 1974
62. Donoghue E, Kirman B, Bullmore GH: Some factors affecting age of walking in a mentally retarded population. Dev Med Child Neurol 18:71, 1976
63. Shapiro BK, Accardo PJ, Capute AJ: Factors affecting walking in a profoundly retarded population. Dev Med Child Neurol 21:369, 1979
64. Molnar GE: Motor deficit of retarded infants and young children. Arch Phys Med Rehabil 55:393, 1974
65. Grady A, Gilfoyle E: A developmental theory of somatosensory perception. In Henderson A, Coryell J (eds): The Body Senses and Perceptual Deficit. Boston University, Boston, 1973
66. Montgomery P, Gauger J: Sensory dysfunction in children who toe walk. Phys Ther 58:1195, 1978
67. Bertoti DB: Effect of short leg casting on ambulation in children with cerebral palsy. Phys Ther 66:1522, 1986
68. Montgomery PC, Richter E: Sensorimotor Integration for the Developmentally Disabled Child: A Handbook. Western Psychological Services, Los Angeles, 1980
69. Cleland CC, Powell HC, Talkington LW: Death of the profoundly retarded. Ment Retard 9:36, 1971
70. Chaney RH: Respiratory complications in the profoundly retarded compared to those in less retarded. In Schwartz JD, Eyman PC, Cleland CC, O'Grady R (eds): The Profoundly Mentally Retarded. Vol. IX. Western Research Conference, Austin, TX, 1978
71. Barnard K: Nursing child assessment feeding scale. Nursing Child Assessment Satellite Training. Kathryn Barnard, University of Washington, School of Nursing, Child Development and Mental Retardation Center, Seattle, 1985
72. Morris SE, Klein MD: Pre-Feeding Skills: A Comprehensive Resource for Feeding Development. Therapy Skill Builders, Tucson, AZ, 1987
73. Rothman JG: Effects of respiratory exercises on the vital capacity and forced expiratory volume in children with cerebral palsy. Phys Ther 58:421, 1978

74. Bjure J, Berg K: Dynamic and static lung volumes of school children with cerebral palsy. Acta Paediatr Scand Suppl 204:35, 1970
75. Langley MB: A developmental approach to the use of toys for facilitation of environmental control. Phys Occup Ther Pediatr 10(2):83, 1990
76. Presperin J: Seating systems: the therapist and rehabilitation engineering team. Phys Occup Ther Pediatr 10(2):17, 1990
77. Wilson JM: Selection and use of adaptive equipment for children. Totline 6:4, 1980
78. Bergen AF, Colangelo C: Positioning the Client With Central Nervous System Deficits: The Wheelchair and Other Adapted Equipment. Valhalla Rehabilitation Publications, Valhalla, NY, 1982
79. Jacques K, Fraser BA, Hensinger RN, Phelps JA: A Professional's Guide: Physical Management of Multiple Handicaps. Paul H Brookes Publishing Co, Baltimore, 1987
80. Bergen A: Selected Equipment for Pediatric Rehabilitation. Blythdale Children's Hospital, Valhalla, NY, 1974
81. Slominski A: Please Help Us Help Ourselves: Inexpensive Adapted Equipment for the Handicapped. Cerebral Palsy Clinic, Indiana University Medical Center, Indianapolis, 1970
82. Robinault I: Functional aides for the multiply handicapped. Harper & Row, New York, 1973
83. Dubose RF, Deni K: Easily Constructed Adaptive and Assistive Equipment. The Council for Exceptional Children, Reston, VA, 1980
84. Capecchi J: Skater sled for retarded persons. Phys Ther 58:181, 1978
85. Webster's New Collegiate Dictionary. Merriam, Springfield, MA, 1979
86. Hutt ML, Gibby RG: The Mentally Retarded Child: Development, Training and Education. 4th Ed. Allyn and Bacon, Boston, 1979
87. MacLean W, Baumeister A: Observational analysis of the stereotyped mannerisms of a developmentally delayed infant. Appl Res Ment Retard 2:257, 1981
88. Scherzer AL, Mike V, Ilson J: Physical therapy as a determinant of change in the cerebral palsied infant. Pediatrics 58:47, 1976
89. Sommerfeld S, Fraser BA, Hensinger RN, Beresford CV: Evaluation of physical therapy service for severely mentally impaired students with cerebral palsy. Phys Ther 61:338, 1981
90. Bry PM, Nawas MM: Is reinforcement necessary for the development of a generalized imitation operant in severly and profoundly retarded children? Am J Ment Deficiency 76:658, 1972
91. Westervelt VD, Luiselli JK: Establishing standing and walking behavior in a physically handicapped, retarded child. Phys Ther 55:761, 1975
92. Sparling J: The transdisciplinary approach with the developmentally delayed child. Phys Occup Ther Pediatr 1(2):3, 1980
93. Kielhofner G, Miyake S: The therapeutic use of play with mentally retarded adults. Am J Occup Ther 35:375, 1981
94. Godfrey B, Kephart N: Movement Patterns and Motor Education. Appleton-Century-Crofts, New York, 1969
95. Chaney C, Kephart N: Motoric Aids to Perceptual Training. Merrill, Columbus, OH, 1971
96. Kephart N: The Slow Learner in the Classroom. 2nd Ed. Merrill, Columbus, OH, 1968
97. Cratty BJ, Martin MM: Perceptual Motor Efficiency in Children. Lea & Febiger, Philadelphia, 1974

98. Cratty BJ: Motor Activity and the Education of Retardates. Lea & Febiger, Philadelphia, 1974

99. Cratty BJ: The use of movement activities in the education of retarded children. p. 311. In Pearson PH, Williams CE (eds): Physical Therapy Services in the Developmental Disabilities. Charles C Thomas, Springfield, IL, 1972

100. Ostrosky KM: Facilitation vs motor control. Clin Management 10:34, 1990

101. Carr JH, Shepherd RB: The motor learning model for rehabilitation. p. 31. In Carr JH, Shepherd RB, Gordon J et al (eds): Movement Science: Foundations for Physical Therapy in Rehabilitation. Aspen Publishers, Rockville, MD, 1987

102. Bobath K, Bobath B: Diagnosis and assessment of cerebral palsy. p. 31. In Pearson PH, Williams CE (eds): Physical Therapy Services in the Developmental Disabilities. Charles C Thomas, Springfield, IL, 1972

103. Semans S: The Bobath concept in treatment of neurological disorders: a neurodevelopmental treatment. Am J Phys Med 46:732, 1967

104. Stockmeyer SA: An interpretation of the approach of Rood to the treatment of neuromuscular dysfunction. Am J Phys Med 46:900, 1967

105. Stockmeyer SA: A sensorimotor approach to treatment. p. 186. In Pearson PH, Williams CE (eds): Physical Therapy Services in the Developmental Disabilities. Charles C Thomas, Springfield, IL, 1972

106. Ginsburg H, Opper S: Piaget's Theory of Intellectual Development. Prentice-Hall, Englewood Cliffs, NJ, 1969

107. Bradley-Johnson S, Friedrich DD, Wyrembelske AR: Exploratory behavior in Down's syndrome and normal infants. Appl Res Ment Retard 2:213, 1981

108. Montgomery P, Richter E: Effect of sensory integrative therapy on the neuromotor development of retarded children. Phys Ther 57:799, 1977

109. Norton Y: Neurodevelopment and sensory integration for the profoundly retarded multiply handicapped child. Am J Occup Ther 29, 1975

110. Clark FA, Miller LR, Thomas JA et al: A comparison of operant and sensory integrative methods on developmental parameters in profoundly retarded adults. Am J Occup Ther 32:86, 1978

111. Webb RC: Sensory-motor training of the profoundly retarded. Am J Ment Defic 74, 1969

112. Ottenbacher K: Developmental implications of clinically applied vestibular stimulation: a review. Phys Ther 63(3):1, 1983

113. Ottenbacher K, Short MA, Watson PJ: The effects of a clinically applied program of vestibular stimulation on the neuromotor performance of children with severe developmental disorders. Phys Occup Ther Pediatr 1(3):1, 1981

114. Magrun WM, Ottenbacher K, McCue S et al: Effects of vestibular stimulation on the spontaneous use of verbal language in developmentally delayed children. Am J Occup Ther 35:101, 1981

115. Bright T, Bittick K, Fleeman B: Reduction of self-injurious behavior using sensory integrative techniques. Am J Occup Ther 35:167, 1981

116. Evans RG: The reduction of hyperactive behavior in three profoundly retarded adolescents through increased stimulation. American Association for the Education of S & P Hand Rev 4:259, 1979

117. Page D: Neuromuscular reflex therapy as an approach to patient care. Am J Phys Med 46:816, 1967

118. Delacato CH: The Diagnosis and Treatment of Speech and Reading Problems. Charles C Thomas, Springfield, IL, 1963

119. Doman RJ, Spitz EB, Zucman E et al: Children with severe brain injuries. Neurologic organization in terms of mobility. JAMA 174:157, 1960

120. Cohen HJ, Birch HG, Taft LT: Some considerations for evaluating the Doman-Delacato "patterning" method. Pediatrics 45:302, 1970
121. Sparrow S, Zigler E: Evaluation of a patterning treatment for retarded children. Pediatrics 62:137, 1978
122. Zigler E: A plea to end the use of the patterning treatment for retarded children. Am J Orthopsychiatry 51:388, 1981
123. Position on Doman-Delacato Treatment. House of Delegates (HOD 06-87-09-15), American Physical Therapy Association Annual Conference, June 1989
124. Skinner BF: Science and Human Behavior. Macmillan, New York, 1953
125. Bragg JH, Houser C, Schumaker J: Behavior modification in the treatment of children with cerebral palsy. Phys Ther 55:860, 1975
126. Banks SP: Behavior therapy with a boy who had never learned to walk. Psychother Theory Res Pract 5:150, 1968
127. Chandler LS, Adams MA: Multiply handicapped child motivated for ambulation through behavior modification. Case report. Phys Ther 52:399, 1972
128. Hester SB: Effects of behavior modification on the standing and walking deficiencies of a profoundly retarded child. Case report. Phys Ther 61:807, 1980
129. Kolderie ML: Behavior modification in the treatment of children with cerebral palsy. Phys Ther 51:1083, 1971
130. Loynd J, Barclay A: A case study in developing ambulation in a profoundly retarded child. Behav Res Ther 8:207, 1970
131. Miller H, Patton M, Henton K: Behavior modification in a profoundly retarded child: a case report. Behav Ther 2:375, 1971
132. Rice HK, McDaniel MW, Denney SL: Operant conditioning techniques for use in the physical rehabilitation of the multiply handicapped retarded patients. Phys Ther 48:342, 1968
133. Garber NB: Operant procedures to eliminate drooling behavior in a cerebral palsied adolescent. Dev Med Child Neurol 13:641, 1971
134. O'Brien F, Azrin T, Bugle C: Training profoundly retarded children to stop crawling. J Appl Behav Anal 5:131, 1972
135. Vukelich R, Hake DF: Reduction of dangerously aggressive behavior in a severely retarded resident through a combination of positive reinforcement procedures. J Appl Behav Anal 4:215, 1971
136. Corte HE, Wolf MM, Locke BJ: A comparison of procedures for eliminating self-injurious behavior of retarded adolescents. J Appl Behav Anal 4:201, 1971
137. Luiselli JK: Controlling self-inflicted biting of a retarded child by the differential reinforcement of other behavior. Psychol Rep 42:435, 1978
138. Barret R, Matson J, Shapiro E et al: A comparison of punishment and DRO procedures for treating the stereotypic behavior of mentally retarded children. Appl Res Ment Retard 2:247, 1981
139. Alberto PA, Troutman AC: Applied Behavioral Analysis for Teachers-Influencing Student Performance. 2nd Ed. Charles E Merrill, Columbus, OH, 1987
140. Levin J, Scherfenberg L: Selection and Use of Simple Technology in Home, School, Work, and Community Settings. ABLENET, Minneapolis, MN, 1987
141. Burkhart LJ: Homemade Battery Powered Toys and Educational Devices for Severely Handicapped Children. Linda J. Burkhart, 8503 Rhode Island Ave, College Park, MD 20740, 1985
142. Burkhart LJ: More Homemade Battery Powered Toys and Educational Devices

for Severely Handicapped Children. Linda J. Burkhart, 8503 Rhode Island Ave, College Park, MD 20740, 1985

143. Ball TS, McCrady RE, Hard AD: Automated reinforcement of head posture in two cerebral palsied retarded children. Percept Mot Skills 40:619, 1975

144. Silverstein L: Biofeedback with young cerebral palsied children. p. 142. In Feingold B, Bank C (eds): Developmental Disabilities of Early Childhood. Charles C Thomas, Springfield, IL, 1978

145. Maloney FP, Kurtz PA: The use of a mercury switch head control device in profoundly retarded, multiply handicapped children. Phys Occup Ther Pediatr 2(4):11, 1982

146. Leiper CI, Miller A, Lang J et al: Sensory feedback for head control in cerebral palsy. Phys Ther 61:512, 1981

147. Ball TS, Combs T, Rugh J et al: Automated range of motion training with two cerebral palsied retarded young men. Ment Retard 15:47, 1977

148. Skrotzky K, Gallenstein JS, Osternig LR: Effects of electromyographic feedback training on motor control in spastic cerebral palsy. Phys Ther 58:547, 1978

149. Ball TS, McCrady RE: Automated finger praxis training with a cerebral palsied retarded adolescent. Ment Retard 13:41, 1975

150. Frielander BZ, Kamin P, Hesse GW: Operant therapy for prehension disabilities in moderately and severely retarded young children. Train Sch Bull (Vinel) 71:101, 1974

151. Whitman TL, Scibak JW, Reid DH: Behavior Modification With the Severely and Profoundly Retarded: Research and Application, Academic Press, San Diego, 1983

152. Clark FA, Shuer J: A clarification of sensory integrative therapy and its application to programming with retarded people. Ment Retard 6, 1978

153. Ayres AJ: Southern California Postrotary Nystagmus Test. Western Psychological Services, Los Angeles, 1975

154. McClure JT, Moss RA, McPeters JW et al: Reduction of hand mouthing by a boy with profound mental retardation. Ment Retard 24(4):219, 1986

155. Perske R, Clifton A, McLean B et al (eds): Mealtimes for Severely and Profoundly Handicapped Persons: New Concepts and Attitudes. 2nd Ed. University Park Press, Baltimore, 1986

156. Eyman RK, Miller C: Introduction: a demographic overview of severe and profound mental retardation. In Meyers CE (ed): Quality of Life in Severely and Profoundly Mentally Retarded People: Research Foundations for Improvement. American Association for Mental Retardation, Washington, DC, 1978

157. Denhoff E: Current status of infant stimulation or enrichment programs for children with developmental disabilities. Pediatrics 67:32, 1981

158. Crocker AC, Cushna B: Pediatric decisions in children with serious mental retardation. Pediatr Clin North Am 19:413, 1972

159. Anderson RM, Greer JG, Smith RM: Educating the Severely and Profoundly Retarded. University Park Press, Baltimore, 1976

160. Gottlief J: Improving attitudes toward children by using group discussion. Except Child 47:106, 1979

161. Kitano M, Chan KS: Taking the role of retarded children: effects of familiarity and similarity. Am J Ment Defic 83:37, 1978

162. Westervelt VD, Turnbull AP: Children's attitudes toward physically handicapped peers and intervention approaches for attitude change. Phys Ther 60:896, 1980

163. Gilfoyle EM, Gliner JA: Attitudes toward handicapped children: impact of an educational program. Phys Occup Ther Pediatr 5(4):27, 1985
164. Aiello B: Information brochure. The Kids On the Block, Inc. The Washington Bldg, Suite 510, Washington, DC, 20005, 1980
165. Levine SB (ed): Books for children and adolescents. A special book review section. Phys Occup Ther Pediatr 9(4):85, 1989

10 | Cerebral Palsy

Janet M. Wilson

Cerebral palsy (CP) may be the most common pediatric neurologic problem referred to physical therapists and, at the same time, may represent the least well-defined and least understood pediatric neurologic problem. It is important, first, to understand that the term CP is a description, not a specific diagnosis, of the clinical sequelae resulting from a nonprogressive encephalopathy whose etiology may be pre-, peri-, or postnatal.[1] Cerebral palsy is characterized by sensorimotor dysfunction, which has as its expression abnormal muscle tone and abnormal posture and movement. While CP is caused by a static encephalopathy, the symptoms often appear to be progressive because it affects a changing organism in which a developing, albeit abnormal, central nervous system (CNS) attempts to direct and control other maturing systems, including the musculoskeletal structures. The expression of the disorder can appear worse as the child grows, develops, and attempts to compensate for abnormality while confronting the force of gravity in every effort to move. Cerebral palsy is a developmental disorder affecting the total development of the child either directly, relating to sensorimotor function, or indirectly through associated problems. As a developmental disorder, CP has varying effects on children at different stages of development as well as at different chronologic ages. Although the hallmark of CP is motor dysfunction, various other problems frequently coexist, including sensory impairments, retrolental fibroplasia, nystagmus, strabismus, seizure disorders, mental retardation, behavior disorders, learning disabilities, sensory integrative dysfunction, speech and language disorders, or oral–dental disorders.[2]

PREVALENCE AND ETIOLOGY

Because CP is neither a reportable disease nor a diagnostic entity, prevalence figures in the literature vary.[3-8] Much of the variation arises from the lack of uniform criteria for diagnosis, sample selection and size, and age at

301

time of outcome assessment. A figure of 2.0 per 1,000 live births represents an average of data from prevalence studies reported in a review by Hagberg.[9] The notion of a steady reduction in CP prevalence rates corresponding to improved neonatal care is not sustained by the available evidence. Reported changes in rates vary from one country to another as well as within cities and counties within a single country.[4,6] In recent years, neonatal mortality rates for low birth weight infants have declined in neonatal intensive care units; however, considerable variation exists in the reported rates of handicaps in these surviving children.[5]

Etiologic factors underlying CP are usually grouped into pre-, peri-, and postnatal categories.[10] Prenatal factors are hereditary or genetic conditions; prenatal infections including viral (rubella, herpes), bacterial, and parasitic (toxoplasmosis); fetal anoxia caused by hemorrhage from premature separation of the placenta or maldevelopment of the placenta; Rh incompatibility including erythroblastosis fetalis, hemolytic anemia, and hyperbilirubinemia; metabolic disorders such as maternal diabetes and toxemia of pregnancy; and developmental deficits, which include maldevelopment of the brain, vascular, and skeletal structures.

Perinatal factors include rupture of brain blood vessels or compression of the brain during prolonged or difficult labor, and asphyxia caused by drug sedation, distress of labor, premature separation of the placenta, and placenta previa or related to prematurity.

Postnatal factors leading to CP include vascular accidents and intracranial hemorrhage, head trauma, brain infections including bacterial or viral encephalopathies, toxic conditions such as lead poisoning, anoxia from drowning or cardiac arrest, seizures, and tumors. Most children with CP are noted to have multiple etiologies, with intra- and periventricular bleeds or difficulty maintaining adequate oxygenation because of prematurity being the most common associated factors.[10] Certain etiologic factors predispose to specific clinical types of CP. For example, O'Reilly and Walentynowicz showed in their study of 2,004 children that prematurity or multiple births accounted for 55 percent of children with spastic diplegia while anoxia, respiratory distress, and erythroblastosis fetalis accounted for 63 percent of the athetoid children.[10]

The clinical picture resulting from hemorrhagic or ischemic brain damage differs depending on the postconceptional age of the infant at the time of the insult.[11,12] The clinical picture of spastic diplegia in the very young, premature infant results from ischemic damage to descending motor pathways in the internal capsule that control the motoneurons to muscles of the legs and trunk. Intraventricular bleeds in the immature infant may cause destruction of the germinal matrix surrounding the cerebral ventricles and result in hydrocephalus. Birth asphyxia in the term infant results in a variety of patterns of damage depending on the extent to which systemic blood pressure and cerebral blood flow are maintained. The clinical picture ranges from spastic quadriplegia or hemiplegia to choreoathetosis.[12,13]

Changes in obstetric management and neonatal intensive care have altered the percentages in the various etiologic categories. For example, O'Reilly and

Walentynowicz[10] and Churchill and colleagues[14] report increasing incidence of spastic diplegia related to the problems of prematurity, a decrease in athetosis related to erythroblastosis fetalis, and a decrease in hemiplegia associated with cesarian section. Pape and Wigglesworth,[12] however, believe that the incidence of uncomplicated periventricular leukomalacia resulting in clinical spastic diplegia is decreasing with improved management of hypothermia, nutrition, and apnea. In the surviving very low birth weight infants, an increased frequency of severe multiple defects, including spastic quadriplegia, hemiplegia, and severe mental retardation, is related to massive periventricular lesions.

CLASSIFICATION

Classification of CP by clinical types was adopted by the American Academy for Cerebral Palsy (now the American Academy for Cerebral Palsy and Developmental Medicine) and remains the most widely used system of classification.[15] This system, based on a description of topographic distribution of the tone and movement disorder, is useful to physical therapists because it provides a picture of the child's motor problem. Appendix 1 of this chapter summarizes this classification of CP. Although this system is well recognized, it is limited in two aspects. First, it does not take into account changes that occur during development of the child with CP. For this reason, it is possible for an infant to be described as having hypotonic CP, and, at 1 year, as he or she begins to crawl and sit, to be described as a spastic diplegic, while at 4 years, as he or she pulls to stand, attempts to walk, manipulates toys, and struggles with self-care, the child may be described as a spastic quadriplegic. None of these descriptions are wrong. This child actually presented quite differently at various developmental stages and chronologic ages. Yet, the changing "diagnosis" leads to confusion and mistrust between the parents and the professionals and lack of credibility among professionals.

Another system of classification, described by Quinton and Wilson,[16] classifies children with CP according to tonus and changing motor patterns. Quinton classifies CP by the development of the child's tone and movement as he or she changes over time with position and movement against gravity. This classification serves three functions: it allows the examiner to (1) recognize normal and abnormal changes in tone and movement as the child grows and develops, (2) observe the progression of symptoms of motor dysfunction and determine which child is recovering from an initial brain insult and which one is developing increasing symptoms of motor dysfunction, and (3) determine if treatment is effectively changing the child's movements to more normal patterns.

A second problem of classifying CP according to clinical types is the inability to provide clues for reliable prognosis. This problem is addressed in a classification system proposed by Milani-Comparetti and Gidoni.[17,18] This classification is divided into three syndromes: regression, defect, and disharmony syndromes.

The regression syndromes are abnormalities of movement identical with patterns seen in the early stages of normal fetal development, hence the term. The primary characteristic of these syndromes is limited variety of movement resulting from the overpowering influence of the early fetal movement patterns. The defect syndrome is characterized by lack of postural control. This syndrome is often associated with severe mental retardation. The disharmony syndrome is characterized by disorganized movement, but without any limitation in the variety of movement patterns available.

To some extent, choice of a system of classification of CP depends on the reasons for describing the child. Classifications of CP that focus on progression of symptoms as the child moves against the force of gravity may provide more information to the physical therapist who is interested in how movement changes (normally and abnormally) and how movement patterns can be affected by treatment. The traditional classification by topographic distribution of tone and abnormal movement does not have this inherent component.

DIAGNOSIS AND PROGNOSIS

In addition to the problems of classifying and describing children with CP, the problems of accurate identification and prediction of the extent of motor dysfunction are well known. Retrospective studies have emphasized a history of pre- and perinatal complications, including prematurity,[19,20] the presence of a number of abnormal neurologic findings in the neonatal period,[21-23] abnormal tone and maintained primitive reflexes,[24-26] failure of development of the postural reflex mechanism, and delayed developmental milestones,[2,25,26] as precursors or indications of the diagnosis of CNS dysfunction in children. Paine and colleagues[27] followed the natural history of a large number of abnormal infants and described the appearance of abnormal tone, persistent primitive reflexes, and delay in the postural reactions in this population. Data from the Collaborative Perinatal Project, in which 53,600 singleton infants born between 1959 and 1969 were periodically examined and followed for 7 years, have been published.[3,28] This study has provided much additional information regarding specific signs as predictors of CP. Ellenberg and Nelson[3] report the combination of low birth weight and hypertonus at 4 months as highly predictive of CP at 7 years. They also report that the additional presence of delayed motor milestones at 4 months strengthens the accuracy of this prediction. Campbell and Wilhelm[29,30] have reported their initial data from a longitudinal prospective study of infants at high risk for CNS dysfunction during the first year of life and found primitive reflexes and increased tone to be evident for long periods of time in the high-risk infants, but they were not related to motor outcome at 2 years unless very strong or very delayed in resolving. Again, delayed motor milestones in the first 6 months were highly predictive of poor outcome, although not necessarily of CP, at 2 years of age. While clinical data are accumulating, the task of early identification as it affects the prognosis of any specific child remains difficult, especially in the case of children with mild CNS dysfunction who may not be identified in infancy.

To compound the problem of accurate early identification, modern neonatal care and intensive care nurseries are rapidly changing the distribution of types of infants who survive severe birth trauma with major motor deficits. The actual incidence of infants surviving with handicaps ranges from 10 percent in inborn units to 30 to 40 percent in outborn units.[31-33] Follow-up studies confirm that the most immature infants and those requiring ventilatory support have the highest risk of neurodevelopmental sequelae.[31,32,34] Initial reports on the neurodevelopmental outcome of infants surviving neonatal intraventricular hemorrhage documented by computed tomographic brain scan or sequential ultrasound show similar incidences of neurologic defects.[35-37] Although this information is important for medical management, it actually contributes to the frustration of parents and therapists who have been told by well-informed pediatricians that a specific child will be likely to recover from early insult. In approximately 75 percent of the cases, the physician is correct and, fortunately, most children do develop normally; however, because of the inability to predict which children will fall into the approximately 25 percent who do not recover, the family may experience continued uncertainty and frustration in managing the child, loss of confidence in their own parenting skills, delay in involvement in intervention programs, and loss of confidence in the medical community if an unfavorable diagnosis is finally established.

Accurate diagnosis of CP at a young age is important for economic, social, emotional, and medical reasons. Because the value of early intervention has not been clearly established, accurate identification is essential for evaluation of the independent effects of treatment and maturation.

The question regarding prognosis most frequently asked of the physical therapist is, "Will my child walk?" Predicting walking for children with CP is a difficult and often unrewarding task. Consequently, therapists should be cautious about making predictions regarding ambulation potential because the outcome may either be better or worse than the initial presenting symptoms suggest.[38]

Some children who appear to be only "mildly" involved (i.e., show good reciprocal movements of their legs and the ability to stand with support at 12 months) may develop more severe problems as they struggle with the force of gravity, and walking may be delayed until the age of 5 or 6 years.[39] Some babies who appear to be severely affected following a difficult birth and perinatal course may make a good recovery and achieve motor milestones at a nearly normal rate.[40]

Several investigators have described the development of ambulation in children with various types of CP.[41-47] Molnar and Gordon reported that 78 percent of a sample of 233 children achieved some degree of functional walking.[41] Largo and colleagues found that the type of CP and the severity of tonal abnormalities were correlated with the development of locomotion skills.[43] The mean ages for attaining all forms of locomotion (crawling, creeping, cruising, and walking) were higher in a group of preterm infants with CP than in either normal preterm or full-term infants.

Molnar and associates found that the type and severity of CP were useful guides in predicting ambulation.[41,44,46] Most children with spastic hemiplegia walked by 2 years, and all walked by 3 years. Children with ataxia attained walking later, but all walked by 8 years. Children with spastic diplegia had a generally favorable outcome: 65 percent walked unassisted, 20 percent required assistive devices, and an additional 15 percent relied on wheelchairs and did not walk. Of the ambulators, the majority walked by 3 years. Children with spastic quadriplegia had the most variable outcome: only 63 percent ambulated independently or with assistive devices. Of children with athetosis, 75 percent became ambulatory, with or without aids. In separate studies, Badell-Ribera,[42] Molnar,[44] and Watt and colleagues[45] found that sitting by 2 years was a good predictive sign of eventual ambulation.

Other investigators have tried to link the potential for walking to motor patterns specific to CP. Bleck used the persistence of five primary tonic reflexes and absence of two postural reactions as indicators of eventual walking.[46] Molnar and Gordon found that 27 of 99 infants with CP had persistent primary reflexes at 12 months of age; of these children, only 22 percent ultimately walked.[41] Watt and colleagues also correlated persistent primitive reflexes and onset of postural reactions with the ability to ambulate.[45] The presence of primitive reflexes at 2 years was significantly associated with nonambulatory status at 8 years.

Various aspects of motor control have been shown to correlate with delayed onset of walking, but the relative contributions to achievement of ambulation of persistent primary reflexes, absent postural reactions, control of sitting, and clinical type of CP cannot be determined. Additional factors, including motivation, intelligence, interest, self-image, spatial abilities, family interest, support systems, and barrier-free school and home environments are all important considerations in the final outcome of ambulation.

MEDICAL MANAGEMENT

Pharmaceutical Management

Various drugs, including meprobamate, mephenesia, and benzodiazepines, have been used over the years to reduce spasticity or control involuntary movement in the child with CP. Most recently, baclofen, a gamma aminobutyric acid derivative, has been shown to be an effective inhibitor of mono- and polysynaptic reflexes and gamma motoneuron activity in decerebrate animals and a facilitator of Renshaw cell activity.[48]

Baclofen has been shown to be useful in the control of spinal and cerebral spasticity in adults.[49] More recently, studies have been done to determine the effectiveness of oral baclofen in reducing spasticity in children with spastic CP. Milla and Jackson[48] and McKinlay and associates[50] examined the effects of baclofen in double-blind crossover trials. Both groups examined 20 children between 2 and 16 years of age with spastic CP. Milla and Jackson[48] found that baclofen was significantly more effective than placebo in reducing spasticity in children with CP. Active movement showed significant improvement and resistance to passive movement decreased. McKinlay and colleagues,[50] however, did not find any significant benefits from baclofen on post-trial examination. Both groups reported side effects of hypotonia, sedation, enuresis, and attention problems.

Young[51] reported on an open trial of oral baclofen in 27 children between 4 months and 12 years of age with spastic CP. He found that baclofen was beneficial in spastic diplegia in improving mobility and ability to wear orthoses. He cautioned that although independent mobility improved, the gait pattern did not because tonal distribution contributing to scissoring was unchanged by baclofen. The drug was ineffective in mixed types of CP or in children with fixed deformities.

Minford and colleagues[52] assessed gait by polarized light goniometry in 15 hemiplegic children between 4 and 15 years of age prior to and following a 4- to 6-week treatment with baclofen. Each child was matched for age and sex with a normal child. A statistically significant decrease in hip and knee flexion at the toe-off phase of the gait cycle was found in both legs of experimental group children. Of the nine children who showed the greatest change on goniometric assessment, five showed obvious clinical improvement as well. Again, side effects of transient sedation, enuresis, and deterioration in behavior and concentration were reported, and the investigators suggest that oral baclofen should be used with caution and careful supervision.

Baclofen can be supplied intrathecally as well as orally. Recently, several investigators have explored the use of intrathecal baclofen in children and adults with CP.[53,54] An intrathecal catheter and drug infusion pump are placed at the level of T12 to L1. Significantly higher spinal concentrations can be obtained with fewer unwanted side effects.

Five studies assessing the use of baclofen on spasticity resulting from supraspinal injury or CP[53,55–58] have found desirable clinical effects. In the three double-blind crossover design studies, outcomes assessed included severity of spasticity, tonus, range of motion (ROM), deep tendon reflexes, spasm, ability to respond to therapy, walking, self-help, and manual dexterity. The results included significant improvement in reduction of spasticity and spasm and improved manual dexterity, ease of care, and ability to respond to therapy.

The two single-subject studies[57,58] used electromyography (EMG) to study the effects of baclofen on hyperactivity of muscles. One study[57] reported that effects were seen within minutes in the lower extremities. In the upper extremities, however, muscle activity initially increased and required 4 to 6 hours to decrease to an activity level similar to that in the legs. The other study reported significant reduction in spasticity in the involved side of a hemiplegic patient, while no weakness or decrease of function was noted in the uninvolved extremities despite the high intrathecal dosage of baclofen.[58]

Dantrolene sodium has also been used to control spasticity in children with CP. Joynt and Leonard[59] reported a double-blind study of 20 children comparing the effects of dantrolene sodium suspension and a placebo. The drug was physiologically active in reducing the force of muscle contraction in response to peripheral nerve stimulation, but objective functional improvement as measured by multiple performance tests, including tests of mobility and manual dexterity, was not found.

In addition to drugs that affect spasticity, intramuscular alcohol has been used for temporary reduction in spasticity. Carpenter and Sietz[60] reported on the use of intramuscular alcohol injection in 211 patients between the ages of 18 months and 16 years. They found the procedure to be ineffective for athetosis, rigidity, or ataxia, or when contracture was involved. The gastrocnemius-soleus muscle group had the highest predictable reduction of tone from the alcohol injection.

In selected cases, with careful monitoring, pharmaceutical management may be beneficial for assessment periods or for management of a specific problem related to overcoming spasticity.

Orthopedic Surgery

Orthopedic surgery is an important aspect of the management of the child with CP. The current literature describes procedures for the upper extremities, spine, and lower extremities.[61,62] The orthopedic literature is extensive; however, most of the reports are descriptive rather than evaluative. The ages, types, and severity of involvement as well as detailed descriptions of the surgical procedures are mentioned. Postoperative results are usually described in general terms of increased function, improved posture, or improved cosmesis and hygiene, without providing details regarding how the results are obtained or how they correlate with preoperative status.

In articles on surgery of the upper extremity and hand, only House and colleagues[63] describe the evaluation of various upper extremity surgical procedures. In 56 children with CP, they compared each patient's pre- and postoperative functional status measured on a functional classification scale devised by themselves. They found that patients with a markedly impaired hand showed greatest functional improvement on their scale of functional skills. IQ did not seem to play a very important role in predicting results. Normal sensibility was important, but not as useful as voluntary control in predicting outcome. Although the functional scale was an attempt to provide quantitative data, no evidence exists to suggest that this scale actually represents the levels of acquisition of hand skills in the CP population.

All of the articles reviewed indicated that outcome of surgical treatment of spastic patients was more predictable than in children with athetosis. Patients with hemiplegic CP made up the great majority of children for whom upper extremity surgery was indicated. Age and IQ were reportedly not as important as they once were thought to be, so long as the child was old enough and capable of cooperating with the program. Goals for hand surgery generally include improved function and activities of daily living (ADL) and improved cosmesis and hygiene.[63–65]

Hoffer and colleagues[66] indicate that the most difficult factors to document for surgical decision making are the control and phasic activity of various muscles. These investigators suggest that dynamic EMG using needle electrodes can be used to document muscle control and phasic activity. The EMG results in 21 patients showed that in CP, muscles are phase dependent and will not change phase; thus, it is important to transfer a muscle that will operate in the appropriate phase for its intended function. If the EMG demonstrated that target muscles were continuously active throughout the grasp-release cycle, lengthening of these muscles, rather than transfer, was indicated.

Surgical management of scoliosis in children with CP may be the most difficult problem facing the orthopedic surgeon. Because of the many other problems of CP, scoliosis treatment by conventional means is difficult and presents many postsurgical management problems.[67] Harrington rod instrumentation requires prolonged postoperative management in a body cast, a treatment difficult for the child with CP to tolerate. Bonnett and associates[68] and MacEwen[69] reported poor correction overall as well as various postoperative problems of pseudoarthroses, instrument failures, pressure sores, and poor tolerance to casts. Bonnett and colleagues[68] also described treatment with Dwyer instrumentation and anterior fusion, and again reported pseudoarthrosis and broken cables as problems. Allen and Ferguson[70] reported problems, including pressure sores, of managing patients in a body jacket. They also reported 10 patients with CP who had L-rod instrumentation in which L-shaped steel rods were secured by a sublaminar wire at each vertebra. The advantage of this procedure is that the wire fixation was sufficiently secure so that there was generally no need for a patient to wear a postoperative plaster cast or orthosis.

Surgical management of the lower extremities ranges from tenotomies, muscle lengthenings, and muscle transplants to osteotomies, neurectomies, and fusions. The results reported are equally variable. Truscelli and colleagues[71] suggest that the variation in long-term results of elongation of the tendoachilles depends on differences in underlying pathophysiology rather than differences in surgical techniques. They suggest that there may be a reduction in the number or length of the sarcomeres, resulting in varying outcome of muscle lengthening and immobilization.

Castle and associates[72] suggest that abnormalities in the muscle may contribute to variation in surgical outcome. On biopsies of various muscles in the extremities of 85 patients undergoing surgery, they demonstrated various degrees and combinations of types I and II muscle fiber atrophy and hypertrophy. These investigators believe that a muscle showing type II fiber atrophy or type I hypertrophy will not be appropriately functional if transplanted, but may only serve as a dynamic tenodesis. The normal type II fiber component of a muscle seems to be required for reeducation of the transplant, and the health of type

II fibers appears to serve as an indicator of the quality of neuronal activation of the muscle.

Many investigators compare the results of one surgical method to another. Root and Spero[73] compared adductor tenotomy with hip adductor transfer in a 10-year study of 102 patients. With an average of 3.8 years at follow-up, these investigators reported that although the adductor transfer operation takes longer and is associated with a higher incidence of postoperative problems, the transferred muscle provided better pelvic stability, decreased hip flexion contractures, and reduced hip instability in comparison to tenotomized muscle.

Orthopedic surgery is considered essential treatment in many children with CP; however, a lack of uniform criteria exists for selection, surgical intervention procedures, and outcome assessment. Studies that incorporate the essential elements of research design are notably absent from the literature, and a need exists for systematic longitudinal data on the effectiveness of orthopedic surgical intervention for children with CP.

Neurosurgery

Cooper and associates[74] introduced chronic electric stimulation of the cerebellum to reduce spasticity and improve motor function in patients with CP. Numerous articles on this technique have been written, but controversy remains over its effectiveness.[75–78] Double-blind studies have produced little support for the stated effects of cerebellar stimulation.

Penn and Etzel[77] reported on the effects of chronic electric stimulation of the cerebellum in 14 patients with CP who were studied prospectively for 1 to 44 months; 11 showed improvement in motor function. However, a double-blind test of 10 patients off and on stimulation for an average of 8 weeks produced no significant changes; thus, the functional changes may not have been the result of a cerebellar stimulation.[79]

Gahm and associates[80] used a double-blind crossover technique to assess the value of chronic cerebellar stimulation in eight children or adolescents with CP. Improvements in speech, reduced spasticity, and increased mental alertness occurred during placebo periods as often as with stimulation. Whittaker[81] also used a double-blind crossover experiment with 3-week periods of on–off intervention and was unable to document any changes in function.

Chronic cerebellar stimulation for CP remains a controversial procedure, difficult to evaluate objectively because of the complexity of the symptoms in CP. The clinical syndrome varies over time, and the patients undergoing the procedure and their families are highly motivated to change. Tests of neurophysiologic function, spasticity, and motor skills have suggested that changes occur, but double-blind evaluations have not provided supportive data.[82]

Peacock and Staudt recently introduced a procedure, termed *selective dorsal rhizotomy* (SDR), as a neurosurgical method to permanently reduce spasticity in children with CP.[83] This procedure involves limited laminectomy from L2 to L5. The dorsal roots are separated from the ventral roots. Each dorsal root is divided into its rootlets, then each is stimulated electrically. Those rootlets associated with an abnormal EMG response, as evidenced by incremental EMG pattern, ipsilatural or contralateral spread to muscle groups other than the one stimulated, or clonus, are divided. Those associated with a normal EMG response are left intact.

In 1989, Peacock and associates[84] reported the outcome of surgery in 60 children between the ages of 20 months and 19 years. Patients whose function improved most dramatically were purely spastic and intelligent, were most affected in the lower extremities, had some degree of forward locomotion, and could sidesit independent of hand support. All children received intensive physical therapy following the operation.

Arens and colleagues reported on 5-year outcome of 51 children with spastic CP who had undergone SDR between 1981 and 1984.[85] Reduction of tone was maintained in all cases. Functional gains were greater in children less than 8 years of age. Sensory disturbances were minimal and there was no evidence of spinal instability.

Berman reported on 29 patients who were assessed 2 days before and 4 months after surgery.[86] Each patient served as his or her own control. Berman developed clinical scales to quantify the degree of muscle tone and the ability to initiate and inhibit voluntary movement, joint stiffness, and functional movement. Consistent reduction in spasticity was reported in all muscle groups innervated from L1 to S1. The extent of functional improvement depended on the extent of the initial disability. Those who had some ambulatory skills made greater improvements than those who were nonambulatory. All children received physical therapy.

Wilson[87] reported similar results in seven cases operated on at the University of Virginia between May 1987 and May 1988. Each child was assessed prior to surgery and at 6 weeks, 6 months, and 1 year after surgery. Functional changes and increasing independence in ambulation were reported in five children with spastic diplegia who could sit and had some method of forward locomotion prior to surgery. Finally, three studies of gait following SDR showed improved ROM during swing and stance at the hip and knee, changes in foot–floor contact patterns, and changes in the temporal variability of gait.[88–90]

Although more controlled research is needed, SDR appears to be a viable option for children with spastic CP in whom spasticity primarily interferes with walking and functional movement. Selective dorsal rhizotomy successfully reduces spasticity and, with intensive physical therapy, results in improved function.

PHYSICAL THERAPY ASSESSMENT

The interdisciplinary, multidisciplinary, or transdisciplinary team approach is the current standard of practice for assessment of CP.[91,92] The components of the team may vary depending on the child's age, developmental level, and degree of involvement, the system of service delivery, and the physical setting. The physical therapist may select either norm- or criterion-referenced tests. A norm-referenced test is one in which a child's performance is compared against the performance of other children and is usually standardized. A criterion-referenced test compares a child's performance to a predetermined behavioral criterion and reports the child's performance in terms of what the child can do. Examples are the Vulpe Assessment Battery and the Learning Accomplishment Profile. These tests are often not standardized. Both types of tests are important in different ways and are used depending on what information is to be gained from the assessment process.[93] The physical therapy assessment is designed to collect information systematically and objectively, to serve as a baseline for function at a given time, and to aid in evaluating the change resulting from applying a specific intervention. For example, a presurgical assessment must include specific information on muscle strength and joint ROM, while an assessment for the purpose of planning physical therapy needs to include those areas that are the focus of intervention.

The description of assessment in this chapter will focus on the importance of collecting data for program planning. Only the sensorimotor components of the assessment will be presented in depth. The actual method of assessment of movement dysfunction in CP depends to some extent on the theoretic framework, training, and experience of the individual therapist; however, most investigators describe the following components as essential in the motor assessment of children with CP[94-97]: (1) muscle tone, (2) voluntary and automatic posture and movement patterns, (3) strength, (4) ROM, and (5) balance.

Muscle Tone

Abnormalities of muscle tone have been found to be consistent as well as predictive findings in young children who are at risk for CP, as well as hallmarks of children described as having CP.[3,98,99]

Investigators have attempted to define and measure spasticity and muscle tone in many ways; however, interrater reliability in clinical settings is very low according to Kathrein.[100] The difficulty of assessing muscle tone in developing children is compounded by the fact that muscle tone normally changes drastically in the premature infant as development progresses through the first year of life. Saint-Anne Dargassies[101] has described the changes in muscle tone in the normally maturing premature infant and uses this method of evaluating their distribution of tone. Amiel-Tison[102] has used a similar method of assessing tone in small-for-dates infants.

Most examiners assess resistance of a muscle as passive movement is imposed by the examiner[103-109]; however, others recommend that measures of muscle tone should capture the effect of tone on the adaptability of muscles during active movement as well.[96,110] It is often important in treatment to determine in what ways spasticity interferes with execution of movement. The following criteria can be applied when assessing passive or active tone in children with CP.

1. *Severe hypotonia*

   Active: inability to resist gravity, lack of concontraction at proximal joints for stability, weakness, limited voluntary movements

   Passive: joint hyperextensibility, no resistance to movement imposed by examiner, full or excessive passive ROM

2. *Moderate hypotonia*

   Active: decreased tone primarily in axial muscles and proximal muscles of the extremities; interferes with rate of development and length of time a posture can be sustained

   Passive: mild resistance to movement when imposed by examiner in distal parts of extremities only; joint hyperextensibility at elbows and knees

3. *Mild hypotonia*

   Active: decreased tone interferes with axial muscle cocontractions, delays initiation of movement against gravity, and reduces speed of adjustment to postural change

   Passive: mild resistance in proximal as well as distal segments; full passive ROM

4. *Normal tone*

   Active: quick and immediate postural adjustment during movement; ability to use muscles in synergic and reciprocal patterns for stability and mobility depends on task of the moment

   Passive: body parts resist displacement, momentarily maintain new posture when placed in space, and can rapidly follow changing movements imposed by examiner

5. *Mild hypertonus*

   Active: increased tone causes delay in postural adjustment; poor coordination, slowness of movement

   Passive: Resistance to change of posture in part of or throughout the range; poor ability to accommodate to passive movements

6. *Moderate hypertonus*

   Active: increased tone limits speed, coordination, variety of movement patterns, and active ROM

   Passive: resistance to change of posture throughout the range; limited passive ROM at some joints

7. *Severe hypertonus*

   Active: severe stiffness of muscles in stereotypic patterns limits active ROM; little or no ability to move against gravity; very limited patterns of movement

   Passive: passive ROM limited; unable to overcome resistance of muscle to complete full range

8. *Intermittent tone*

   Active: occasional and unpredictable resistance to postural changes alternating with normal adjustment; may have difficulty initiating active movement or sustaining posture

Passive: unpredictable resistance to imposed movements alternating with complete absence of resistance

In addition to describing active and passive tone, the following areas are addressed in the assessment.

Distribution of Tone

Muscle tone in one part of the body is described relative to other body parts. Generally, the head, neck, and trunk tone is compared with that in the extremities, the right side compared with the left, the upper extremities compared with the lower extremities, and the distal parts of the extremities compared with the proximal parts. Any asymmetries, including facial asymmetries, are also described.

Tone Under Stimulation

Changes in tone with speaking, laughing, crying, excitement, change in environment, and play are noticed. This information is particularly important to a therapist when planning treatment. For example, a child who gets very stiff when asked to talk should not be engaged in complicated language games during difficult movement activities.

Interactions of Tone and Movement Patterns

The interdependent relationship between muscle tone and movement patterns has been described by several investigators.[111,112] This section gives the therapist the opportunity to comment on the influence tone has on movement in various positions in which the force of gravity must be resisted. Some children get much stiffer when they attempt to move, and the degree of tone at rest does not correlate well with the interference experienced during movement. Other children become less stiff with movement. Although movement will not be the only factor affecting the child's tone, treatment planning requires that the therapist know what to expect when the child begins moving. If a child is stiff (or floppy) prior to beginning treatment, and gets stiffer with movement, the therapist will need to find positions and movements that do not increase tone and alter speed and stimulation to accommodate tone changes. In addition, some children will be much more able to manage movement without abnormal tone change in some positions against gravity than in others. By observing the interaction of tone and movement in various positions, the therapist will be able to decide which positions give the child the greatest opportunity for producing the most normal quality of movement.

Effect of Sensory Input on Tone

The therapist needs to note the effect of pressure and touch on tonus of the child. Some children have a low threshold to tactile input, so they are unable to inhibit motor response to exteroceptive stimuli. Children who have not been treated are often fearful of movement and become quite stiff when handled. In addition, the therapist will note the influence of speed, direction, and force of vestibular input on the changing patterns of the child's tone. In an initial assessment, it is important to attempt to find the amount and type of sensory input and movement a child can tolerate while maintaining relatively normal muscle tone.

Postural Alignment and Patterns of Weight-Bearing

The child should be encouraged through play to assume as many postures requiring resistance to the force of gravity as possible. Given a comfortable situation and adequate time, a child will do what he or she can do. It is possible to gain a representative sample of a child's motor behavior only if the child is cooperative and unthreatened. The examiner should question the parent as to whether observations represent typical behavior. In each position, the therapist looks for common components that are normal or abnormal. One can either describe each position and then later analyze common problematic patterns (see Wilson, "Analysis of Posture and Mobility," in *Vulpe Assessment Battery*[113]), or note repeating abnormal postural alignment as the child moves. For example, rounded upper back in four-point, sit, and kneeling positions; weight on right side in sitting and standing positions; or weight on fisted hands in prone on elbows, prone on hands, or four-point position. The focus is on the repetition of abnormal components of posture, not the position itself, because consistent patterns will be more predictive of future development and potential orthopedic problems.

This section of the assessment also includes description of the patterns of weight-bearing, noting how the child shifts and bears weight in anticipation of movement in each position. The inability to shift weight initially in the direction opposite the anticipated movement is frequently seen in children with CP. Symmetry or asymmetry in weight-bearing is noted because persistent asymmetric weight-bearing to one side limits movement of that side and can contribute to development of structural scoliosis and other orthopedic problems. Often, the side that appears most stable for weight-bearing is, in fact, the more spastic side; once tone is reduced in treatment or through surgery, it may turn out to be the less stable side.

In addition, the therapist should note the child's ability to adapt to the weight-bearing surface. The child often cannot conform to the surface, but has very limited weight-bearing patterns that will then limit movement.

Motor Control

Children with CP move in patterns that are more or less predictable based on the clinical description, age, extent of involvement, and their own movement experience.[114] This information makes it possible to anticipate how a child's existing control of posture and movement will influence, either positively or negatively, his or her continued development.

Information on motor control is gathered as a child moves spontaneously during an examination and includes the following data.

Normal and Abnormal Movement

It is important to note how the child moves, emphasizing both normal and abnormal movement patterns. A mildly involved diplegic child may move quite normally in lower level developmental positions and only show abnormal movement patterns when standing and walking. Knowing the position in which the child has basically normal control of movement aides selection of positions to be used in treatment. In addition to describing how the child moves, one should note the frequency with which a movement pattern is performed. For example, does the child *always* support on the left side and reach out with the right? Does the child *always* get to sitting by moving over the left side or pull to stand with the right leg placed forward? This information is valuable both for planning treatment as well as for predicting future outcome.

Finally, this section of the assessment includes identification of primitive movement patterns. Many infants and young children with CP who have had little experience of movement retain motor patterns typical of younger children. It is important to differentiate between truly abnormal patterns and patterns that are only immature, because primitive patterns can be easily modified in therapy if treatment begins before the patterns become established habits.

Initiation and Inhibition of Movement

The inability to initiate movement with the body part appropriate for the task causes distortion in control of movement patterns. Hemiplegic children often initiate movement with the sound side. The diplegic child often initiates movement with the head, neck, upper trunk, or arms, while the legs follow through quite passively. Some children attempt to initiate movement with the same side (or extremity) they are using for weight-bearing or support. In addition, speed of initiation and effort of movements are noted. Many children show long latency of response, which can be confused with lack of understanding directions rather than related to the motor control problem. Excessive effort to initiate movement may contribute to poor general exercise endurance.

This section also evaluates the child's ability to inhibit a movement on command once the movement is started. Many children are unable to stop, slow, or reverse a movement once it begins. This results in poor grading of agonists and antagonists for smooth reciprocal movements.

Asymmetries of Movement

Assessment of asymmetry includes observation of differences in amount of movement and stability of one side versus the other, the extremities versus the trunk, one extremity from another, or parts of the extremities relative to each other (proximal versus distal). Asymmetries between the two sides of the body are easy to detect in hemiplegic children, but are also commonly found in spastic diplegic and athetoid children.[113] Asymmetries may change with position and stress, as well as with development. Facial asymmetries during talking or eating should be recorded.

Effects of Sensory Input on Posture and Movement

Just as it is important to know the effect sensory input has on tone, the therapist also needs to know the effect of exteroceptive or proprioceptive input on posture and movement. Some children are extremely sensitive to auditory or visual stimuli to the point that loud or sudden auditory input or bright visual input may affect their ability to maintain balance in a position. Some children are almost immobilized by multisensory stimulation because they are unable to attend and respond to appropriate cues for movement.

Associated Reactions

Increased tone in certain parts of the body is caused by movement in other body parts. These reactions are clear in hemiplegia,[113] but are also seen in the lower extremities in diplegia. The presence of associated reactions indicates lack of disassociation of muscular activity of one body part from that in another and is one sign of increased tone occurring with movement.

Associative Movement

Mirror movements, either partial or complete, in the paired contralateral extremity are frequently observed in normally developing preschool and early school-aged children. The persistence or overpowering nature of these associative movements in children with CP prevents them from performing different functions with their two hands, as exemplified by the child who always drops an object held in one hand when trying to release an object in the other hand, or by the child who cannot release an object with one hand while holding something with the other. The predominance of these reactions prevents co-ordinated, reciprocal hand use.

Influence of Developmental Reflexes on Motor Control

Primitive Reflexes

Molnar[115] has described the differences in motor behavior of children with CP and those with mental retardation. She postulates that the motor deficit of retarded infants is related to disturbance in the postural reflex mechanism, while the motor deficit found in children with CP is related to both the persistence of primitive reflexes and a disturbance in the postural reflex mechanism.

The persistence of primitive reflexes as an influence on movement in CP has been described by many researchers.[113–118] If these early reflex patterns dominate the child's movement, the child will have little variety of movement, decreased ability to isolate movement in a body part, and inability to inhibit the effect of exteroceptive and proprioceptive input on motor responses. For example, one may see that the only way a child can extend one arm is by initiating it with a head turn toward that arm. The influence of the asymmetric tonic neck reflex prevents other variations of arm extension and disassociation of movements of the head from those at the shoulders. Recognizing the influence of primitive reflex patterns during spontaneous movement requires close observation and a great deal of experience. If the tester records the way a child moves in the second part of the assessment (Patterns of Posture and Movement), examination of the recurring patterns may reveal consistent influence of the primitive reflexes. The importance of recognizing whether arm extension with head turning is in fact the persistence of the asymmetric tonic reflex, or a visual problem or habit pattern, is clearly important in treatment and educational planning. Habit patterns often can be modified through a behavioral modification approach, a visual problem can be corrected with lenses or surgery, while a persistent asymmetric tonic neck reflex can be modified only with maturation and perhaps through specific handling techniques.

Developmental reflex testing provides information on how a child responds to specific sensory input applied in a systematic way. Reflex testing, positions, and procedures have been described by Fiorentino,[116] Wilson,[117] Capute and associates,[118] and Barnes and associates.[119] These criterion-referenced tests provide for test–retest comparison of a child, but none have normative data available. For the severely involved child who has little voluntary or spontaneous movement, a reflex test will determine if movement can be elicited through proprioceptive and exteroceptive stimulation. For less-involved children, a specific reflex test may not be necessary, but will aid the examiner's ability to recognize the more subtle way that reflexes interfere with motor control.

Balance and Postural Reactions

This part of the assessment includes evaluation of the postural reactions of equilibrium, righting, and protective extension, which are primarily responsible for a child's ability to gain and maintain mobile posture against the force of gravity and gain the freedom of movement necessary to develop highly skilled activities. Most children with CP have at least some components of the postural reflexes, but poorly developed reactions interfere with posture and balance in upright positions and limit the child's movement repertoire. A child who has poor equilibrium reactions in sitting will frequently place one hand on the floor in a protective response, thereby limiting two-hand use for dressing or play. A child who is posturally insecure will often develop one way to perform a task, and his or her movements will be stereotyped and limited in variety. Fisher[120] reports that a developmental sequence is evident in the quality of equilibrium responses and that it is possible to distinguish between delayed responses and abnormal responses. Comments regarding the quality of righting, equilibrium, and protective responses as they relate to speed, direction, force, frequency, and duration of the stimulus, as well as the quality of response in different positions, are provided.

Muscle Strength

Strength is probably the single most difficult area to assess in children with CP because of the many developmental, biomechanical, and neuromuscular factors that influence the child's ability to demonstrate the power to initiate, complete, or repeat a movement. Traditional methods of isolating a single muscle's ability to resist the force of gravity or perform against a resisting force are not effective in these children. The physical therapist, however, is often asked to assess strength preoperatively, to determine if orthopedic surgery or neurosurgery can be effective, and postoperatively, to demonstrate change in strength and movement patterns.[62,84]

Strength can be assessed in children with CP in functional developmental positions using movements that the child has demonstrated that he or she can perform. The therapist must keep in mind the muscle group (e.g., hip extensors) or specific muscle that is to be tested. I suggest that each assessment test include the following components:

1. Isometric power: the ability to hold a position against the force of gravity or a known resistance. Most often the muscle is tested by applying force in its shortened range. In children with CP, it is often important to test ability to hold a mid-range position as well.
2. Isotonic power: the ability of the muscle to move through its range with resistance applied throughout.
   Eccentric power: the ability to resist a force as a muscle is lengthened.

Concentric power: the ability to resist a force as the muscle is shortened.

3. Repetitive power: the ability to produce adequate power for 10 repetitions.

4. Speed of contraction: the ability of a muscle to quickly adapt throughout the range.

For example, hamstrings can be tested for isometric power if the child is placed supine, legs in hooklying with arms across the chest, and asked to make a bridge by raising hips off floor. Eccentric and concentric power can be tested if the child is placed on hands and feet with weight distributed across metatarsal heads and wrists and asked to slowly bend knees to gain hands–knees position and return to hands–feet position. Repetitive power can be tested in the same position by asking for 10 repetitions. The positions and movements selected can be used in test–retest situations or before and after surgery to monitor progress.

It is important to know, prior to testing strength, the available ROM and how spasticity may limit the movement. These factors complicate strength testing and require the therapist's creativity in factoring out confounding variables.

Range of Motion, Contractures, and Deformities

One of the primary effects of treatment for children with CP might well be prevention of contractures and deformities. This part of the assessment includes recording of joint ROM, contractures, and deformities. Joint ROM should be measured with a goniometer. The position for testing should be recorded because tone or reflexes may influence the child's passive or active ROM.[121,122] To compare results over time, the same test position must be used each time. This section includes information on the potential influence of current posture and movement on future development of deformities and contractures. For example, if a child sits between his heels, he is at risk for hip adductor contractures and medial femoral torsion.

Developmental Skills

Children with CP experience delays in motor development. It is particularly difficult to apply motor age equivalents to children with CP because their development is uneven. Often, however, this information is requested by educational programs for placement and is sometimes used to document the success of therapeutic programs. General level of development is also important in planning treatment programs because the developmental milestones represent the functional goals of a therapeutic program. Assessment of developmental level includes gross and fine motor skills the child performs independently regardless of the pattern of movement. This section also includes notation of the influence of tone, reflexes, and abnormal movement on the level of skills. Some children show delays that are even greater than would be expected based on evaluation of tone, reflexes, or abnormal movements because of a significant degree of mental retardation. It is important to identify the strongest influences on limitations of functional skills because the therapist must adjust the methods and expectations for goal achievement according to the findings.

The influence of handling on the level of skills should also be recorded. Providing minimal support for balance often allows a child to pull to stand even though the child cannot perform the task independently. This information is important for determining later progress and potential for independence. Vulpe developed a Performance Analysis Scale that allows the examiner to rate the child's ability to perform skills based on the type of assistance the child needs to accomplish the task.[114] The Performance Analysis Scale can be used to show progress indicating a greater degree of independence in task completion, even if the child is not performing new, higher level skills in a retest situation. Such information can be beneficial in demonstrating improvement in severely involved children who cannot be expected to show progress using standard tests.

Oral Motor Functions

Many children with CP have a history of oral dysfunction that includes feeding problems, persistent primitive oral reflexes, respiratory problems, drooling, and delayed or abnormal vocalization. As part of the motor assessment, this section includes information regarding the child's oral history, present oral function, and influence of tone, posture, and movement on overall oral functions. If oral motor dysfunction is severe, a separate oral motor assessment should be done. Comprehensive assessment has been described by Morris.[123,124]

Splinting and Surgery

If the child has splints, braces, or casts or has had surgery, these are noted in the assessment. First, there is a description of surgical procedures and their influence on the child's current movement. Second, notes are made of splints, braces, and casts, including how long they are worn and for what purposes they are worn, and movement with and without appliances is described.

Adaptive Equipment and Assistive Devices

Descriptions of adaptive equipment, assistive devices, or mobility aides used to increase function and independence are included in the assessment. Appropriate mobility aids can alter a child's gait pattern and promote independence in walking.[125] Depending on the setting, data may be gathered by asking the parents about the child's function with and without equipment.

Other Areas of Development

Analysis of the basic sensory functions and behavioral and physiologic characteristics are also recorded, but will not be discussed in this chapter.

Summary of Assessment

The assessment summary includes a list of the child's strengths. This may include information regarding both internal and external resources, intelligence, interest, attention, cooperativeness, self-concept, sensorimotor skills, and activities of daily living as they apply to the specific child. The family's size, interest, level of understanding of the child's abilities and disabilities, time and energy available for interaction and therapy, and financial resources may be noted. Following a list of strengths, problems are noted. The procedure of enumerating strengths and problems allows the reader to focus on how the strengths can be used to facilitate development in the problem areas and facilitates integration of all aspects of the child's functional abilities.

Listing the problems leads directly to a list of goals for therapy and of treatment methods designed specifically to meet the goals listed. In the following section, a sample of how the evaluation and problems list are integrated with a treatment plan is illustrated.

PLANNING TREATMENT

Treatment for the child with CP must be individualized based on the child's specific problems, age, degree of involvement, intelligence, associated problems, and family involvement; however, certain guidelines are important to follow if treatment is to remain effective over time.

1. *Treatment goals are designed to meet specific problems.* These will vary with age and extent of symptoms at onset of treatment.
2. *Treatment goals must be changed with changes in the presenting problem.* For example, an infant with hemiplegia may initially present with hypotonicity in the upper extremity and by 6 to 8 months present with hypertonicity once he or she begins to move against gravity.[114] The goal therefore changes from increasing tone in the involved upper extremity to decreasing tone in the involved upper extremity.
3. *Treatment methods and techniques change with the child's age, need for independence and function, as well as motor symptoms.* A young baby enjoys being held for play, therapy, dressing, and feeding. A natural environ-

ment is mother's lap and a great deal of baby treatment can effectively take place there. Because a 2-year-old needs to develop independence, dressing can be done on a bench or chair (with appropriate support) and treatment requires much more mobility, exploration, and self initiation. A 10-year-old needs to function independently. Treatment changes to provide the child with methods to monitor his or her own movements, maintain ROM, and perform movement independently. Teenagers are assisted in finding methods through recreation to integrate movement into their lifestyle.

4. *Families need to be given information regarding the child's problem and treatment as they are able to understand and assimilate the information.* The role of the family in treatment is described in detail in the section on family involvement in this chapter.

5. *Suggestions to the family should be as practical as possible*, remembering that parents have responsibilities toward their other children and to each other as well as to their handicapped child.

6. *Therapy should be designed to provide active response from the child.* Passive movement is less effective in producing changes in tone or movement patterns. Active movement does not necessarily mean voluntary movement. For example, postural reactions performed automatically require a great amount of strength and endurance.

7. *Whenever possible, movement should be initiated by the child.* Control of movement is maintained by the therapist, but the child should lead the treatment and initiate the activity.

8. *Repetition is an important component in motor learning.* Motor activities repeated throughout the session and in functional ways at home have a better chance of becoming part of the child's habitual repertoire.

9. *The environment should be conducive to cooperative participation and support of the child's efforts.* Because therapy will be an active part of a CP child's life, it should be pleasurable. If the child enjoys movement, he or she will be more inclined to make movement, through exercise and recreation, part of his or her lifestyle.

10. *Treatment must be geared to the functions the child needs as the child grows and develops.* Functions used in activities of daily living, including dressing, feeding, and personal grooming, are important therapeutic techniques.

11. *Play should be integrated into therapy to provide motivation and purpose to reinforce and direct movement responses.* Play must be carefully monitored during treatment so that it does not overstimulate the child and interfere with the desired movement response or produce abnormal tone.

12. *Sensory stimulation must be integrated with motor output.* Loud or vigorous auditory and visual stimuli can be used to call attention and produce forceful movement. Multisensory stimuli, however, should not be used with highly distractible or emotionally volatile children. Tactile or vestibular hypersensitivity or hyposensitivity can have a profound effect on the movement outcome. Changing the type and level of sensory input can have a direct effect on improving the quality of motor response.

13. *Therapy should be designed to use the child's strengths to build on*

problem areas. If a child has good imaginary play and language skills, story telling can focus the child's attention and imaginary play can provide a framework for moving.

14. *A single treatment progresses from positions in which the child has the most normal tone and movement to ones that are more challenging*. Within each treatment session a child should have the opportunity to work in various developmental positions appropriate to his or her age, but the progression from one position to another must be carefully controlled so that as the child is challenged by the force of gravity he or she continues to produce movement with normal postural tone. Treatment should end with positions and activities that are functional for the child and that provide a cooldown period after a vigorous exercise session.

15. *Movement in one position prepares for movements in another*. Through experience with an individual child, the therapist will find positions and activities that change tone and provide greater variety in the child's movements. These activities are used early in a treatment session to give the child the feeling for control in positions in which movement is easier prior to attempting movement in positions that are difficult or new for the child.

16. *As a child is able to perform movements independently, the therapist provides time in a treatment for the child to move freely*. It is important for the child to feel movement produced through his or her own efforts without the control of the therapist. Only in this way will the child incorporate these movements into daily living.

17. *Individual treatment sessions should be designed to evaluate the effectiveness of treatment within the session*. This can be done informally by motivating the child to demonstrate an activity, movement, or posture at the beginning of treatment and again at the end to determine if changes have occurred or through more formalized methods (see Treatment Evaluation). Knowing that change has occurred is motivating to the child and reinforcing for the therapist.

18. *Physical therapy treatment should be coordinated with all other medical and educational disciplines involved with the child*. Treatment should be integrated with the goals and methods of occupational and speech therapy, orthopedic management, and educational and home management. While the roles of these disciplines are very important in the total management of the child, they will not be discussed in this chapter. At different times in the child's life, the focus and importance of the various disciplines will change so that one discipline will have a higher priority than another. Interdisciplinary communication is essential to maintain a consistent approach to meeting the changing needs of the child and the family.

ILLUSTRATION OF TREATMENT

To illustrate how these principles of treatment are integrated into a specific program, a case study is presented, following the child from assessment through a treatment progression and treatment evaluation.

Summary of Assessment

Michael A. is a 3-year 1-month-old boy, born 10 weeks prematurely, who has a history of respiratory distress syndrome. He presents with the moderate to severe spastic diplegic type of CP. The following summarizes his strengths and problem areas:

Strengths

1. Intelligent, cooperative, inquisitive child. No standardized testing done to date.
2. Uses speech to express wants and desires.
3. Motivated to move.
4. Not fearful of movement.
5. Normal vision and hearing.
6. Supportive, intelligent family, interested and able to provide appropriate care.

Problem Areas

1. Abnormal tone: increased extensor tone more on left than right, lower extremities more than trunk and upper extremities, distal parts more than proximal parts. Poor cocontraction in trunk muscles with intermittent extensor tone.
2. Abnormal sensory responses: heightened response to tactile stimulus; unanticipated touch produces generalized extensor response.
3. Abnormal patterns of movement: Michael's lower extremities are dominated by extension and adduction of the hips and plantar flexion at the ankles. Movement is initiated primarily from head and shoulders. More movement on the right side. More stability with abnormal tone on left side.
4. Persistent primitive reflexes: limited variety of movements; asymmetric tonic neck reflex influences posture of upper extremities.
5. Delayed postural reactions: all components of the postural reactions are disturbed, preventing movement and maintenance of posture against the force of gravity. Inadequate postural reactions inhibit weight shift and ability to maintain or regain normal postural alignment, and produce isolated movements of body parts. Often, the primitive reflex patterns override Michael's postural reactions, so balance is inadequate in any position.
6. Oral motor dysfunction: Michael has slowly articulated single words and phrases. His voice is very low in volume. Open mouth posture is seen frequently in association with maintaining antigravity postures or stress in movement. Occasional drooling is observed.
7. Delay in motor development: Michael's independent gross motor development is at approximately a 6-month level; fine motor, 18 months to 2

years; and activities of daily living skills, 12 to 15 months. These delays are clearly related to motor dysfunction.

8. Limited ROM: this child's active range is often limited by tone. Passive range is limited to 65 degrees in hamstrings, 60 degrees in hip adductors, and to neutral in gastrocnemius-soleus muscle group bilaterally.

Figures 10-1 to 10-4 illustrate Michael's problems.

Treatment Goals

Based on the problems described and illustrated in the assessment summary, the following immediate goals for therapy were established:

1. Change amount and distribution of abnormal tone
    a. Decrease excessive extensor tone in lower extremities
    b. Increase cocontraction patterns in trunk and shoulder girdle
    c. Decrease tone in distal muscles, plantar flexion of feet, and flexion of hands
2. Develop symmetry in weight-bearing through upper and lower extremities for normal posture alignment
3. Develop greater variety of movement patterns, particularly in the trunk and lower extremities
4. Develop rotation within the body axis to assist with transitions from one position to another
5. Develop weight shift through upper extremities for weight-bearing while reaching out, and in the lower extremities in preparation for locomotion
6. Initiate movement with appropriate body parts for the task of the moment; for example, ability to use one part for movement while using another for weight-bearing and stability
7. Develop better disassociation of movements of one body part from another for coordinated movements
8. Develop postural adaptations and alignment to improve equilibrium in all positions
9. Develop better freedom of movement to decrease influence of primitive reflexes seen with stress
10. Increase upper thoracic extension to prevent possible structural deformities
11. Provide opportunities for age-appropriate skills of self-help, play, and locomotion

Figures 10-5 to 10-12 show a progression of treatment activities designed to meet the goals described. Photographs were taken in a single treatment session. (See pages 329 to 333.)

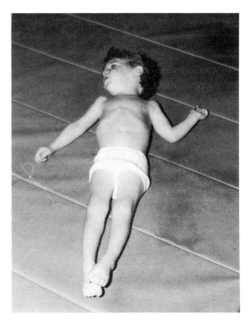

Fig. 10-1. Supine: extensor tone evident more in lower extremities, more in distal parts. Asymmetric tonic neck reflex posturing assumed with head turning. Flaring of ribs indicates inactivity of abdominal muscles.

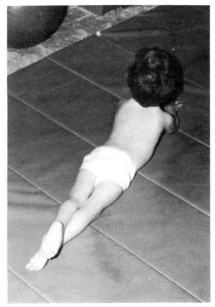

Fig. 10-2. Prone on elbows: movement initiated from head and shoulders. Legs still dominated by extension, adduction, and plantar flexion. Limited equilibrium prevents good alignment. Can maintain position only if center of gravity is kept well within base of support.

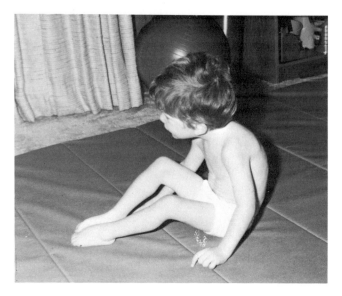

Fig. 10-3.   Placed in sitting: Michael cannot assume sitting. Placed in sitting extensor tone evident in lower trunk and hips pulling him back onto sacrum. Hamstring spasticity contributes to hip extension and knee flexion. Plantar flexion persists. Lack of equilibrium evidenced by hands on floor to maintain position. Upper trunk and neck flexion in attempt to counteract excessive hip extension and bring center of gravity forward over base of support. Weight primarily on left side.

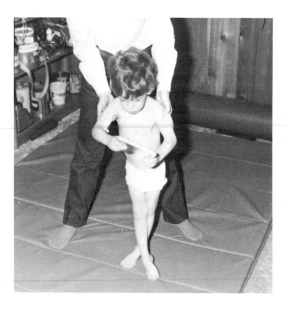

Fig. 10-4.   Supported in standing: throughout assessment posture, tone and available active patterns for movement are almost unchanged. Unable to align body in upright position. No equilibrium.

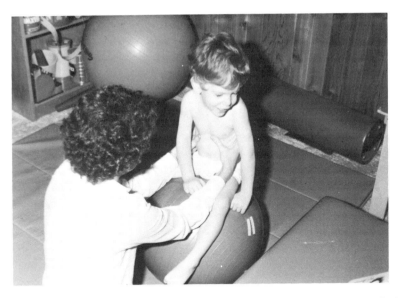

Fig. 10-5. Therapy begins on a ball. Therapist's forearms inhibit adduction while hands facilitate trunk alignment, symmetric weight-bearing, and increased tone in trunk. Slow movement on the ball reduces extensor hypertonus while preparing for movement. This activity is designed to meet treatment goals 1, 2, 4 to 6, and 11.

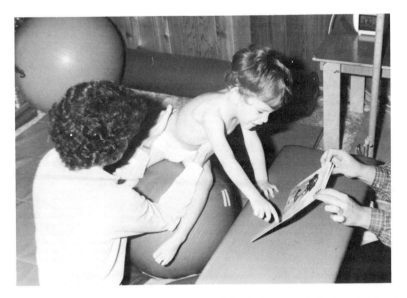

Fig. 10-6. Once tone is more appropriate, activity is begun to left since Michael takes weight more easily on left and can produce movement while maintaining normal tone. This will prepare for rotation and weight-bearing on right. Therapist facilitates trunk rotation while weight-bearing through left hip, continuing to inhibit adduction. This activity is designed to meet treatment goals 1 to 6 and 11.

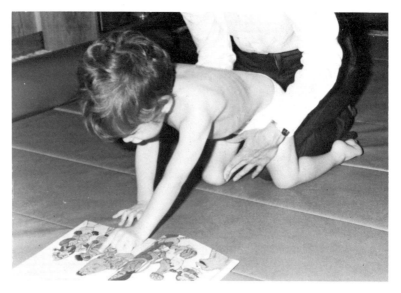

Fig. 10-7. In a more stable hands–knees position, right hand shows less stress: weight shift forward and back is facilitated by reaching out to identify characters in the book. Lateral weight shift is facilitated at pelvis by therapist's hand. This activity is designed for treatment goals 1, 3, 6 to 10, and 11.

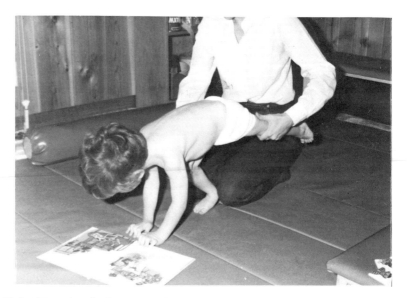

Fig. 10-8. From hands–knees position, Michael is brought onto right foot with left leg extended, requiring flexion of right leg with weight-bearing and extension of left leg. This is a very difficult position for Michael to assume or maintain because of his inability to adapt to positions requiring a high degree of disassociated movements while maintaining equilibrium over a very narrow base of support. This activity is designed for treatment goals 1, 3, 6 to 10, and 11.

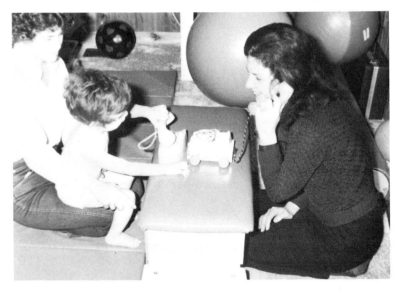

Fig. 10-9. Now that extensor tone in the lower extremities is reduced and trunk tone is increased, play activities are incorporated with moving to standing. Initially sitting in good alignment, Michael has a phone conversation with his mother. This activity is designed for treatment goals 1 to 9 and 11.

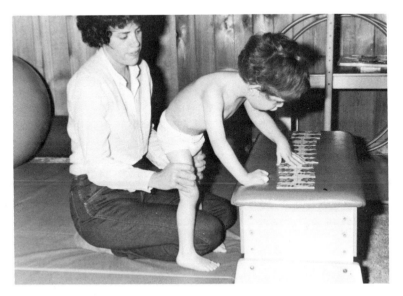

Fig. 10-10. By positioning toys on a low support surface, Michael stands with legs extended and trunk leaning forward. This keeps his weight forward over his feet while preventing excessive extension and adduction of his legs. This activity is designed for treatment goals 1 to 9 and 11.

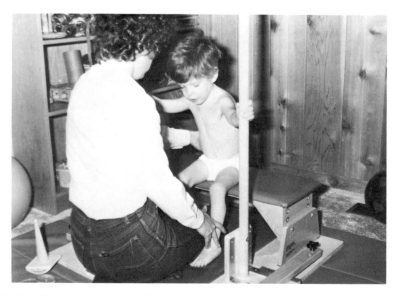

Fig. 10-11.   To prevent increased flexor tone in the upper extremities, which accompanies pulling with the arms, Michael uses parallel poles that maintain the shoulders at 90 degrees flexion and abduction, elbows extended, and forearms supinated. This will assist him in shifting his weight forward over his feet as he comes to stand. This activity is designed for treatment goals 1 to 5, 8, and 9.

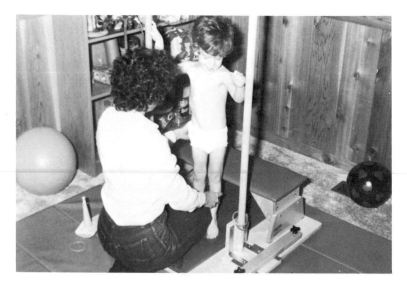

Fig. 10-12.   In standing, trunk alignment is facilitated by the therapist's hand on the hip extensors. In this position, Michael still has excessive extensor tone in the lower extremities, but body and head alignment are good and balance is sufficient that he can let go with one hand at a time to drop rings over the top of a stick (compare with Fig. 10-4). These activities represent a typical treatment session. This activity is designed for treatment goals 1 to 5, 8, and 9.

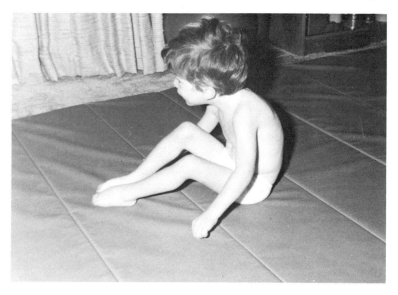

Fig. 10-13. This picture was taken prior to beginning the treatment session illustrated in the previous series of pictures. It illustrates well the problems described in the assessment summary: abnormal extensor tone with compensatory abnormal alignment, lack of equilibrium, and delayed development.

Treatment Evaluation

Informal evaluations can be made during treatment if the therapist observes a particular skill, movement, or position prior to treatment, later in treatment (compare standing alignment in Fig. 10-4 with posture during therapy in Fig. 10-12), and again at the end of treatment. By observing changes in tone, posture, and movement, it is possible to assess whether the goals for treatment are appropriate, whether the methods selected are meeting these goals, and what problems continue to exist. Figure 10-13 was taken prior to therapy and demonstrates Michael's problem in independent sitting; this contrasts with Figure 10-14, which was taken at the end of the treatment session.

FAMILY INVOLVEMENT

Involvement of the family in the intervention program for a child with CP is an important aspect of treatment. To be effective in involving the family in an intervention program, physical therapists must recognize that a family consists of a system of relationships. The needs of the family and their resources to cope with these needs change over time, reflecting both continuity of family development as well as changes in structure and function of the family unit.[126]

When planning the home management aspect of the sensorimotor program,

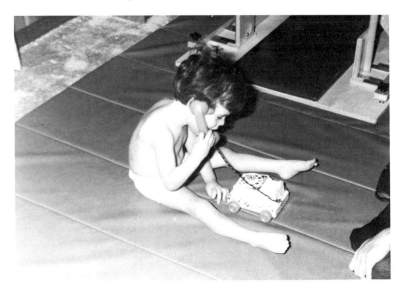

Fig. 10-14. After 1 hour of therapy, extensor tone in the legs is decreased, allowing a posture of hip flexion, abduction, and knee extension. With a wider base of support and his weight more evenly distributed, Michael can free one hand for play. Problems still persist. Extensor tone dominates pelvic posture and lack of cocontraction in the trunk prevents the pelvis being maintained in vertical position so that compensatory upper trunk flexion persists. These problems will continue to be addressed in therapy and home management.

the therapist must recognize and accept that children grow up in different sub-cultures that have their own values, expectations, patterns of interpersonal relationships, manners, and styles of intellectual operations and communications.[127] Programs for groups of culturally distinct or economically disadvantaged families have been notable failures when planned by white middle-class professionals, partly because of the lack of attention to individual needs and failure to understand attitudes of the group to be served.[128] The therapist must ask the parents what *they* would like to know about the child and what they would like to be able to do for him or her. Redman-Bentley,[129] in a study of 66 parents of children diagnosed with physical or mental disabilities or developmental delay, found that parents of young handicapped children do have specific needs and priorities as well as expectations of professionals with whom they were involved. She reported that parents wanted a more active role in the rehabilitation process of their handicapped children, a say in decisions concerning their child's program, as well as information regarding test results and changes in the child's progress and program.

Recognizing and responding to the parents' needs may require the therapist to reorder priorities to initiate realistic plans for meeting the family's goals. According to Schaefer,[130] the most effective way to influence the development of children is to provide professional support for parental care of children. The family spends the greatest amount of time with the child; therefore, keeping the total child in mind, it makes sense to teach the parents to understand normal and abnormal development and make use of the available knowledge about care and management that is pertinent to their child. When beginning home management, it is important, when appropriate, to imitate the interactive style of the parents rather than require that the parents give up their accustomed methods of handling their child to follow a prescribed approach that may be incompatible with their own natural style. The parents can learn child care routines that will reinforce and maximize the child's skills while continuing to feel adequate as parents.[91] The parent who is taught basic concepts of development and who understands general principles of intervention is better equipped to generalize handling techniques to accommodate various situations that arise as the child grows and develops, as well as to assimilate these methods of management into their own parenting style.

Evidence is accumulating that the child's own parents are the best choice as caregivers to facilitate long-term gains. If, however, the internal and external resources of the family are inadequate to provide an optimal learning environment, a parent surrogate can be substituted if the person can provide a stable, stimulating situation.[131] Extended family members and day care personnel are common sources of help.

Some of the success of the home management aspect of the intervention program depends on how effectively the parent is instructed. I previously reported a project that involved teaching 16 families of severely motor-handicapped children various activities to be done at home.[132] The initial interaction of the parents with the therapist and the therapist's attitude and concern were as important to the overall performance of the parents as the actual method of written or oral instructions. Redman-Bentley[129] also found that the professional's personal traits were important. Parents preferred a professional who was honest and knowledgeable, and who listened to information provided by the parents. The physical therapist must realize, in deciding which daily care routines or therapeutic techniques should be included as part of the home program, that parents represent the entire range of social, emotional, and intellectual behaviors. Some parents have high intellect, good motor skills, and learn easily, but children sometimes have parents who are retarded, emotionally disturbed, alcoholic, or preoccupied with basic physiologic or financial needs.

Many therapists have a preconceived notion that managing a child with CP places additional stress on the family, but the validity of this statement is unclear from the literature. Lonsdale[133] interviewed the parents of 60 developmentally delayed children about their reactions and the effect of the child on family relationships. More than half the parents interviewed reported marriage difficulties resulting from the birth of the handicapped child.[133] This is consistent with the findings reported by Gath.[134] High rates of physical and mental ill health among parents of handicapped children have been reported both by McMichael[135] and by Tizard and Grad.[136] Reports by Butler and colleagues[137] and Burden[138] have also stressed the likelihood of mental ill health in mothers.

On the other hand, the majority of studies reviewed by Dunlap and Hollingsworth[139] did not support the perception that the handicapped member has a substantial effect on family life. Wishart and colleagues[140] compared the reports of regular family activities obtained from parents of developmentally delayed children and from parents of normal children acting as controls. These results showed little difference between the control and handicapped groups, and the presence of a delayed child in the family did not appear to change the family routine to any large extent. This study did not include families with children with significant motor handicaps. A comparison of families with children who have different degrees of physical and mental dysfunction may provide more information regarding the effects of motorically handicapped children on family routines and activities.

Simeonsson and McHale[141] reviewed the effects of a handicapped child on sibling relationships. This review demonstrates that there is a great diversity of effects on the sibling relationship. Some studies showed that the presence of a handicapped child in a family results in problems of adjustment and development for siblings,[142] while other studies indicate that siblings of handicapped children may benefit from their experience and are often well adjusted.[133,143,144]

What are the implications for the therapist? First, the therapist should not assume that the presence of a handicapped child necessarily disturbs the structure, function, or development of the family unit. However the handicapped child is perceived by his or her own family, parents are able to accommodate the problems of raising a child with a handicapping condition to a considerable extent, assuming a successful parenting role with their child.

Second, the therapist must be able to achieve effective parent involvement as appropriate for the individual family. Therapists should not have preconceived ideas about what parents should do for their children, but should rather accept what a parent can do for their child and capitalize on these abilities. Scherzer and Tscharnuter[91] state that, whenever possible, family involvement should go beyond intervention methods of home management to include treatment procedures, but that the therapist must help the parents put the home management program into the proper perspective so as not to disturb the parent-child relationship or the family unit and its functions. Focusing attention exclusively on the infant's disabilities may hamper rather than foster overall development and place undue focus on the parent's inability to parent the handicapped child. All efforts must be made, rather, to stress the competencies of the child and the parents.

Third, handling techniques must be adapted to the skills of the parents and may consequently differ from the techniques and standards the therapist applies to the same activity. Some parents have the time, energy, and skills to carry out complicated therapeutic techniques on a regular basis, while other families will need constant instruction and support to modify feeding, dressing, or daily care routines.

Fourth, while there is no prescribed method to assure successful teaching, methods of instruction include demonstration, written programs, verbal instructions, repetition, and continual support. The intensity of instruction and need to adhere to a systematic teaching method will vary from family to family. The therapist must be able to evaluate the family's resources and vary the style of instruction, as well as goals for the home program, to meet the current level of skill, knowledge, and attitudes of the family.

Finally, the individual family's involvement in a home program varies. First, it may vary based on when they have their initial contact with the intervention program. Parents who have a young baby with suspected CNS dysfunction may not initially see the infant as different from other babies. All babies need to be dressed, bathed, diapered, and loved. The parents, therefore, may not see the need to change their method of caring for their infant, particularly if the child is comfortable in the present interaction and protests with imposition of new positions and movements. Parents who first begin therapy with an 18-month-old child diagnosed with CP may be quite anxious to have activities to do at home to "help their child walk" or achieve some other obviously delayed motor milestone.

The family's involvement with a home program varies with the age of the child. Babies, toddlers, and preschool children generally spend a great deal of time with their own parents and are usually assisted with daily care routines. Parents have the opportunity to provide continued input for facilitating activities involving dressing, feeding, and self-care, as well as functional motor skills. A school-aged child has a greater need for independence and may refuse assistance from a parent once they have discovered some way to accomplish the task independently. At this point, the parents may be more involved with transporting the child to after-school activities and assisting with homework, and, in their need to be parents, are realistically less involved with therapeutic intervention. Home programs for preteens and teenagers often involve instructing the child to carry out mobilizing techniques independent of adult assistance or stressing recreational activities that encourage mobility and reinforce functional movement. The home management program does not decrease as the child grows older; however, the goals, activities, and persons responsible for the program must change if it is to remain an effective method of intervention. As an example, Figures 10-15 and 10-16 illustrate some of the activities included in Michael A.'s home program, which includes activities to position for self-help skills (Fig. 10-15 illustrates dressing), play and use of adaptive equipment to promote social interaction with family (Fig. 10-16) and independent mobility.

ADJUNCTS TO THERAPY

Tone-Reducing Casts

Short leg tone-inhibiting casts are designed to maintain normal alignment of the foot and ankle while inhibiting toe grasp as a habitual or compensatory stabilizing effort. They are currently used as an adjunct in therapy and during

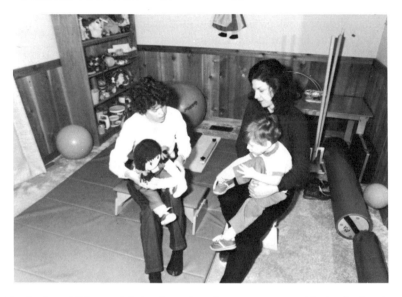

Fig. 10-15. In addition to Michael's active therapy program, his family has been instructed in positioning and assisting with daily care, which reinforces his therapeutic goals. Here, Michael's mother learns to facilitate trunk rotation and disassociated movements of one leg from the other while Michael assists with undressing.

selected intervals of treatment and management at home and school. Sussman and Cusick[145] described the basic hypotheses in the use of tone-reducing casts. First, extending the toes inhibits the plantar grasp response. Second, firm fixation of the subtalar joint provides a stable base to reduce tone and facilitate mobility of the hips, knees, and trunk. Third, prevention of ankle dorsiflexion inhibits use of extensor thrust. As a result, tone-reducing casts allow development of desirable movement components of the trunk, hips, and knees with relatively full mobility during standing and walking.

Cusick and Sussman[146] described the use of tone-reducing casts with 145 children over a 46-month period. They developed specific criteria for patient selection, considerations for treatment, and follow-up. The casts were not used to correct foot deformity or to reduce contracture at the foot or ankle; they were implemented when passive foot and ankle range was complete and only during a closely supervised program of positioning and movement training when it was believed that gains in movement control could be made faster or sooner if the foot was stabilized in good alignment. The majority of cases were children with spastic CP; however, use of casts with hypotonia and mixed athetoid-spastic CP was also reported.

Embry[147] presented a preliminary report on a study designed to evaluate the effectiveness of inhibitory casts when used concurrently with a neuro-developmental approach to children with CP. Ten matched pairs of subjects between the ages of 6 months and 5 years were selected to receive 8 weeks of

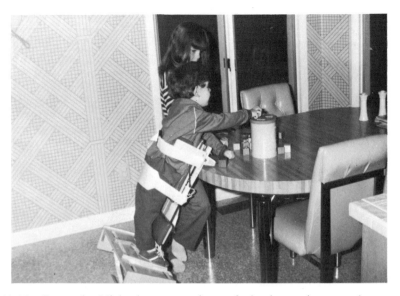

Fig. 10-16. Presently, Michael uses two pieces of adaptive equipment at home to provide him with a larger variety of movement patterns. This prone stander is attached to the kitchen table so that Michael can stand and play with his sister. Since he does not need to take weight on his hands to balance or support in standing, his hands are free for play.

treatment. The experimental group wore casts during weight-bearing activities in treatment and at home. Data on step length, stride length, foot angle, walking base, and symmetry of gait were obtained from a weight-sensitive paper. While the data were not analyzed statistically at the time of reporting, early findings based on a small number of subjects appeared to support the effectiveness of inhibitory casting in achieving improved ambulation when used concurrently with a neurodevelopmental treatment approach. Figures 10-17 to 10-19 demonstrate the differences in postural alignment, tone, and independence in balance and movement achieved during therapy when tone-reduction casts were used with Michael A.

Use of Adaptive Equipment

Adaptive equipment has become an integral part of therapeutic, educational, and home management programs for preschool children with motor dysfunction resulting from CNS deficit.[96,97,148–150] Attempts have been made to document changes in posture or function in children using adaptive equipment.

Nwaobi and colleagues[151] reported a study designed to determine whether tonic myoelectric activity of low-back extensors of children with spastic CP

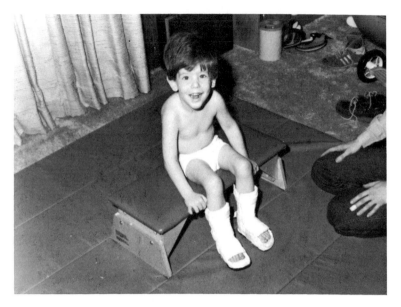

Fig. 10-17.   With casts on, Michael sits with better alignment and hip abduction.

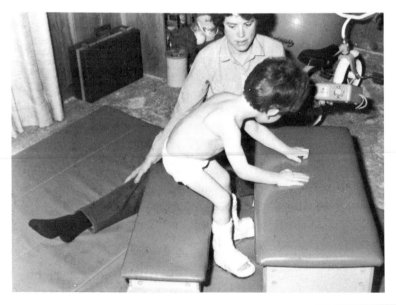

Fig. 10-18.   Michael is able to move from standing to sitting independently, keeping his weight forward over his feet as he lowers himself to the bench. Still unable to balance in standing, it is necessary for Michael to use the bench for support.

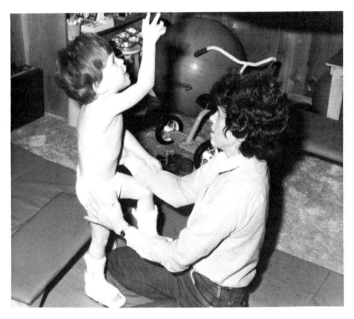

Fig. 10-19. Disassociation of the movements of the lower extremities is now possible. Michael can take weight on the right leg while maintaining hip and trunk alignment. The left leg is forward and flexed in preparation for stepping. The therapist facilitated weight shift and balance reactions.

changed in response to changes in seating. Electromyograms recorded less electric activity when the seat surface elevation was 0 degree and the backrest was 90 degrees.

In a single-case study design, Cristarella[152] compared the sitting posture of a normal 3-year-old child with the sitting posture of a child with spastic CP of the same age. While seated in small chairs, the children were filmed during play, and line drawings were made from a frame selected at random. In the normal child, the angles at the hips, knees, and ankles approximated 90 degrees, while the child with CP showed significantly less than 90 degrees at the same joints. Spinal alignment was also compared. In the normal child, the pelvis was vertical and the spine showed normal curves. In the child with CP, the upper spine was excessively rounded and the pelvis was not vertical. The child with CP was then placed in a straddle position on a special chair that provided hip abduction. Film analysis showed that the joint measurements of hip and knee flexion and ankle dorsiflexion were much closer to 90 degrees, and the spinal curves approximated those of the normal subject. These studies suggest that tone and postural alignment can be influenced by adaptive equipment.

Hulme and colleagues[153] reported on the results of a survey constructed to assess the benefits of adaptive equipment used in homes of primarily non-ambulatory, multiply handicapped clients ranging from 1 to 68 years of age. Significant improvements were noted in social interactions and motor coordination. Adaptive chairs were the most consistently used types of equipment. A significant increase in independent eating and drinking was also found, along with a significant decrease in the time needed to eat a meal and the time the client spent in the bedroom. In the areas of social interaction, there was significant improvement in the number of times the client left the home and an increased variety of places visited by the client in the community.

In general, the current literature describes the selection, construction, and uses of various commercially available as well as custom-designed products to solve a particular problem of positioning, mobility, or activities of daily living function.[154–166]

Selection of Adaptive Equipment

Adaptive equipment should be carefully selected in consultation with a physical or occupational therapist to make certain that it meets the goals for which it is intended. Adaptive equipment is used to meet the following goals:

1. Adaptive equipment is used in homes to provide greater opportunities for independence in activities of daily living. By properly positioning a child so that he or she feels secure and motivated to practice newly acquired skills, many children are able to participate in feeding, toileting, or other self-help skills.[148,167]

2. To prevent contractures and deformities by positioning a child to prevent the deforming influence while encouraging active movement.[154,168]

3. To provide greater variety of movement experiences and prevent habit patterns that limit the development of normal variations of posture and movement.[148]

4. To reinforce normal movement components, providing an opportunity for more normal alignment, weight shift, and postural adjustment during functional movement.[125,154,169–171]

5. To increase the child's opportunity to participate in social interaction and educational programs.

6. To provide mobility and encourage exploration. This is often the goal of providing adapted standard or electric wheelchairs for children who have no means of mobilization or whose movements are so slow that the effort is not worth the goal toward which the movement is directed.

Appropriate equipment provides enough support so that the child can direct his or her energies toward participation in the educational or social environment rather than exclusively toward maintaining posture. This reason alone may warrent the use of adaptive equipment for severely handicapped children.[150,172,173] Severely handicapped children are often unable to experience any degree of interaction or independence in school, recreation centers, or shopping areas without the assistance of adaptive chairs.[172]

Adaptive equipment, whether individually designed or commercially available, must meet the needs of the child as he or she grows, gains better control of posture and movement, and develops educational and daily living skills. Several books are available on planning, designing, and building adaptive equipment.[148,154,174–178] Appropriate selected adaptive equipment allows movement and encourages the child to make postural adaptations necessary in any given situation. It should not restrict the child's movements, but rather increase the child's possibilities to practice and use movements that he or she is developing.

EVALUATION OF OUTCOME

Evaluating treatment presents a dilemma to those involved in treating children with CP. The dilemma exists because therapists hold a strong belief, on the one hand, that early intervention is essential and effective and, on the other hand, documenting effectiveness is difficult because of the complex problems characterizing this population. The dilemma is heightened by the fact that the state-of-the-art of evaluation of patients with CP is not far advanced and results of clinical studies present confusing and sometimes contradictory results.[179] The confusion is partly caused by differences among studies in the subject selection, sample size, criteria for diagnosis, rigorousness of experimental design, and methods of evaluating and documenting change.

However, parents and consumer groups as well as granting agencies increasingly demand accountability. While it may not yet be possible to rigidly apply scales and measurements to quantify program results, efforts must be made to document and compare various strategies of intervention. Numerous measurements of effectiveness have been used to determine the long-term effect of treatment. These measurements include assessment of general motor development,[180,181] standardized scales,[182] maturation of developmental reflexes,[183,184] increase in passive joint ROM,[183,185] age of onset of walking and quality of gait,[98,185] improvements in home management,[186] and changes in functional abilities.[181,185] Many studies have used multiple evaluation measurements because it is not clear in which realms changes can be expected.

Individual case histories and case review series have been used to evaluate the effectiveness of therapy. Paine[185] presents a case review follow-up study of 117 patients comparing treated with nontreated children from 1930 to 1950. The treated and untreated groups were comparable as to type, severity of involvement, and intelligence. Outcome assessments included gait, hand use, presence of contracture, and frequency of orthopedic surgery. The data presented suggest that intensive physical therapy of the type available from 1930 to 1950 had its chief effect on the patient with moderately severe spastic hemiparesis or quadriparesis, who developed a better gait if treated and had fewer contractures. Among the athetoids, no difference in gait or hand function in the treated group was found. Some data suggested that children with spastic CP who began treatment prior to 2 years of age had better gait, fewer contractures, and less orthopedic surgery. No evidence suggested that early treatment was beneficial in athetosis.

Köng[98] performed clinical case reviews of 96 patients receiving a specific therapeutic approach (Bobath) for at least 1 year. Degree of involvement at the end of the treatment period provided the only basis for comparison. Degree of involvement prior to treatment was not described. After 1 to 4 years of treatment, 53 (75 percent) had a normal gait and showed only minimal neurologic signs. No specific test instruments for outcome measures were described. No controls were used.

Several attempts have been made to use a more standard study design involving a control group. Hochleitner compared groups of children with and without Bobath therapy.[187] Direct matching of the two groups was not attempted; diagnoses varied, as did severity and associated disabilities. Results demonstrated significant reduction in degree of disability among the treated group in comparison with the control group. Specific outcome measurements were not described.

Wright and Nicholson[184] studied 47 spastic children under 6 years of age selected at random for immediate treatment, delayed treatment, or no treatment groups. This study showed no evidence after 1 year that physical therapy affected the range of dorsiflexion of the ankle or abduction of the hip, or that it had any effect on the retention or loss of primitive reflexes.

Scherzer and colleagues[186] used a double-blind design to study the effects of physical therapy on 22 children with CP who were younger than 18 months of age. The treatment group received a combination of several modalities of neurodevelopmental physical therapy and the control group received passive ROM exercises. Assignment to group was by random selection. Group matching was not attempted with such a small sample size. The treatment group showed significant improvement in all areas evaluated, including motor development, social maturity, and ease of home management.

Sommerfeld and associates[183] compared the effect of two methods of providing physical therapy services in 19 severely mentally impaired students with CP. In a school setting, the students were paired and assigned to either a direct therapy group or a supervised therapy management group. A group of 10 students from a school in which there was no physical therapy available served as a control comparison. The results of this study showed no significant differences in maturity of development reflexes, gross motor skills, or passive joint ROM among students placed in direct, supervised, or comparison groups.

Several studies have attempted to compare the effectiveness of one method of intervention with another. Sparrow and Zigler[182] used three groups, each with 15 profoundly retarded institutionalized children, to evaluate a modification of the sensorimotor patterning treatment (developed at the Institutes for the Achievement of Human Potential [IAHP]). The treatment group received a program developed after the IAHP method; a matched group participated in motivational activities for the same duration and intensity. A no-treatment group received standard care of the institution. A wide variety of behavioral measurements were used. On the majority of measurements, no differences in post-test performance among the three groups were found. All three groups showed some improvement in performance between the beginning and end of the study.

d'Avignon and colleagues[188] studied three groups of children who showed signs of CNS dysfunction prior to 6 months of age to compare the effectiveness of early physical therapy according to Bobath or Vojta versus a control group. Of the total 30 children, an evaluation at 33 months to 6 years showed 15 children with CP and 15 who were considered normal. Vojta's criteria for "complicated" CP (with sensory problems, seizures, or mental retardation) and "uncomplicated" CP were used for comparison among the three groups. The difference in distribution of these types was not significant. The intervention for the treated groups is not clearly described and the control group received "a less strictly performed and combined form of physiotherapy."

Abdel-Salam and colleagues[189] compared the effects of physical therapy on seven children with infantile spastic CP with seven children with postencephalitic spastic paralysis. Both groups received the same therapeutic intervention. After 4 months, the group with infantile spastic CP showed more significant improvement in function, as measured by decreased time to begin a movement and increased tempo of the movement, as well as improvement in activities of daily living and perceptual motor performance (as measured by tests devised by the researchers) than did the group with postencephalitic spastic paralysis.

In addition to evaluating the long-term effects of treatment, it is valuable to document the immediate effects. Using a single-case study design, Watube and associates[190] used serial photographs to document changes in posture and gait in a spastic diplegic child during the course of a single treatment session. Palisano,[191] using a single-case design, used surface electrode EMG recordings to demonstrate changes in the phase of muscle activity during gait of a 10-year-old child with spastic diplegia following a 1-hour treatment session using neurodevelopmental techniques (Bobath). In both of these studies, changes in gait could be identified immediately after therapy. When combined with temporal information to coordinate the electric activity with particular phases in the gait cycle, EMG is able to provide information on dynamic patterns of muscular activity during walking.[192–194] It cannot, however, adequately record the force generated by muscle activity. Cinematography has been combined with EMG to provide information on joint displacement, velocity, and acceleration.[195,196] Letts and colleagues[197] used videotape analysis and EMG to obtain similar information.

Holt[198] advocated the use of EMG in children with CP as early as 1966. He noted that the action of a muscle during a functional activity may be different from its action in response to conscious effort, and that a muscle's state of activity could not be reliably predicted from observation or clinical examination alone. Perry and associates[122] confirmed these findings. In the evaluation of 23 ambulatory children with spastic diplegia, muscle activity patterns during gait could not be anticipated based on muscle activity in muscle test positions. While it is not possible for most clinics to use EMG during clinical treatment, this method of evaluation has been shown to provide objective data for evaluating change in children with CP, as well as for making decisions regarding orthopedic surgery.

The need to document changes and progress in children as a function of specified intervention still exists as a primary problem in evaluating effectiveness of treatment.

CONCLUSION

The treatment of the child with CP presents an ongoing challenge and commitment by the physical therapist for several reasons. First, intensive care of newborn infants is changing this population and their presenting symptoms. Second, earlier identification and recognition of motor dysfunction brings the child to therapy at a much younger age; and third, better understanding of normal and abnormal development provides the therapist with greater possibilities for planning treatment. The physical therapist must be prepared to deal with all aspects of motor dysfunction and the associated problems of CP as well as all aspects of normal child development in order to continue effective treatment as the child grows and develops. However, there remains a lack of systematic, longitudinal data on the development of handicapped children and on strategies to measure developmental changes related to programming. Therapists who believe that intervention is effective and essential must assume the professional responsibility to document treatment methodology and changes in motor outcomes. Only through objectively documenting these changes will the treatment of children with CP advance. As caring professionals, we have ahead of us the important task of documenting support for our strong commitment to the improvement of function in physically handicapped children.

REFERENCES

1. Bax MC: Terminology and classification of cerebral palsy. Dev Med Child Neurol 6:295, 1964
2. Bobath K: A neurological basis for the treatment of cerebral palsy. Clin Dev Med 75: 1980
3. Ellenberg J, Nelson K: Early recognition of infants at high risk for cerebral palsy: examination at age four months. Dev Med Child Neurol 23:705, 1981
4. Dale A, Stanley FJ: An epidemiological study of cerebral palsy in Western Australia, 1956–1975. II: Spastic cerebral palsy and perinatal factors. Dev Med Child Neurol 22:13, 1980
5. Hagberg B, Hagberg G, Ingemar O: Gains and hazards of intensive neonatal care: an analysis from Swedish cerebral palsy epidemiology. Dev Med Child Neurol 24:13, 1982
6. Stanley FJ, Hobbs MST: Neonatal mortality and cerebral palsy: the impact of neonatal intensive care. Aust Paediatr J 16:35, 1980
7. Kiely J, Paneth N, Zena S et al: Cerebral palsy and newborn care. I: Secular trends in cerebral palsy. Dev Med Child Neurol 23:533, 1981

8. Lagergren J: Children with motor handicaps. Epidemiological medical and socio-paediatric aspects of motor handicapped children in a Swedish country. Acta Paediatr Scand Suppl 8:289, 1981

9. Hagberg B: The epidemiological panorama of major neuropaediatric handicaps in Sweden. p. 111. In Apley J (ed): Care of the Handicapped Child. Clinics in Developmental Medicine. No. 67. JB Lippincott, Philadelphia, 1978

10. O'Reilly D, Walentynowicz J: Etiological factors in cerebral palsy: an historical review. Dev Med Child Neurol 23:633, 1981

11. Koch B, Braillier D, Eng G et al: Computerized tomography in cerebral palsied children. Dev Med Child Neurol 22:595, 1980

12. Pape K, Wigglesworth J: Haemorrhage, ischaemia and the perinatal brain. Clin Dev Med 69/70, 1979

13. Hill A, Volpe J: Seizures, hypoxic-ischemic brain injury and intraventricular hemorrhage in the newborn. Ann Neurol 10:109, 1981

14. Churchill J, Masland RL, Naylor AA et al: The etiology of cerebral palsy in preterm infants. Dev Med Child Neurol 16:143, 1974

15. Minear WI: A classification of cerebral palsy. Pediatrics 18:841, 1956

16. Quinton MB, Wilson JM: Competition of movement patterns applied to the development of infants. p. 164. In Slaton DS, Wilson JM (eds): Caring for Special Babies. University of North Carolina, Chapel Hill, 1983

17. Milani-Comparetti A, Gidoni EA: Pattern analysis of motor development and its disorder. Dev Med Child Neurol 9:625, 1967

18. Milani-Comparetti A: Pattern analysis of normal and abnormal development: the fetus, the newborn, the child. p. 1. In Slaton D (ed): Development of Movement in Infancy. University of North Carolina, Chapel Hill, 1980

19. Crothers B, Paine RS: The Natural History of Cerebral Palsy. Harvard University Press, Cambridge, MA, 1959

20. del Mundo Vallarta J, Robb JP: A follow-up study of newborn infants with perinatal complications: determination of etiology and predictive value of abnormal histories and neurological signs. Neurology 14:413, 1964

21. Prechtl HFR: Prognostic value of neurological signs in the newborn infant. Proc R Soc Med 58:3, 1965

22. Stanley FJ: Spastic cerebral palsy: changes in birthweight and gestational age. Early Hum Dev 5(2):167, 1981

23. Ziegler AL, Calame A, Marchand C et al: Cerebral distress in full-term newborns and its prognostic value. A follow-up study of 90 infants. Helv Paediatr Acta 31:299, 1976

24. Amiel-Tison C: Birth injury as a cause of brain dysfunction in full-term newborns. Adv Perinat Neurol 1:57, 1978

25. Capute AJ: Identifying cerebral palsy in infancy through a study of primitive reflex profiles. Pediatr Ann 8:589, 1979

26. Ingram TTS: The new approach to early diagnosis of handicaps in childhood. Dev Med Child Neurol 11:279, 1969

27. Paine RS, Brazelton TB, Donovan DE et al: Evolution of postural reflexes in normal infants and in the presence of chronic brain syndrome. Neurology 14:1036, 1964

28. Nelson KB, Ellenberg JH: Neonatal signs as predictors of cerebral palsy. Pediatrics 64:225, 1979

29. Campbell SK, Wilhelm IJ: Developmental sequence in infants at high risk for central nervous system dysfunction: the recovery process in the first year of life.

p. 90. In Stack J (ed): The Special Infant: An Interdisciplinary Approach to the Optimal Development of Infants. Human Sciences Press, New York, 1982

30. Campbell S, Wilhelm I: Development of infants at risk for central nervous system dysfunction: progress report. p. 96. In Slaton DS, Wilson JM (eds): Caring for Special Babies. University of North Carolina, Chapel Hill, 1983

31. Thompson T, Reynolds J: The results of intensive care therapy for neonates. I. Overall neonatal mortality rate II. Neonatal mortality rates and long-term prognosis for low birth weight neonates. J Perinat Med 5:59, 1977

32. Fitzhardinge PM: Follow-up studies in the low birth weight infant. Clin Perinatol 3:503, 1976

33. Stewart A, Turcan D, Rawlings G et al: Outcome for infants at high risk for major handicap. Ciba Found Symp 59:151, 1978

34. Kamper J: Long-term prognosis of infants with severe idiopathic respiratory distress syndrome I. Neurological and mental outcome. Acta Paediatr Scand 67:61, 1978

35. Rajani K, Goetzman BW, Kelso GF et al: Prognosis of intracranial hemorrhage in neonates. Surg Neurol 13:433, 1980

36. Williamson WD, Desmond MM, Wilson GS et al: Early neurodevelopmental outcome of low birth weight infant surviving neonatal intraventricular hemorrhage. J Perinat Med 10:34, 1982

37. Krishnamoorthy KS, Shannon DC, DeLong GR et al: Neurologic sequelae in the survivors of neonatal intraventricular hemorrhage. Pediatrics 64:233, 1979

38. Wilson J: Developing ambulation skills. p. 83. In Connolly B, Montgomery P (eds): Therapeutic Exercise in Developmental Disabilities. Chattanooga Corp, Chattanooga, 1987

39. Holt KS: Review: the assessment of walking in children with particular reference to cerebral palsy. Child Care Health Dev 7:281, 1981

40. Campbell Sk, Wilhelm IJ: Developmental sequence in infants at high risk for central nervous system dysfunction: the recovery process in the first year of life. p. 90. In Stack J (ed): The Special Infant: An Interdisciplinary Approach to the Optimal Developmental of Infants. Human Sciences Press, New York, 1982

41. Molnar GE, Gordon SU: Cerebral palsy: predictive value of selected signs for early prognostication of motor function. Arch Phys Med Rehabil 56:153, 1976

42. Badell-Ribera A: Cerebral palsy: postural-locomotor prognosis in spastic diplegia. Arch Phys Med Rehabil 66:614, 1985

43. Largo RH, Molenari L, Weber M et al: Early development of locomotion: significances of prematurity, cerebral palsy and sex. Dev Med Child Neurol 27:183, 1985

44. Molnar GE: Cerebral palsy: prognosis and how to judge it. Pediatr Ann 8:596, 1979

45. Watt JM, Robertson CMT, Grace MGA: Early prognosis for ambulation of neonatal intensive care survivors with cerebral palsy. Dev Med Child Neurol 31(6):766, 1989

46. Bleck EE: Locomotor prognosis in cerebral palsy. Dev Med Child Neurol 17:18, 1975

47. Molnar GE: Cerebral palsy. p. 420. In Molnar GE (ed): Pediatric Rehabilitation. Williams & Wilkins, Baltimore, 1985

48. Milla PT, Jackson ADM: A controlled trial of baclofen in children with cerebral palsy. J Intern Med Res 5:398, 1977

49. Hudgson P, Weightman D: Baclofen in the treatment of spasticity. Br Med J 4:15, 1971

50. McKinlay I, Hyde E, Gordon N: Baclofin—a team approach to drug evaluation of spasticity in childhood. Scott Med J Suppl 1:526, 1980

51. Young JA: Clinical experience in the use of baclofen in children with spastic cerebral palsy: a further report. Scott Med J Suppl 1:523, 1980

52. Minford A, Brown JK, Minns RA et al: The effect of baclofen on the gait of hemiplegic children assessed by means of polarized light goniometry. Scott Med J Suppl 1:529, 1980

53. Armstrong R, Steinbok P, Farrell M et al: Continuous intrathecal baclofen for the treatment of severe spasticity. Presented at the AACPDM Annual Meeting, October 1989

54. Penn R, Kroin JS: Intrathecal baclofen in the long term management of severe spasticity. p. 325. In Park TS, Phillips LH, Peacock WJ (eds): Neurosurgery: State of the Arts Review 4(2). Hanley and Belfus, Philadelphia, 1989

55. van Hemert JCJ: Spasticity: Disordered Motor Function; A Double-blind Comparison of Baclofen and Placebo in Patients With Spasticity of Cerebral Origin. Year Book Medical Publishers, Chicago, 1980

56. Milla PH, Jackson ADM: A controlled trial of baclofen in children with cerebral palsy. J Int Med Res 5:398, 1977

57. Muller H, Zierski J, Dralle D et al: The effects of intrathecal baclofen on electrical muscle activity in spasticity. J Neurol 234(5):348, 1987

58. Latash M, Penn R, Corcos D et al: Effects of intrathecal baclofen on voluntary motor control in spastic paresis. J Neurosurg 72:388, 1990

59. Joynt R, Leonard J: Dantrolene sodium suspension in treatment of spastic cerebral palsy. Dev Med Child Neurol 22:755, 1980

60. Carpenter E, Sietz D: Intramuscular alcohol as an aid in management of spastic cerebral palsy. Dev Med Child Neurol 22:497, 1980

61. Samilson R (ed): Orthopaedic Aspects of Cerebral Palsy. Clin Dev Med 52/53, 1975

62. Bleck EE: Orthopedic Management of Cerebral Palsy. WB Saunders, Philadelphia, 1979

63. House JH, Gwathmey FW, Fidler MO: A dynamic approach to thumb-in-palm deformity in cerebral palsy. Evaluation and results in 56 patients. J Bone Joint Surg 63A:216, 1981

64. Goldner LJ: The upper extremity in cerebral palsy. p. 221. In Samilson RL (ed): Orthopaedic Aspects of Cerebral Palsy. Clinics in Developmental Medicine. No. 52/53. JB Lippincott, Philadelphia, 1975

65. Zancolli EA, Zancolli ER: Surgical management of the hemiplegic spastic hand in cerebral palsy. Surg Clin North Am 61:2 395, 1981

66. Hoffer MM, Perry J, Melkonian GJ: Dynamic electromyography and decision making for surgery in the upper extremity of patients with cerebral palsy. J Hand Surg 4:424, 1979

67. Bleck E: Deformities of the spine and pelvis in cerebral palsy. In Samilson R (ed): Orthopaedic Aspects of Cerebral Palsy. JB Lippincott, Philadelphia, 1975

68. Bonnett C, Brown JC, Grow T: Thoracolumbar scoliosis in cerebral palsy. Results of surgical treatment. J Bone Joint Surg 58:328, 1976

69. MacEwen GD: Operative treatment of scoliosis in cerebral palsy. Reconstr Surg Traumatol 13:58, 1972

70. Allen BL, Ferguson RL: L-rod instrumentation for scoliosis in cerebral palsy. J Pediatr Orthop 2:87, 1982

71. Truscelli D, Lespargot A, Tardieu G: Variation in the long-term results of elon-

gation of the tendo achillis in children with cerebral palsy. J Bone Joint Surg 61B:466, 1979

72. Castle ME, Reyman TA, Schneider M: Pathology of spastic muscle in cerebral palsy. Clin Orthop 142:223, 1979
73. Root L, Spero CR: Hip adductor transfer compared with adductor tenotomy in cerebral palsy. J Bone Joint Surg 63A:767, 1981
74. Cooper IS, Riklan M, Amin I et al: Chronic cerebellar stimulation in cerebral palsy. Neurology 26:744, 1976
75. Davis R, Barolat-Romana G, Engle H: Chronic cerebellar stimulation for cerebral palsy: five year study. Acta Neurochir Suppl (Wien) 30:317, 1980
76. Ivan LP: Chronic cerebellar stimulation in cerebral palsy. Appl Neurophysiol 45:51, 1982
77. Penn RD, Etzel ML: Chronic cerebellar stimulation and developmental reflexes. J Neurosurg 46:506, 1977
78. Wong PKH, Hoffman HJ, Froese AB et al: Cerebellar stimulation in the management of cerebral palsy: clinical and physiological studies. J Neurosurg 5:217, 1979
79. Penn RD, Myklebust BM, Gottlieb GL et al: Chronic cerebellar stimulation for cerebral palsy. Prospective and double-blind studies. J Neurosurg 53(2):160, 1980
80. Gahm NH, Russman BS, Cerciello RL et al: Chronic cerebellar stimulation for cerebral palsy: a double-blind study. Neurology 31:87, 1981
81. Whittaker CK: Cerebellar stimulation for cerebral palsy. J Neurosurg 52:648, 1980
82. Penn RD: Chronic cerebellar stimulation for cerebral palsy. A review. Neurosurgery 10(1):116, 1982
83. Peacock WJ, Staudt L: Selective dorsal rhizotomy: history and results. p. 403. In Park TS, Phillips LH, Peacock WJ (eds): Neurosurgery: State of the Arts Reviews 4(2). Hanley and Belfus, Philadelphia, 1989
84. Peacock WJ, Arens LJ, Berman B: Cerebral palsy spasticity: selective dorsal rhizotomy. Pediatr Neurosci 13:61, 1987
85. Arens LJ, Peacock WJ, Peter J: Selective dorsal rhizotomy: a long-term follow-up study. Childs Nerv Syst 5:148, 1989
86. Berman B: Selective posterior rhizotomy: does it do any good? p. 431. In Park TS, Phillips LH, Peacock WJ (eds): Neurosurgery: State of the Arts Reviews 4(2). Hanley and Belfus, Philadelphia, 1989
87. Wilson J: Outpatient based physical therapy program for children with cerebral palsy undergoing selective dorsal rhizotomy. p. 417. In Park TS, Phillips LH, Peacock WJ (eds): Neurosurgery: State of the Arts Reviews 4(2). Hanley and Belfuss, Philadelphia, 1989
88. Vaughn CL, Berman B, Peacock WJ, Eldridge NE: Gait analysis and rhizotomy: past experiences and future considerations. p. 445. In Park TS, Phillips LH, Peacock WJ (eds): Neurosurgery: State of the Arts Reviews 4(2). Hanley and Belfus, Philadelphia, 1989
89. Perry J, Adams J: Foot-floor contact patterns following selective dorsal rhizotomy. Presented at the Annual Meeting, AACPDM, October 1989
90. Kobltsky S, Mason D, Giuliani C: The effects of dorsal rhizotomy on standing posture and the temporal characteristics of gait of children with cerebral palsy. Presented at the AACPDM Annual Meeting, October 1989
91. Scherzer A, Tscharnuter I: Early Diagnosis and Therapy in Cerebral Palsy. Pediatric Habilitation. Vol. 3. Marcel Dekker, New York, 1982
92. Sparling JW: The transdisciplinary approach with the developmentally delayed child. Phys Occup Ther Pediatr 1:3, 1980

93. Johnson J: Preface to developing norm-referenced standardized tests. Phys Occup Ther Pediatr 9(1):xiii, 1989
94. Levine MS, Trost-Miller T: Minimal diagnostic criteria for cerebral palsy: a single-blind study. Dev Med Child Neurol 23:114, 1981
95. Bobath K: The normal posture reflex mechanism and its deviation in children with cerebral palsy. Physiotherapy 11:1, 1971
96. Shepherd RB: Physiotherapy in Paediatrics. 2nd Ed. Heinemann, London, 1980
97. Farber SD: Neurorehabilitation, A Multisensory Approach. WB Saunders, Philadelphia, 1982
98. Kong E: Very early treatment of cerebral palsy. Dev Med Child Neurol 8:198, 1966
99. Hoessly M: Normal and abnormal movement patterns in the newborn and young infant. Physiotherapy 65:372, 1979
100. Kathrein JE: Interrater reliability in the assessment of muscle tone of infants and children. Phys Occup Ther Pediatr 10(1):27, 1990
101. Saint-Anne Dargassies S: Neurological Development in the Full-term and Premature Neonate. Excerpta Medica, New York, 1977
102. Amiel-Tison C: Neurological evaluation of the maturity of newborn infants. Arch Dis Child 43:89, 1968
103. McKinly JC, Berkowitz NJ: Quantitative studies on human muscle tonus: a description of methods. Arch Neurol Psychol 19:1036, 1928
104. Stillwell DM, Gersten JW: Effect of ischemia and curare on spasticity. Arch Phys Med 37:533, 1956
105. Ashworth B: Preliminary trial of carisoprodol in multiple sclerosis. Practitioner 192:540, 1964
106. Chandler LS, Andrews MS, Swanson MW: The Movement Assessment of Infants. Movement Assessment of Infants, Rolling Bay, WA, 1980
107. Brazelton TB: Neonatal Behavioral Assessment Scale. Clin Dev Med 50, 1973
108. Dubowitz L, Dubowitz V: The Neurological Assessment of the Preterm and Full-term Newborn Infant. Clinics in Developmental Medicine. Vol. 79. JB Lippincott, Philadelphia, 1981
109. Prechtl H: The Neurological Examination of the Full-Term Newborn Infant. Ed. 2. Clinics in Developmental Medicine. No. 63. JB Lippincott, Philadelphia, 1977
110. Chan SWY: Motor and sensory deficits following a stroke: relevance to a comprehensive evaluation. Physiother Can 38:29, 1986
111. Bly L: The components of normal movement during the first year of life. p. 85. In Slaton D (ed): Development of Movement in Infancy. University of North Carolina, Chapel Hill, 1980
112. Provost B: Normal development from birth to four months: extended use of the NBAS-K. Part I. Phys Occup Ther Pediatr 1:39, 1980
113. Vulpe S: Vulpe Assessment Battery. NIMR, Toronto, 1977
114. Bobath B, Bobath K: Motor Development in the Different Types of Cerebral Palsy. Heinemann, New York, 1975
115. Molnar G: Motor deficit of retarded infants and young children. Arch Phys Med 55:393, 1974
116. Fiorentino MR: Reflex Testing Methods for Evaluating Central Nervous System Development. 2nd Ed. Charles C Thomas, Springfield, IL, 1973
117. Wilson J: Developmental Reflex Test. p. 335. In Vulpe S (ed): Vulpe Assessment Battery. NIMR, Toronto, 1977
118. Capute AJ, Accardo PJ, Vining EP et al: Primitive Reflex Profile. University Park Press, Baltimore, 1978

119. Barnes M, Crutchfield C, Heriza C: The Neurophysiological Basis of Patient Treatment. Reflexes in Motor Development. Stokesville Publishing, Morgantown, WV, 1978

120. Fisher AG: Objective assessment of the quality of response during equilibrium tasks. Phys Occup Ther Pediatr 9(3):57, 1989

121. Perry J: Rehabilitation of spasticity. p. 87. In Feldman RG, Young RR, Koella WP (eds): Spasticity: Disordered Motor Control. Year Book Medical Publishing, Chicago, 1980

122. Perry J, Hoffer MM, Antonelli MS et al: Electromyography before and after surgery for hip deformity in children with cerebral palsy. J Bone Joint Surg 48A:201, 1976

123. Morris SE: Assessment and treatment of children with oral motor dysfunction. p. 106. In Wilson JM (ed): Oral-Motor Function and Dysfunction in Children. University of North Carolina, Chapel Hill, 1977

124. Morris SE: The Normal Acquisition of Oral Feeding Skills: Implications for Assessment and Treatment. Therapeutic Media, Central Islip, NY, 1982

125. Levangie PK, Chimera M, Johnston M et al: The effects of posterior rolling walkers vs. the standard rolling walker on gait characteristics of children with spastic cerebral palsy. Phys Occup Ther Pediatr 9(4):1, 1989

126. Simeonsson RJ, Simeonsson NE: Parenting handicapped children: psychological perspectives. In Paul J (ed): Parents of Handicapped Children. Holt, Rinehart, & Winston, New York, 1981

127. Lambie D, Bond J, Welkart DP: Home Teaching With Mothers and Infants, the Ypsilanti-Carnegie Infant Education Project. High/Scope Educational Research Foundation, Ypsilanti, MI, 1974

128. Campbell S, Wilson J: Planning infant learning programs. Phys Ther 56(12):1347, 1976

129. Redman-Bentley D: Parent expectations for professionals providing services to their handicapped children. Phys Occup Ther Pediatr 2(1):13, 1982

130. Schaefer E: Evaluating intervention effects on children, parents and professionals. p. 85. In Wilson J (ed): Planning and Evaluating Developmental Programs. 2nd Ed. University of North Carolina, Chapel Hill, 1979

131. Etaugh C: Effects of maternal employment on children: a review of recent research. Merrill-Palmer Q Behav Dev 20:71, 1974

132. Wilson J: Help your child—a home management program for children with CNS dysfunction. p. 194. In Wilson J (ed): Infants at Risk: Medical and Therapeutic Management. 2nd Ed. University of North Carolina, Chapel Hill, 1981

133. Lonsdale G: Family life with a handicapped child: the parents speak. Child Care Health Dev 4:99, 1978

134. Gath A: The impact of an abnormal child upon the parents. Br J Psychiatry 130:405, 1977

135. McMichael J: Handicap. A Study of Physically Handicapped Children and Their Families. Staples Press, London, 1971

136. Tizard J, Grad JC: The Mentally Handicapped and Their Families. Maudsley Monograph No. 7, London, 1961

137. Butler N, Gill R, Pomeroy D et al: Handicapped Children—Their Homes and Life Styles. Department of Child Health, University of Bristol, 1978

138. Burden RL: Measuring the effects of stress on the mothers of handicapped infants. Must depression always follow? Child Care Health Dev 6:111, 1980

139. Dunlap WR, Hollingsworth JS: How does a handicapped child affect the family? Implications for practitioners. Fam Coord 26(3):286, 1977

140. Wishart MC, Bidder RT, Gray OP: Parents' report of family life with a developmentally delayed child. Child Care Health Dev 7:267, 1981

141. Simeonsson RJ, McHale SM: Review: research on handicapped children: sibling relationships. Child Care Health Dev 7:153, 1981

142. Tew B, Laurence KM: Mothers, brothers and sisters of patients with spina bifida. Dev Med Child Neurol 15(6):69, 1973

143. Caldwell BM, Guze SB: A study of the adjustment of parents and siblings of institutionalized and non-institutionalized retarded children. Am J Ment Defic 64:845, 1960

144. Grossman FK: Brothers and Sisters of Retarded Children: An Exploratory Study. Syracuse University Press, Syracuse, 1972

145. Sussman M, Cusick B: Preliminary report: the role of short-leg, tone reducing casts as an adjunct to physical therapy of patients with cerebral palsy. Johns Hopkins Med J 145:112, 1979

146. Cusick B, Sussman M: Short leg casts: their role in the management of cerebral palsy. Phys Occup Ther Pediatr 2:93, 1982

147. Embry O: Preliminary report: inhibitive tone casts used in connection with neurodevelopmental treatment. NDT Newsletter, August 1982

148. Finnie N: Handling the Young Cerebral Palsied Child at Home. 2nd Ed. Dutton, New York, 1975

149. Conner FP, Williamson GG, Siepp JM: The First Three Years: A Curriculum Guide for Infants and Toddlers With Sensorimotor and Other Developmental Disabilities. Appendix A. Columbia University Press, New York, 1978

150. Fraser B, Galka G, Hensinger RN: Gross Motor Management of Severely Multiply Impaired Students. Vol. 1: Evaluation Guide. University Park Press, Baltimore, 1980

151. Nwaobi OM, Burbaker CE, Cusick B et al: Electromyographic investigation of extensor activity in cerebral palsied children in different seating positions. Dev Med Child Neurol 25:2, 175, 1983

152. Cristarella M: Comparison of straddling and sitting apparatus for the spastic cerebral-palsied child. Am J Occup Ther 29(5):273, 1975

153. Hulme JB, Poor R, Schillein M et al: Perceived behavioral changes observed with adaptive seating devices and training programs for multihandicapped, developmentally disabled individuals. Phys Ther 63:2204, 1983

154. Bergen A, Colangelo C: Positioning the Client With CNS Deficits: The Wheelchair and Other Adaptive Equipment. Valhalla Rehabilitation Publishers, Valhalla, NY, 1982

155. Breed A, Ibler I: The motorized wheelchair: new freedom, new responsibility, and new problems. Dev Med Child Neurol 24:366, 1982

156. Carlson J, Winter R: The 'Gillette' sitting support orthosis for nonambulatory children with severe cerebral palsy or advanced muscular dystrophy. Minn Med 61(8):469, 1978

157. Carmick J: High chair adaption. Totline 7(4):15, 1981

158. Carrington E: A seating position for a cerebral palsied child. Am J Occup Ther 32(3):179, 1978

159. Coletti T, Weaver J, Jacquard S: Adaptive kneeler for handicapped children. Phys Ther 59:886, 1979

160. Dunkel R, Trefler E: Seating for cerebral palsied children—the Sleek Seat. Phys Ther 57:524, 1977

161. Gajdosik C, Gajdosik R: Spool roll for positioning the child prone. Phys Ther 61:1288, 1981

162. Ivey A, Roblyer DD: Rollermobile for children with cerebral palsy. Phys Ther 60:1162, 1980

163. Ottenbacher K, Malter R, Weckwerth L: Toilet seat arrangement for children with neuromotor dysfunction. Am J Occup Ther 33(3):193, 1979

164. Susko G, Rice H, Williams J: Orthopedic cart for severely handicapped persons. Phys Ther 56:1132, 1976

165. Trefler E, Hanks S, Huggins P et al: A modular seating system for cerebral palsied children. Dev Med Child Neurol 20:199, 1978

166. Wilbur S: Foam rubber sidelying support for children with cerebral palsy. Phys Ther 55(12):1345, 1975

167. Wilson J: Selection and use of adaptive equipment for preschool children. p. 171. In McLaurin S (ed): The Preschool Special Child. University of North Carolina, Chapel Hill, 1982

168. Rang M, Douglas G, Bennet G et al: Seating for children with cerebral palsy. J Pediatr Orthop 1:279, 1981

169. DiCarlo C, Forbis A: A chair for the child with hypertonic CNS dysfunction. Phys Ther 56(10):1151, 1977

170. Logan L, Byers-Henkley K, Ciccone C: Anterior vs posterior walkers for children with cerebral palsy: a gait analysis study. Presented at the AACPDM Annual Meeting, October 1987

171. Howell-Garvey V, Tylkowski CM, Kates D et al: The influence of walkers on the gait of children with cerebral palsy. Presented at the AACPDM Annual Meeting, October 1987

172. Hulme JB, Gallacher MA, Hulme RD: The Montana Adaptive Equipment Project: A cost efficient model for the delivery of adaptive equipment services in rural settings. Phy Occup Ther Pediatr 1:59, 1981

173. Sontag ED (ed): Educational Programming for the Severely and Profoundly Handicapped. CEC, Boothwyn, 1977

174. Except Child, suppl. 9(1):4, 1979

175. Hofmann R: How to Build Special Furniture and Equipment for Handicapped Children. Charles C Thomas, Springfield, IL, 1970

176. Lowman E, Klinger J: Aids to Independent Living. McGraw-Hill, New York, 1969

177. Macey P: Mobilizing Multiply Handicapped Children: A Manual for the Design and Construction of Modified Wheelchairs. University of Kansas, Lawrence, 1974

178. Robinault I (ed): Functional Aids for the Multiply Handicapped. Harper & Row, Hagerstown, MD, 1973

179. Simeonsson RJ, Cooper DH, Scheiner AP: A review and analysis of the effectiveness of early intervention programs. Pediatrics 69:635, 1982

180. Ingram AJ, Withers E, Speltz E: Role of intensive physical and occupational therapy in the treatment of cerebral palsy: testing and results. Arch Phys Med Rehabil 40:429, 1959

181. Footh WK, Kogan KL: Measuring the effectiveness of physical therapy in the treatment of cerebral palsy. J Am Phys Ther Assoc 867, 1963

182. Sparrow S, Zigler E: Evaluation of a patterning treatment for retarded children. Pediatrics 62(2):137, 1978

183. Sommerfeld D, Fraser B, Hensinger RN et al: Evaluation of physical therapy service for severely mentally impaired students with cerebral palsy. Phys Ther 61(3):338, 1981

184. Wright T, Nicholson J: Physiotherapy for the spastic child: an evaluation. Dev Med Child Neurol 15:146, 1973

185. Paine R: On the treatment of cerebral palsy—the outcome of 177 patients, 74 totally untreated. Pediatrics 29:605, 1962
186. Scherzer A, Mike V, Ilson J: Physical therapy as a determinant of change in the cerebral palsied infant. Pediatrics 58:47, 1976
187. Hochleitner M: Vergleichende Untersuchung von Kinder mit zerebraler Bewegungsstörng, mit und ohme neurophysiologischer Frühtherapie. Oesterr Aerzt 32:1108, 1977
188. d'Avignon M, Noren L, Arman T: Early physiotherapy ad modum Vojta or Bobath in infants with suspected neuromotor disturbance. Neuropaediatrics 12:232, 1981
189. Abdel-Salam E, Maraghi S, Tawfik M: Evaluation of physical therapy techniques in the management of cerebral palsy. J Egypt Med Assoc 61:531, 1978
190. Watube S, Otabe T, Kii K et al: Improving the walking patterns of a spastic diplegic child. Totline 7(1):14, 1981
191. Palisano RJ: Investigation of Electromyographic Gait Analysis as a Method of Evaluating the Effects of Neurodevelopmental Treatment in a Child With Cerebral Palsy. Master's Thesis. Division of Physical Therapy, School of Medicine, University of North Carolina, Chapel Hill, 1981
192. Chong KC, Vojnic CD, Quanbury AO et al: The assessment of the internal rotation gait in cerebral palsy. Clin Orthop 132:145, 1978
193. Perry J, Hopper M, Giovan P et al: Gait analysis of the triceps surae in cerebral palsy. J Bone Joint Surg 56A:511, 1974
194. Woltering H, Guth V, Abbink F: Electromyographic investigations of gait in cerebral palsied children. Electromyogr Clin Neurophysiol 19:519, 1979
195. Sutherland DH, Schottstaedt ER, Larsen LJ et al: Clinical and electromyographic study of seven spastic children with internal rotation gait. J Bone Joint Surg 51A:1070, 1969
196. Sutherland DH, Cooper L: Crouch gait in spastic diplegia. Orthop Trans 1:76, 1977
197. Letts RM, Winter DA, Quanbury M: Locomotion studies as an aid in clinical assessment of child gait. Can Med Assoc J 112:1091, 1975
198. Holt KS: Facts and fallacies about neuromuscular function in cerebral palsy as revealed by electromyography. Dev Med Child Neurol 8:255, 1966

APPENDIX 10-1

Classification of Cerebral Palsy by Topographical Distribution of Tone and Abnormal Movement

Spasticity is characterized by increased muscle tone, stereotyped and limited patterns of movement, decreased active and passive ROM, the tendency to develop contractures and deformities, the persistence of primitive and tonic reflexes, and poor development of the postural reflex mechanism.

Spastic hemiplegia is the most common type of spastic CP.[1]

Characteristics

1. One side of the body shows abnormal muscle tone and movement.
2. The entire side of the body is involved, including the face, neck, and trunk, as well as the extremities. The upper extremity is significantly more involved than the lower extremity. There is no preference for side.[2]

3.   Often strabismus, oral motor dysfunction, somatosensory dysfunction (akinesia, astereognosis), and perceptual and learning disorders are associated problems.

4.   Sensory deficit may be as detrimental to ultimate function as spasticity and motor deficit.

5.   The child often ignores the involved side and uses the sound side for activities and weight-bearing (Fig. 10A-1).[3]

6.   Seizures often develop as the child grows older.[4]

Spastic diplegia is most frequently related to problems of prematurity, with increasing prevalence.[5,6]

Characteristics

1.   The total body is affected, with greater involvement in trunk and lower extremities than upper extremities and face (Fig. 10A-2).

2.   Often the child has associated bilateral esotropia, along with oral motor and speech problems.

3.   Often one side is more involved than the other (double hemiplegia), particularly in the lower extremities.

Spastic quadriplegia is often related to birth asphyxia in term infants[5] or grade 3 and 4 intraventricular bleeds in very immature infants.[7,8]

Characteristics

1.   The total child is involved—head, neck, trunk, and arms equally or more involved than legs.

2.   The infant often presents first with hypotonia.

3.   If the disorder is severe, tone dominates the child's posture and movement, either totally extended (Fig. 10A-3A) or totally flexed (Fig. 10A-3B). The ability to move against gravity is very slight.

4.   Associated problems include vision, hearing defects, seizures, mental retardation, and oral motor problems.

5.   Often the involvement is asymmetrical, leading to contractures and deformities, particularly scoliosis and dislocation of the hip on the more involved side.[9]

Athetosis (dyskinetic syndromes) is related to erythroblastosis and birth asphyxia.[1]

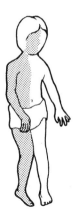

Fig. 10A-1. Right spastic hemiplegia.

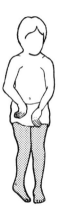

Fig. 10A-2. Spastic diplegia.

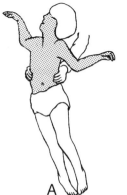
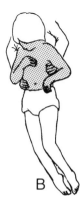

Fig. 10A-3. Spastic quadriplegia.

A   B

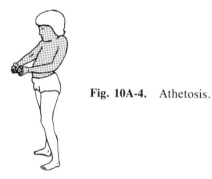

Fig. 10A-4.   Athetosis.

Types of Dyskinetic Syndromes

1. *Nontension athetoid*: involuntary movements without increased muscle tone
2. *Dystonic athetoid*: abnormal positioning of limbs, head, and trunk with unpredictable increased tone
3. *Choreoathetoid*: involuntary, unpredictable small movements of the distal parts of the extremities
4. *Tension athetoid*: increased muscle tone, which actually blocks involuntary movements

Characteristics

1. Muscle tone is variable.
2. Purposeful movement is poorly executed and coordinated.
3. The child lacks the ability to sustain postural alignment (Fig. 10A-4).
4. Involvement is often asymmetric.
5. Tonic reflexes dominate posture.[10]
6. Hypotonia precedes onset of athetosis.
7. Involuntary, unpredictable movements are exaggerated by voluntary movement, postural adjustments, changes in emotions and anxiety or speech.[11]
8. The child usually has severely impaired speech, poor respiratory control, and other oral motor problems. High-frequency hearing loss is common.

Ataxia is associated with developmental deficits of the cerebellum.

Characteristics

1. Low postural tone, markedly defective postural function resulting in disturbed equilibrium and cocontraction make sustained control against gravity difficult.[10,12]

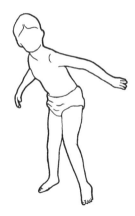

Fig. 10A-5.   Ataxic CP.

    2. Diplegic distribution affects trunk and legs more than arms and hands.

    3. Balance is poor when standing and walking; stance and gait are wide-based (Fig. 10A-5).

    4. Intention to use the hands produces tremor.

    5. Movement is uncoordinated for both gross and fine motor tasks.

    6. Stress or attempts to speed up movement increases incoordination.

    7. Spastic diplegia or athetosis is often concomitant.

    8. Ataxia often follows the initial stage of hypotonia.

    9. Associated problems include nystagmus, poor eye tracking, and delayed and poorly articulated speech.

Flaccid, hypotonia is often a transient stage in the evolution of athetosis or spasticity.[13]

Characteristics

    1. The child has decreased muscle tone, real or apparent weakness, and increased ROM, but has little power to move against gravity.

    2. Excessive joint flexibility is indicative of severe hypotonia.

    3. The child lies in "frog-leg" position when placed on back (Fig. 10A-6A).

    4. If the child develops enough tone to sit up, he often stabilizes the body with the hands and sits between the legs to provide a wider base of support and accommodate for postural instability in the trunk (Fig. 10A-6B).

Mixed types is the term used most commonly to indicate spastic diplegia mixed with athetosis, but it may be used to describe any child who does not fit the characterizations described above.

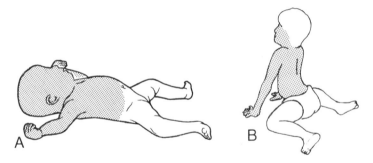

Fig. 10A-6. Atonic CP. **(A)** Supine. **(B)** Sitting.

References

1. O'Reilly D, Walenlynowicz J: Etiological factors in cerebral palsy: a historical review. Dev Med Child Neurol 23:633, 1981
2. Michaelis R, Rooschuz B, Dopfer R: Prenatal origins of congenital spastic hemiparesis. Early Hum Dev 4(3):243, 1980
3. Knutsson E: Muscle activation patterns of gait in spastic hemiparesis, paraparesis and cerebral palsy. Scand J Rehabil Med Suppl 7:47, 1980
4. Cohen ME, Duffner PK: Prognostic indicators in hemiparetic cerebral palsy. Ann Neurol 9:353, 1981
5. Bennett FC, Chandler LS, Robinson NM et al: Spastic diplegia in premature infants, etiologic and diagnostic consideration. Am J Dis Child 135:732, 1981
6. Russell EM: Correlation between birth weight and the clinical findings on diplegia. Arch Dis Child 35:548, 1960
7. Pape K, Wigglesworth J: Haemorrhage, ischemia and the perinatal brain. Clin Dev Med 69/70, 1979
8. Scott H: Outcome of very severe birth asphyxia. Arch Dis Child 51:712, 1976
9. Bleck EE: The hip in cerebral palsy. Orthop Clin North Am 11:79, 1980
10. Carr JH, Shepherd RB: Physiotherapy in Disorders of the Brain. Heinemann, London, 1982
11. Kabat H, McLeod M: Athetosis: Neuromuscular dysfunction and treatment. Arch Phys Med Rehabil 40:285, 1959
12. Hagberg B, Sanner G, Steen M: The dysequilibrium syndrome in cerebral palsy. Acta Paediatr Scand Suppl 61:226, 1972
13. Lesny IA: Follow-up study of hypotonic forms of cerebral palsy. Brain Dev 1(2):87, 1979

11 | Physical Therapy in the Education Setting

Jack Berndt
Ann Falconer

The American Physical Therapy Association (APTA) supports the provision of physical therapy services to children with special needs. Physical therapists have provided services to students with handicaps throughout the history of the profession. Public Law 94-142 (PL 94-142) provides the opportunity for physical therapists and physical therapist assistants to be actively involved in providing services to students with handicaps in educational programs. Public Law 99-457 (PL 99-457) extends this involvement to early intervention services for handicapped infants and toddlers and their families.[1]

HISTORIC BACKGROUND

In 1900, the first public school for "crippled children" in the United States opened in Chicago. At the turn of the century in Chicago, and soon after in several other metropolitan areas, children with physical handicaps were educated in orthopedic divisions of the local school system.[2] These special classes, separate from regular classes, were provided in existing schools; however, it soon became necessary to build separate schools because of overcrowding and the presence of physical barriers. The ethos of the time held that children with sensory and motor deficits should be segregated from their nondisabled peers. Segregation was thought to be in the best interest of the child with a physical handicap who would otherwise have to compete with normal, healthy children.[3-5]

361

Eligibility to attend these special or orthopedic schools was based on a physician's examination. Criteria for admission might include the inability to walk to school and access the building, the need for daily rest periods, the need for adult assistance with activities of daily living or personal care, or the need for ongoing medical care, nursing, or therapy services.[3,6] Children with mental retardation were believed to be noneducable. It was recommended that they be sent to an institution or a private facility.[2,7]

Physical therapy as a profession emerged from World War I. Muscle reeducation exercises were developed during and after the war to rehabilitate disabled veterans.[8] Concurrently (as early as 1915), muscle training techniques were used in the treatment of poliomyelitis.[3,8,9] The majority of children in the early orthopedic schools were handicapped from the aftereffects of infection by the polio virus.

Corrective exercises for students with disabilities initially were taught by physical educators or sometimes by nurses. By the late 1920s, these teachers were required to take additional coursework and be graduates of recognized "physiotherapy" courses.[3,7] During the 1930s, orthopedic care, followed by prescribed therapeutic exercises, became an essential component in these special schools. The treatment center or physical therapy department was equipped with the standard armamentarium of the hospital clinic: infrared and ultraviolet lamps, massage and treatment tables, stall bars, hydrotherapy tanks, and, in some buildings, therapeutic swimming pools.[10,11]

Besides polio, disabling conditions of children with spastic paralysis, tuberculosis of the bone, osteomyelitis, and various congenital disorders were treated. The orthopedic schools were, in fact, rehabilitation centers in which a student's physical needs were addressed first, followed by academic and vocational needs.[4,5]

The Social Security Act of 1935 was one of the first major pieces of federal legislation that affected children with handicaps.[9] Parts of the Act provided state funds for identification and outreach programs for medically at-risk children, especially in rural communities. Medical intervention became available on a widespread basis for the first time.[12]

The expanded medical identification and intervention for increasing numbers of children led to a need for building additional orthopedic schools for follow-up or aftercare. Increased numbers of physical therapists were needed to provide services in the community as well as in the schools.[13,14] Over the next 30 years, special education was defined primarily by the medical treatment model. With few exceptions, children with mental retardation and multiple handicaps continued to be excluded from this country's public school system.[15]

During the 1960s, parents and other advocates began to use the US courts and the legislative process to challenge this exclusionary policy. Parents believed that education is a right of children with disabilities. Their efforts in the right-to-education movement culminated in two important judicial decisions in the early 1970s: (1) Pennsylvania Association for Retarded Children v. Pennsylvania (1971) decreed that mentally retarded children should have access to a free public education[15] and (2) Mills v. Board of Education (1972) further declared "the constitutional right of all children, regardless of an exceptional condition or handicap, to a publically supported education."[16]

Federal legislation followed in 1973 with the passage of Section 504 of the Rehabilitation Act, which provided the first national policy for nondiscrimination on the basis of handicap.[17-20] This law was first implemented in 1978 when the US Department of Health, Education and Welfare (HEW) promulgated the regulations. It affects all programs, including school programs that receive federal monies.

In 1975, The Education for All Handicapped Children Act was passed by the US Congress. This law (PL 94-142) mandated that a free and appropriate education be provided for all handicapped children, in essence, it became a civil rights law as related to the education of children with disabilities. Public Law 94-142 dramatically shifted special education away from the medically defined model of the early orthopedic schools.[20] This law was amended in 1986 (PL 99-457) to include services for infants and toddlers and their families.[21]

THE MULTIDISCIPLINARY TEAM

Requirements of Public Law 94-142

The passage of PL 94-142 resulted in fundamental changes in the way children with disabilities were educated in the public schools. Public Law 94-142 and the regulations and comments found in 34 CRF Ch. III (7-1-88 Edition)[22-26] form the legal foundation for education programs for children with disabilities. In turn, the states via state statute and rule making, have developed the means of implementing the federal law. There are variations among states that interested persons can research through contact with the designated state education agency (SEA).

Public Law 94-142 is inclusive. Handicapped children are entitled to a "free appropriate public education which means special education and related services" provided at public expense [300.1(a), 300.4(a–d)].[22] A child cannot be excluded because of the type or severity of handicap. This *zero exclusion* provision requires the SEA and/or local educational agency (LEA) to develop a plan for every child determined to be educationally handicapped. Federal and state laws and regulations provide for agreements between the SEA and/or LEA and other agencies such as residential or private schools, correctional facilities, or other out-of-district arrangements (300.121, 300.348, 300.400).[22,24]

The LEA has an obligation to identify within its area of service the children who are handicapped and to evaluate their need for special education. The evaluation is done by a multidisciplinary team appointed by a school administrator and including at least one teacher or other specialist with knowledge of the area of suspected disability. The team should include a specialist in each area of suspected disability, as the child must be assessed for all suspected disabilities. If a need for physical therapy is suspected, a physical therapist must be on the team. Consequently, a multidisciplinary team can be very large when a number of disabilities are present or suspected.[24-26]

A referral for evaluation can come from a parent or guardian, teachers, therapists, preschool staff, child-find staff, social workers, community medical persons—any person who has reason to suspect a need. Parents must give consent before the evaluation can start.[26] For physical therapy assessment, state requirements must be met.

Definitions

Handicapped children are children who have been determined by a multidisciplinary team process ". . . as being mentally retarded, hard of hearing, deaf, speech impaired, visually handicapped, seriously emotionally disturbed, orthopedically impaired, other health impaired, deaf-blind, multi-handicapped, or as having specific learning disabilities, who because of those impairments need special education and related services" [300.5(a–b)].[22]

"*Special education* means specially designed instruction, at no cost to the parent, to meet the unique needs of a handicapped child, including classroom instruction, instruction in physical education, home instruction, and instruction in hospitals and institutions" [300.14(a–b)(1–3)].[22] Note that the child's need for special education is couched in terms of instructional needs, not in terms of the child's particular disability or handicap.

"*Related services* means transportation and such developmental, corrective, and other supportive services as are required to assist a handicapped child to benefit from special education, and includes speech pathology and audiology, psychological services, physical and occupational therapy, recreation, early identification and assessment of disabilities in children, counseling services, and medical services for diagnostic or evaluation purposes. The term also includes school health services, social work services in schools, and parent counseling and training" (300.13).[22] That is, for a child with a handicap, the need for physical therapy (and other related services) is defined by how the handicap affects participation in the special education program, not, per se, by the presence of a handicap or a need for physical therapy.

Specially designed instruction is generally defined to include a modified curriculum, adaptive equipment, adaptive physical education, and/or environmental modifications that enhance the learning process. Under the law, physical therapy is not specially designed instruction but, instead, a supportive service related to that instruction.[27]

Protections for the child and parents are spelled out in the law with requirements of the LEA related to notices of the referral, meeting times, areas to be assessed, and names of team members. The parent or guardian must give permission for the evaluation to begin and consent to contact relevant sources of information outside the school district. Rules of confidentiality must be observed (34 CRF 300.503–513, 300.561, 300.562, 300.565).[25]

Other protections require that test materials be free of cultural or racial bias. The team members who are assessing, interpreting, and making recommendations must be skilled in their particular areas and use evaluation and assessment instruments that are valid and unbiased. The child should be assessed using his or her first language, with an interpreter provided for the parents if necessary [34 CRF 300.532(a–f)].[25]

Multidisciplinary Team Functions

The multidisciplinary team serves several functions. It determines whether the child has a handicap in one or more of the areas cited by law. If so, the disability must be found to be handicapping in the educational setting. The next step is to determine whether special educational program(s) are necessary for the child to learn. Positive answers to these three questions are necessary before a child can be offered a special educational program and related services. If the standards of being educationally handicapped and in need of special education are not met, the child is not eligible for related services under PL 94-142.[22]

The assessment can include, as appropriate, ". . . evaluations of health, vision, hearing, social and emotional status, general intelligence, academic performance, communicative status, and motor abilities."[24] The team collects information from a variety of sources, including the school, community, medical providers, and family members. Parents are considered prime sources of information and play an important role in all parts of the process. It is the responsibility of the multidisciplinary team to integrate the information from the individual findings of the team members in a way that will facilitate planning the educational program of the child over the next 3 years. This will form the foundation of the individualized education program (IEP), which spells out the specifics of the programming. Decisions cannot be based on single tests, such as IQ tests, or on general information.

An administrator of the LEA reviews the multidisciplinary team findings and reports. After administrative review and the resolution of resultant questions, the parents or guardians are offered the services agreed upon. The offer typically includes the specific site and program in which the student will be served, a listing of other services, and the names of the persons appointed to the initial IEP team. The parents have a right to appeal any of the decisions or findings of the multidisciplinary team or the administrator.[25] If the parents or guardians accept the offer of placement, the administrator appoints the members of the IEP team.

Other Aspects of the Multidisciplinary Team Process

The multidisciplinary team process must be repeated at least every 3 years; it may be repeated more frequently if a change in the student's status suggests a need for different services than are currently being provided or that special education services are no longer necessary (34 CRF 300.534).[25] A multidisciplinary team may be convened when a child is approaching a natural change in the educational program. A common time for reevaluation based on these natural changes is when the child moves from an early childhood program to a kindergarten.

One of the functions of the team is to determine the least restrictive environment (LRE) for a child. It is required that the special education environment be the "least restrictive" possible for the particular child to learn (34 CRF 300.550).[25]

A "specially designed" program can be provided in many settings. The former limitation to special classes in special schools no longer applies; in fact, it is no longer legal. Instruction can be provided with same-age peers in the context of a regular education class, or in a combination of regular education and self-contained classes. For children who require functionally based programming, education can occur in the "natural" setting: at a job site, shopping mall, grocery store, YMCA, bowling alley, or on the city bus.

Physical Therapists as Members of a Multidisciplinary Team

Therapists are named as members of a multidisciplinary team based on numerous indicators, including diagnosis, history of therapy services, or specific mention of motoric factors in the referral relating to functional deficit or program difficulties. Therapists are always included on reevaluation teams if the student has been receiving school-based therapy services as determined by a prior multidisciplinary team.

Prior to PL 94-142, in many states, physical and occupational therapy have been *programs* and, as such, could stand alone in the determination of need or no need for intervention based on a clinical evaluation and assessment. Therapists could follow established clinical modes of determining what, how, and how much therapy and project the degree of anticipated benefit based on traditional medical model standards.

As a provider of an educationally related service, therapists are required to not only determine a clinical need (the presence of a significant motoric difference or deficit), but then to translate that clinical need into functional terms by describing what impact the deficit has on the child's special education program. The therapist develops a program of treatment that either immediately or predictably meets the requirement of "enabling the child to benefit from the special education program." Expected outcomes are stated and measured in functional terms as well as in clinical terms. This approach to the definition of need, the provision of service, and the determination of expected outcomes delineates the major difference between clinically and school-based therapists.

In summary, to receive educational services in a special education program, a child must (1) have a handicap within the meaning of the law, (2) have a handicap that interferes with the ability to learn, and (3) require specially designed instruction to learn. In addition, to receive physical therapy services, the enabling relationship between physical therapy and the special education program must be demonstrated. A case study will provide an example.

Case Study: Laura

Laura is a 10-year-old girl attending her neighborhood school. A multidisciplinary reevaluation is in process to determine the continuation of special education and related services. Laura is diagnosed as having cerebral palsy because of cerebral hypoxia at birth and mental retardation. She is academically delayed 3 to 4 years as compared with other students of her chronologic age. Laura receives speech therapy for her articulation problems and language delays; receptive language is better than her expressive abilities. She also receives occupational and physical therapy to address global delays in fine and gross motor development.

Laura has received direct and consultative physical therapy services since the age of 18 months. The services were initially provided in the home twice weekly and expanded to her preschool setting when she was 3 years old. Until Laura was 8 years old, she was educated in self-contained classrooms, with mainstreaming into music, art, and physical education. During the past 2 years, Laura has been integrated in the regular education classroom for full days with her same-age peers. She receives support in the classroom from her special educational teacher and teacher instructional assistant.

Laura's previous records describe her as having gross motor problems in the following areas: (1) muscle strength, (2) balance, (3) endurance, (4) motor planning, and (5) posture. Her records further indicate that she takes appropriate risks during play situations, is attentive and not overly distractable, and her behavior, while not always compliant, does not interfere with her education.

Laura has generalized hypotonia. Her gross motor development is commensurate with her cognitive level. Laura is ambulatory, with no significant gait deviations. A postural examination in collaboration with the school nurse revealed slight kyphosis, which Laura could correct on request. There was no evidence of scoliosis or other structural orthopedic deformities. Laura does not use any adapted equipment. She wears glasses to correct her farsightedness.

No standardized testing was performed for this reevaluation, although components of the Bruininks-Oseretsky Test of Motor Proficiency were used to informally assess speed, strength, balance, and upper limb dexterity. The results of this testing show that Laura is able to

1. complete the shuttle run (best time) in 11 seconds,
2. broad jump slightly over 3 feet,
3. balance on the "Bruininks" beam (2 inches wide) for 1 to 2 seconds with her preferred leg and heel–toe walk on the same beam for one to two steps,
4. hit the designated wall target three out of five times, throwing a tennis ball overhand, and
5. catch a tennis ball by trapping it against her chest and consistently catch a volleyball in her hands.

Laura performs sit-ups and push-ups in a modified manner. She handwalks 10 feet while being supported at the knees and is able to maintain a bridge with her trunk for 3 to 5 seconds before arm and hip strength give out. Laura can independently step onto a vestibular board and maintain her balance; when balance is perturbed, she occasionally falls, but protects herself by extending her arms and head. Protective extension is also elicited during balance activities (prone and sitting) using a cylindric bolster.

Laura was also assessed using an ecologic approach (i.e., evaluating her gross motor abilities in functional situations in a variety of environments). She has the strength, balance, and motor planning skill to open heavy doors throughout the school. If necessary, Laura will prop her body against a door, holding it open long enough to pass through. She can safely negotiate the stairs inside and outside the school. Her preferred manner of descending is to use the railings, but she will carefully walk down unassisted if the situation dictates. Laura accesses the school playground, as do her peers, by running down a hill. She is cautious on uneven ground, moving slowly and deliberately as necessary. Her risk-taking is especially evident in her outside play style. She swings independently, climbs the various play structures alone, uses the slide, and is generally very active during her recess time. On the playground, it is apparent that Laura has developed general strategies to compensate for her balance and strength deficits.

During the course of the school year, Laura has developed friendships with two students from her regular education class. They often play together at recess, and she is included in group activities. For example, Laura is unable to jump rope, but she is able to hold onto and twirl the rope for her friends and others.

Laura attends the regular physical education (PE) class with her peers. Activities are modified in this class when necessary. Monthly meetings with the PE teacher provided an opportunity to plan for Laura's adaptations. According to her PE teacher, Laura enjoys class and needs minimal redirecting to help her understand certain tasks. Some modifications include resting when fatigued, alternately running and walking laps, and using a 6-inch wide beam instead of the standard 2-inch beam for balance activities. When appropriate, peers are encouraged to assist Laura. Balance and endurance are concerns, but not problems in this environment.

Laura has received direct and consultative physical therapy services for more than 8 years. Her parents are aware of Laura's need for ongoing exercise to promote better posture and overall health/well-being. They have had mixed success with home exercise programs, opting instead for family recreational activities. As time allows, Laura and her family attend a "family swim" night at the neighborhood high school.

Laura's gross motor development, as referenced to her peers, will continue to be delayed. These delays, however, do not prevent her from optimally functioning in her educational environments. It is important to consider that Laura is a risk-taker, that she enjoys physical activities, is not overly distractable, and appears to be developing the friendships that will enhance her activity level. Her PE teacher routinely modifies curriculum and expectations so that Laura participates in the same or similar activities as other students and is challenged to improve her skills.

In 2 years, Laura will attend the middle school that adjoins her elementary school. This environment is familiar to her and to her therapist. The expectation is that Laura's transition will be a smooth one.

The related service of physical therapy is recommended to be discontinued at this time because

1. Laura is making gains in the identified areas of concern (strength, endurance, balance, motor planning) through programming in various regularly occurring classes and activities,
2. Laura is motivated to actively participate in motoric activities in structured and unstructured settings,
3. Laura has learned self-monitoring skills regarding her motoric strengths and limitations, and
4. Laura's family promotes physical activity outside the school setting.

THE INDIVIDUALIZED EDUCATION PROGRAM

The IEP or written statement of the special education program for a student is developed following procedures outlined by federal and state regulations. In essence, it is a plan of service for the student (34 CRF 300, App. C).[26] The IEP team includes parents/guardians and professionals. Professional membership is determined by the findings of the multidisciplinary team, and a representative of each appropriate discipline is included. If possible, and as appropriate, the student is a member of the IEP team (34 CRF 300.345).[24]

An IEP is developed annually and is a joint effort of the team. It addresses areas identified by the multidisciplinary team as in need of special education and related services.

The IEP has several components, including (34 CRF 300.346)[24–26]

1. a statement of current level of educational performance;
2. a statement of annual goals and objectives associated with those goals;
3. a statement of specific educational services and related services to be provided, and who is responsible for their provision;
4. specific objective criteria, intervention strategies, and evaluation or measurement techniques;
5. a statement of time anticipated to be spent in regular education;
6. a statement of degree of restrictiveness of the educational environment for the upcoming time period and the reasoning for selecting that environment rather than one that is less restrictive, including reasons for removal from the regular education classroom if that is the case;
7. a daily schedule; and

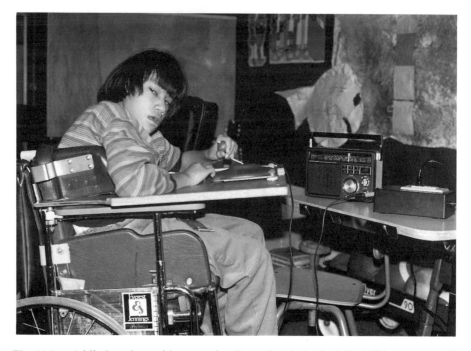

Fig. 11-1. A blind student with severe intellectual and physical disabilities uses a pull-switch to activate a radio. This activity was planned by the IEP team and implemented during a leisure/recreation period. The physical and occupational therapists jointly addressed positioning needs, provided switch adaptations, and instructed others in their use. Once set up, this student can control the radio on her own.

8. a statement of anticipated time of initiation of service and anticipated duration of the service.

As the IEP team designs a plan, the physical therapist will provide an interpretation of the motoric assessment results and describe the therapy interventions that will have an impact on the student's functional motoric capabilities. Specific strategies, treatment techniques, and measurements are a part of this statement. The balance between educational environments is determined as well as how therapists provide service in these settings. If some responsibilities are being "given" to another team member, this person will be identified and a consultation and monitoring plan will be described. For example, an IEP team might identify the use of a switch as a functional motoric goal in the context of a meaningful activity[28] (Fig. 11-1). Figure 11-2 illustrates diagrammatically a switch design that can be used to operate a radio, an electric stapler, or other plug-in devices (not illustrated).

The IEP is a legal document that specifies a plan. Desired outcomes are stated, but the IEP is not a contract that promises the stated outcomes. It is

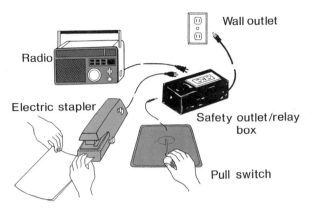

Fig. 11-2. An adapted switch design.

a working document on which the various team members can build or make changes as progress or other changes in status occur (34 CRF 300.349).[24,26]

DELIVERY OF PHYSICAL THERAPY

Types of Service

Public Law 94-142 greatly expanded the types of physical therapy services offered in various educational settings.[29] During the 1980s, states and school districts throughout the country developed policies and procedures describing their approach to the provision of therapy services.[30-33] In 1980, the APTA published an anthology, *Physical Therapy Practice in Educational Environments: Policies, Guidelines, and Background Information*, identifying the types of services physical therapists provide in the schools.[34] Following are synopses of the services described in the 1990 revised edition of this publication.[35]

Screening

Children are surveyed for identification of suspected and previously undetected problems. Written and verbal information is reviewed along with informal observations to determine the need for further assessment. These observations are done in such areas as the playground, gym class, or any of the natural educational settings.

Assessments

An educational related assessment is required in order for a student to receive physical therapy. Eligibility is determined through data collected from observations and testing, which may include formal and informal tests, and is related to the student's educational goals. This information is shared with the multidisciplinary team in the form of a written report.

Program Plan

A therapeutic plan for services is incorporated into the student's IEP and includes statements of long-term goals and short-term objectives.

Intervention (Treatment)

The actual provision of physical therapy services is based on the assessment and approval of the multidisciplinary team. "How to deliver these therapy services" is determined by the therapist and other team members.

Communication

Therapists act as liaisons with various student-related personnel outside the school system. These may include individuals from the medical community (physicians, nurses) as well as other community providers, such as adaptive equipment vendors.

Consultation

Physical therapists are involved in ongoing interactions with parents and school personnel (teachers, teacher assistants, bus drivers, and others) to share general and specific information about a student's physical needs. These interactions can range from simply sharing verbal information regarding a student's disability/handicapping condition to setting up specific therapeutic procedures for teachers and staff to implement on a daily basis. To ensure that these programs are consistent and properly carried out, there are regularly scheduled consultation times.

Education

Besides therapy services for the student, parents and professional staff are educated about a variety of topics (e.g., handicapping conditions, safety issues, and adapted equipment).

Documentation

Physical therapists should be accountable for their services in the educational environment, as they must be in other more traditional "medical" environments: hospitals, nursing homes, and private clinics. This can be achieved through a variety of methods, including establishing a performance data base, recording progress, and writing end-of-year reports.

School-aged children with neurologic dysfunction require a combination of these services. Entry-level as well as experienced medically based pediatric therapists entering the schools are usually familiar with these services, although they initially may lack the skills to decide how their services relate to the student's educational needs. The following are examples of typical dilemmas:

1. Pediatric assessment tools are typically referenced to normal motoric development and do not yield functional performance information.[36]

2. Therapists are trained in direct handling techniques with little or no definitive research to show that neuromotor changes carry over into functional performance.[37,38] Most studies for children with cerebral palsy have measured medically related outcomes (e.g., range of motion [ROM], gross motor milestones, neurologic status) instead of functional outcome changes.

3. Research has not provided definitive answers to the questions of frequency and duration of treatment.[39,40]

4. Consultation is an essential component of school-based physical therapy, although it is not regularly stressed in undergraduate programs.

5. Documentation in the educational environment should be referenced to observable behavioral objectives in a functional context.[41]

Various methods of data collection exist that can assist the therapist in planning for strategies to achieve task-specific objectives and goals.[42] For example, Appendix 11-1 shows an analysis or breakdown of the skills needed to use the playground tire swing (Fig. 11-3). This presents a worksheet or checklist that can be used to assess a student, to develop objectives, and to document progress. Single-subject research designs can provide further documentation of the efficacy of specific treatment strategies.[43,44]

In summary, service delivery decisions are based on the therapist's experience and knowledge in evaluating the needs of each student in collaboration with the parents and other educational staff in light of the school district's policies. Numerous publications are available to provide more information on this important topic.[45–50]

Isolated Versus Integrated Approach

The provision of physical therapy in the educational environment continues to be a topic of much debate and discussion.[42,51] Prior to PL 94-142, therapists generally removed students from their academic programs for assess-

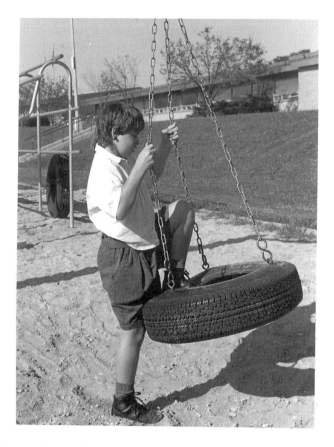

Fig. 11-3.   Student positions body in preparation for climbing onto tire swing.

ments and treatment in the therapy room.[52,53] Although this isolated model of service proved successful for children who had mild handicaps, its efficacy was questionable for students with more severe handicapping conditions. This latter group required more comprehensive educational and therapeutic services. Physical therapists as well as other service providers were forced to reexamine their delivery systems.

An integrated therapy model was initially proposed in 1977 as an alternative to the traditional isolated model of services.[53] In an integrated model, the following are assumed:

1. Assessments should occur in the student's natural environment.
2. Clusters of motor skills are addressed through functional and game activities.
3. Motor skills programs are jointly designed and carried out by teachers,

parents, and therapists. Therapeutic intervention is incorporated throughout the day in a variety of natural settings.

4. Motor skills must be taught or verified as generalizing to the environments in which they naturally occur.

The importance of this model is its recognition that therapy should be viewed within a wide context rather than as short periods of isolated "hands-on" sessions. This concept is illustrated in Figure 11-4, in which a traditional therapy technique is generalized to a playground skill.

Service Modes

Physical therapists in the educational environment provide direct or indirect services. In direct service, the therapist is primarily responsible for the delivery of the intervention. Direct service is hands-on treatment designed to address specific neuromotor problems that have been identified as interfering with the student's education.[35,54] Further implied is an ongoing requirement for professional competence in the use of specific treatment procedures that the therapist cannot release to others. This might include joint mobilization, special handling techniques, or physician-specified exercises for a student following corrective surgery (Fig. 11-5). Treatment principles and programs for children with specific neurologic disabilities are found in the various chapters in this book and will not be further described here.

Direct service can be provided individually (1:1) or to small groups. Grouping may allow the therapist an opportunity to work simultaneously with several students who have similar needs.[54] In settings integrating disabled and nondisabled students, use of groups may facilitate socialization and communication with same-age nondisabled peers by grouping them with a student requiring direct therapy services. The therapist uses an educationally related activity appropriate for all students to promote a therapeutic goal for the individual who requires therapy. The location of this activity may be the therapy room, classroom, gymnasium, playground, or a community site.

Indirect services include monitoring and consultation. These provide a mechanism by which therapists can assist other persons (i.e., teachers, teacher assistants, parents) to carry out programs that have therapeutic benefits for the student.[34,54,55] Indirect services may be defined somewhat differently from one school district to another.

Monitoring involves periodic reviews of a student's physical status or performance ability.[34,54,55] This service style allows a therapist to (1) check for maintenance of achieved skills or educational goals, (2) train and supervise persons providing ongoing therapeutic interventions, and (3) evaluate student changes affecting equipment needs or program modifications. To be effective, monitoring services should be scheduled on a regular basis and occur in the context of the student's educational setting.

Direct and indirect services are not exclusive of one another and are often

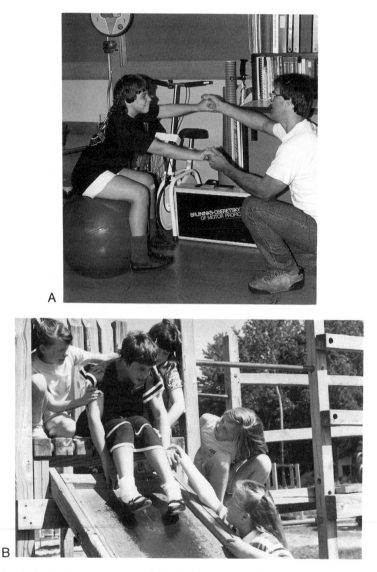

Fig. 11-4. **(A)** Student works on weight-shifting and reaching during direct service in the therapy room. **(B)** The same student uses balance and reaching skills in a functional context. Therapy intervention occurs on the playground as she plays with a group of nondisabled peers.

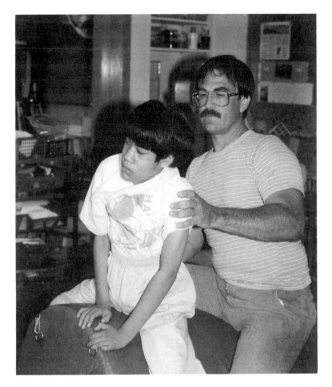

Fig. 11-5. This student has had recent spinal fusion to correct scoliosis. Weight-shifting and balance exercises are being practiced in the therapy room with the physical therapist. Slow progression to resume weight-bearing and assisted walking in other settings is the long-range goal for this student.

carried out concurrently.[34] A student receiving direct therapy usually requires consultation and/or monitoring to ensure that motoric goals are integrated into the various educational programs. Indirect therapy should be designed so that the therapist continues to have regular and ongoing direct interaction with the student. Periodic hands-on contact assures the team that the therapist is up-to-date on the student's status (i.e., motoric, health and safety, positioning/handling, and equipment needs).

Physical therapists in the schools frequently act as consultants, providing a wide array of indirect services. These services may focus on the needs of individual students or be defined as student-related in a broader sense. One style of *consultation* involves making specific recommendations for a single student.[43,54,55] Teachers might suggest the need for adaptive equipment in the classroom or request strategies for working on motoric goals during their instructional times. Figure 11-6 shows a student with severe intellectual and physical disabilities using a standing table in a regular education classroom. The resulting information or recommendations are shared with the appropriate

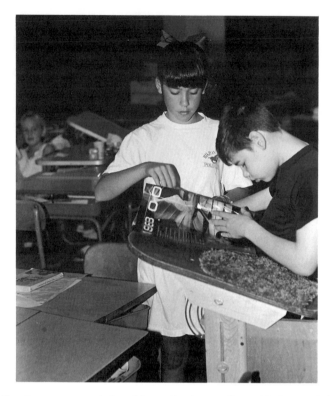

Fig. 11-6. Teachers requested that this student's standing table be used during some of the time he is in the regular education classroom. The teacher's objective is to encourage more social interaction with nondisabled peers. The physical therapy objective for weight-bearing is concurrently being addressed.

personnel having daily contact with the student. The therapist is responsible for providing the equipment or the strategy plan, demonstrating the intervention(s), and periodically reviewing the recommended programming and outcomes. Figure 11-7 shows a blind student with severe intellectual and physical disabilities using a switch during two different functional activities. In both environments, the physical and occupational therapists jointly provided positioning suggestions, initially set up the switch adaptation, and monitored the tasks on a monthly basis.

Consultation is also necessary for the provision of information to the many adults associated with the students.[34,54–56] Information sharing should be both informal and formal through special inservice programs and regularly scheduled team meetings. These programs can educate staff on a variety of topics (e.g., the medical conditions of students with special needs, safe lifting and handling techniques, or recognition of subtle changes in a student's positioning needs and motoric status). On an interpersonal level, inservice programs can provide a forum for adults to exchange ideas and express their concerns. This "give

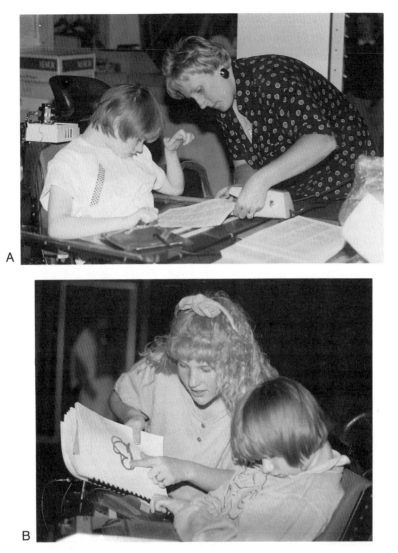

Fig. 11-7. (A) The special education teacher assists the student at a community vocational site. The student is using a pull switch to operate an electric stapler as part of her educational task to staple and file papers. (B) The same student integrated into a regular education leisure reading class. Her educational task is to touch a textured figure in a book. With a verbal cue, she pulls the switch that operates a cassette tape that has a synchronized recorded voice describing the figure. A nondisabled peer volunteered to assist with this task.

and take'' is essential in facilitating the team approach mandated by PL 94-142.[56]

Physical therapists often serve as liaisons between the community and the educational system. They may relay student information to medically oriented personnel, such as physicians, clinic-based therapists, or equipment vendors. Therapists can additionally assist parents and educators by explaining the medical reports on individual students or by accompanying students and parents to clinics.[31] Therapists participate in decision making with community medical personnel, equipment vendors, and architects or contractors. Consultation with caseworkers, parent advocates, and service providers at vocational or recreational sites addresses the student's status in other settings.

Finally, consultation to the school district provides a more general service in which the physical therapist assists in planning for the needs of the system at large. This connotes a service that can be staff- or student-related and of benefit to many. Therapists may be asked to make recommendations for architectural revisions, purchasing special school equipment, and playground safety layout. As a member of a task force, the physical therapist can assist educators in setting up new programs or modifying existing curricula.[31]

Physical therapists are recipients as well as providers of information via consultation. All members of the team have contributions to be made to a successful outcome. Information from the parent is crucial; it gives a view of the child's function and behavior at home and in the community, provides insights regarding motivators and parental expectations, and gives an idea of family priorities. Teacher-provided information is essential to the development and carry through of a related service, and teachers assist the therapist by providing behavioral management information and strategies. Community therapists who treat children (outside of the school system) should be consulted to ensure that their knowledge is incorporated into planning in the educational environment.

Educational Team Models

Public Law 94-142 mandated a team approach to assessment and planning for the student's special educational programming. What was not defined was how to coordinate the various services.[56,57] Two team models of service (multidisciplinary and interdisciplinary) have been described as failing to adequately meet the needs of students with severe handicaps.[51] The multidisciplinary model implies that many disciplines work with a student, but do so in isolation from each other.[57,58] The interdisciplinary approach increases team communication, as professionals meet to plan assessments and discuss findings; however, the actual assessments and resultant intervention provided by each individual discipline may yet occur in isolation from other disciplines.[57,58] These models fail because they are discipline referenced rather than client referenced.[51,59] The student's educational programming does not reflect a collaborative team effort.

The transdisciplinary team model of service has been advocated by numerous investigators[58–61] as the most effective means of integrating educational and therapeutic programming for students with severe handicaps. Many school therapists practice within the general framework of this model, which generally includes the following characteristics:[51,59,61]

1.   Programming must be a joint team effort.
2.   The educational team and parents share their unique expertise with each other.
3.   Assessments relate to the student's functional skills in various environments instead of being referenced only to the discipline performing the assessment.
4.   The responsibilities for education are shared through a "role release" process. Team members are encouraged to release some of their skills to others, so that intervention is continuous and not bound to a single discipline.

An integral component of this model is the program facilitator or manager.[58,60,61] Usually, the teacher is primarily responsible for coordinating the student's overall educational programming. In essence, teachers and their assistants may be providing much of the daily therapy as taught to them by the physical therapist and other personnel (i.e., occupational and speech therapists).

Another model of service with which school therapists may be familiar is actually a combination of the transdisciplinary approach and the integrated therapy model.[62,63] As such, it may represent the ultimate structure in team collaboration. Following the student's assessment, therapists and educators plan and write common goals as a team. The members of each discipline then work to achieve these goals by applying their specific expertise to each problem. Achievement of goals becomes a group responsibility, although each individual must remain accountable for their professional approaches. In this model, instructional strategies are team-designed to take advantage of the student's strengths and accommodate or ameliorate areas of limitation.

Although this model relies on teachers and assistants to integrate daily therapeutic procedures, it is further defined by its flexibility.[63] Direct hands-on interaction with students is encouraged when implemented in contextual educational activities. On occasion, the therapist may be designated as the primary educator, with the teacher and other staff providing consultation. An example of this approach occurs when the educational team decides that "friendship with nondisabled peers" is a goal for a student with disabilities. The team outlines a strategy in which nondisabled students volunteer to participate and adults act as facilitators for potential friendships.[64] The students are encouraged to help plan methods for social interaction. Activities or games are often chosen that involve motor skills, such as soccer/kickball, T ball, or swimming. Because of time constraints on the teacher and the nature of these activities, the therapist might be chosen to direct the weekly program that incorporates motoric objectives within the goal for friendships. Figure 11-8

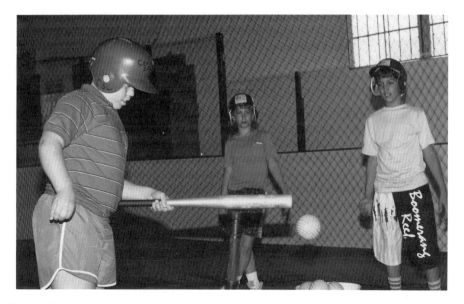

Fig. 11-8. A student with intellectual and physical disabilities, including right hemiplegia, is shown during skilled use of left arm/hand (i.e., hitting a ball off a T). Two students watching are nondisabled classmates who volunteered for a "friendship" program. The physical therapist supervised weekly activities, with assistance from the PE teacher and consultation from other team members.

demonstrates one activity chosen by nondisabled students for this type of educational goal.

Barriers to the Team Approach

Two barriers to the transdisciplinary model are commonly cited in the literature.[65,66] One is related to the training of therapists and educators whose entry level educational programs are vastly different. Their professional belief systems may be at odds and cause problems in establishing program priorities. The medical model of therapeutic intervention dictates an underlying etiology causing a variety of symptoms; once identified, treatment is directed at alleviating the cause. Conversely, educators, with a behavioral background, analyze the student's functional level and direct their intervention to the development of compensatory strategies.

Future physical therapists may not find this barrier to be a major obstacle. Changes in the way physical therapists are educated and the expansion of postuniversity training opportunities both serve to lessen the problems.[67] Current multidisciplinary research in motor control is providing our profession with a new and expanded understanding of human movement. Incorporated in the motor control model is an emphasis on motor skills that have a functional purpose, occur in a behavioral context, and are shaped by specific task demands in natural environments.[68,69] As empiric knowledge expands in this area, we may find that we are more aligned with the concerns of educators than was true in the past. The importance of these emerging theories of motor control was stressed in the recent II STEP conference on this subject and related clinical issues.[70]

Liability has been frequently mentioned as an issue in the context of role-release by therapists of some of their traditional skills.[59,66] How responsible are therapists for potential negligence on the part of nontherapists who are taught to carry out techniques? In reality, this is certainly a concern, but has not become a salient issue. Few cases of liability suits brought against therapists in the school educational environment have been reported,[71] and the authors found no literature on this subject. Therapists should, however, be aware of this potential danger when planning transdisciplinary activities.

Successful Team Strategies

Physical therapists working in a transdisciplinary model can use a variety of strategies for effective service delivery. "Block scheduling" represents one such strategy that allows the flexibility to see one or several students in their different instructional settings. This approach has been described in several recent articles[42,51,63] and will vary depending on the type of student population (i.e., the extent of their individual needs, the therapist's caseload, and the numbers of students with special needs assigned to the same classroom). An example of this kind of scheduling is to set aside half-day blocks for classroom intervention three times a week. The therapist can work with any number of students in the context of their scheduled programming. The remaining 2 days could be planned for individual therapy times. A variation of this approach is to build a "consultation week" into the therapist's monthly schedule. In this model, 1 week each month is designated for indirect service in various settings throughout the educational environment. Block scheduling, however designed, needs to be clearly communicated to the parents and educational personnel because it represents a departure from the traditional locked-in scheduling approach.

Another strategy is to have physical and occupational therapists administratively assigned as members of a team to one or several schools. The additional assignment of a paraprofessional (physical therapist assistant) to this group can define a therapy team within the educational environment.[31]

This model for therapy services has several advantages:

1. It can reduce some of the feeling of isolation long reported in articles about school physical therapy;[72,73] both disciplines have a common background of being trained in the medical environment.

2. Informal communication increases as the two disciplines come into

frequent daily contact. Caseloads are similar for both professionals, providing an opportunity for continual exchange of student information.

3. Many of the daily routines can be implemented by a paraprofessional trained to work closely with both therapists.

4. Teachers often learn to see the student in a holistic manner (i.e., more easily recognizing the interplay between gross and fine motor development as they relate to the individual's learning needs).

Issues that need to be addressed in a therapy team approach include interpersonal concerns, role clarification, and the proper use of a paraprofessional in the educational environment.

PARAPROFESSIONALS

Increasing numbers of physical therapist assistants are being hired by school districts, and can be an extremely valuable addition to the team. Properly used, the physical therapist assistant can enhance the quality of services provided to children.

Wide variation exists among the states in how physical therapist assistants are regulated, in the definition of their scope of practice, and even in whether or not they are recognized as health providers. In some situations, physical therapist assistants are being asked to practice beyond what could be considered ethical. The shortage of therapists certainly increases the chances of this happening, as does the accelerating costs of providing therapy services.

Many basic and fundamental questions must be answered. What is the scope of practice of a physical therapist assistant? Must supervision be on-site or are there circumstances that allow off-site supervision? How frequent should contact with the supervising therapist be? How many assistants can a therapist legitimately supervise before the quality of the delivered service is lost? Many of these questions are fundamental to the profession at large, not just school-based practice.

The following case study demonstrates how a transdisciplinary team, using an integrated therapy model, plans an educational program for a student.

Case Study: James

James is an 8-year-old boy with a diagnosis of cerebral palsy (right spastic hemiplegia) and moderate mental retardation. He is presently integrated 60 percent of the day into a regular second-grade classroom; the remaining time is spent in a "resource room" receiving additional special education that allows close supervision during practice on educational tasks. James uses a one-arm drive wheelchair that he can propel for short distances or maneuver around most obstacles. James is pushed during transitions of long distances or out on the playground. He uses a right ankle/foot orthosis (AFO) and is able to walk 10 to 15 feet with one person providing maximal assistance. Performance is inconsistent and dependent on James' compliance. He assists with transfers into and out of the wheelchair, and has adequate balance to sit at a standard desk or in a regular chair placed close to a table. James uses his right hand primarily as a stabilizer and has good functional use of his left upper extremity.

James' vision and hearing are within functional limits. He responds to verbal cues and communicates by using pictures or line drawings; he also has limited ability to use and respond to sign language. His parents state that he is motivated by looking at magazines or books, likes listening to country and western music, enjoys peer attention, and appears to be interested in watching other children play. James does not like physical activity unless specifically motivated to participate.

James' educational team consists of his special and regular education teachers, the PE teacher, and related services staff: occupational and physical therapists, physical therapist assistant, and speech and language therapist. This group, along with James' parents, have identified the following concerns and environments as being important for James' special education:

Concerns	Environments
Communication	Classroom
Behavior	Resource room
Eating	Hallway
Bathroom/toilet	Art, music, and PE rooms
Mobility	Playground
Socialization	Bathroom
Positioning/handling	Lunchroom
Recreation/leisure	Home

From the list of concerns, the team designed long-term goals that could be integrated into the designated environments. Each discipline was responsible for providing objectives from their area of expertise that could contribute to the success of James' goals.

An example of this planning process follows, and represents one goal for James' IEP:

Goal:

During daily leisure reading times in the classroom, James will choose a book or magazine to look at.

Objectives:

1. Given a verbal cue, James will propel his wheelchair to the book/magazine table 80 percent of the time. (physical therapist)
2. James will independently choose a book 100 percent of the time. (teachers)
3. James will propel himself to the reading table 80 percent of the time. (physical therapist)
4. James will assist in a standing-pivot transfer to the chair 100 percent of the time. (physical therapist)
5. James will ask for assistance by signing "help" if he is unable to turn the pages 60 percent of the time. (occupational and speech and language therapists)
6. James will sign "finish" when book-reading period is over 60 percent of the time. (speech and language therapist and teachers)
7. James will assist in standing and transfering back to his wheelchair 100 percent of the time. (physical therapist)

As noted in the parentheses after each objective, team members remain accountable for their objectives. This educational goal incorporated physical therapist concerns (mobility, positioning, and handling), along with concerns of the teachers and the occupational and speech and language therapists. To initiate this goal, the physical therapist provided consultation services in the classroom. The physical therapist assistant and the teachers and their assistant worked with James to practice transfer techniques. Because the activity was motivating, James was cooperative throughout the task. It was decided that the physical therapist assistant would work with James once a week during the leisure reading period, with carry over otherwise done by the teachers and assistant. The physical therapy direct interaction (monitoring) for this goal was scheduled on a bimonthly basis, with frequent informal communication regarding James' performance status.

Other educational goals can be planned in a similar manner so that James' complete IEP is written as a collaborative team effort reflecting a transdisciplinary and integrated therapy approach to his educational needs.

OTHER ISSUES

Transition to Adult Services

Public Law 94-142 recommends that school districts participate in planning for the transition of students being served in exceptional educational programs to appropriate adult services.[74] In many communities, there is no process for transition from school to adult services, or the process is poorly coordinated, lacks parental involvement, and fails to use a team approach.[75,76] For a variety of reasons, the agencies serving adults are often not available for planning.

Even the number of students leaving the schools and entering adult services may not be communicated to the appropriate adult service funders and providers.

Some districts have formalized the transition process so that team planning occurs in a comprehensive manner. In the Madison (Wisconsin) Metropolitan School District, an individual transition plan (ITP) process was developed for students served by the program for students with mental retardation.[77] The process addresses predictable post-high school needs with the student, parents or guardians, school staff, and adult service agencies. For the past several years, the goal of teachers of students with mental retardation is to have the graduating students trained and working in a stable job position by the end of the last year in school. The need to consider and plan for other components of adult living has also become increasingly apparent.

Development of the ITP for a student is formally initiated 3 years before the student is expected to exit from the school system. Parents and students are asked to develop a vision of what is wanted and necessary for adult living at the time of graduation 3 years in the future. Included in the planning are questions related to job development, living arrangement, financial needs, predictable medical needs, recreation/leisure needs, and further educational planning. The necessary tasks to achieve the desired goals are then identified and a timetable outlining the sequence and responsible persons is set. This is carried out in the context of the IEP meetings over the last 3 years in school and, in a very real sense, controls the content of the IEPs.

Therapists have a crucial role in this planning. Possible considerations in a student's ITP for which physical therapists and/or occupational therapists are primary sources of information or have a performance responsibility include the following:

1. Does the student have a need for continuing therapy?

This is a common question triggered by the knowledge that a student may be on a therapy case load up until graduation, particularly if there is a lack of understanding or a misunderstanding regarding the difference between the clinical service of physical therapy and the educationally related service of physical therapy. It is the responsibility of the physical therapist to define that difference and make recommendations for continued direct service if that is needed or to define what consultation services might be necessary. A common need for consultative or monitoring service is in the area of training caretakers in correct positioning, handling, and lifting techniques and in range of motion home programs with appropriate follow-up monitoring.

In Madison, the adult service agencies have asked that the arrangements for ongoing therapy be in place at the time of graduation to prevent an interruption in service during the transition time. It is not the therapist's responsibility to take the lead in making those arrangements; that is the responsibility of the parent or guardian. However, it is the responsibility of the therapist to convey the need to the parent or guardian, who may then ask for advice and information about possible providers and modes of payment.

2. What degree of physical accessibility is required?

Specific information is provided regarding turning radii for wheelchair access, and the need for ramps, door openers, and access to outdoor amenities (parking lots, patios, trash receptacles). Specific considerations for kitchen and bathroom setups, lifts, and other building adaptations are noted.

3. Will the student have a need for lift-equipped specialized transportation facilities?

4. Are the student's independent mobility skills (which may have been adequate for the school program) sufficient for the larger community environment? Is this a consideration when planning for jobs or recreation/leisure options? What about the student's endurance and sitting tolerance? What are any successfully used strategies to maintain or increase tolerance?

5. What are the needs for equipment maintenance?

Consideration must be given to the student's knowledge and accessibility to equipment vendors who can provide needed repairs.

6. What are the student's skills in medical self-management?

For example, has the student had practice and opportunity to independently contact and make arrangements with community providers for wheelchair maintenance? Is the student able to reliably report pain or discomfort? Is the student able to direct another in the "how's" of providing necessary assistance?

7. Is the student involved in specific fitness programs? Are the programs available in community facilities? Are there restrictions that should be observed that go beyond general guidelines for such programs? If the student requires a specially designed program, is that information available in written form or on audio or video tape for continued future use by the student? How can a specially designed program be monitored and changed if needed?

The following case study is an example of how the physical therapist participates in the ITP process.

Case Study: Betty

Betty is a young woman, aged 20 years, who lives with her parents. Betty and her parents have decided that she should move from the family home to another living arrangement in the community. They would like to have Betty live in an apartment with a roommate and a live-in attendant. Betty is physically disabled and mentally retarded.

Betty has attended public schools since the age of 3 years. Since enrollment in public school, she has received direct, monitoring, and consultative physical and occupational therapy. Recent physical therapy objectives have included maintenance of range of motion, improvement of head control, and improvement of the ability to relax and initiate movement from a relaxed state. Occupational therapy goals have related to improvement of feeding abilities, improvement of ability to interact within the environment, and improvement of partial participation in activities of daily living. Indirect goals have included monitoring of orthopedic status, monitoring of equipment, selection of a new wheelchair with adaptations, and consultation with school and institution staff. These objectives have related to academic goals in the areas of vocational training, development of domestic skills (personal and home-related skills), recreational and leisure time skills and interests, and development of a capability to function in the community.

The county has a range of programs available: an evaluation of Betty must determine her eligibility and her needs if eligible for services. Factors considered include issues of least restrictive environment, health and medical issues, and cost issues.

For Betty, the decision has been made that she is a candidate for community living. She is healthy and medically stable; she does not require the degree of structure that would be provided by an institution (the institution is more restrictive than she needs). The questions of the cost of supporting her in the community must be answered. An important component of the cost question has to do with the number of caretakers needed at the same time. Does she need one or two persons to lift, bathe, and otherwise provide physical care? What level of therapy services will she require?

Betty has a diagnosis of cerebral palsy (mixed athetoid and spastic) and moderate to severe retardation. She is a dependent wheelchair user. Until a year ago, she used a Mulholland chair, which she had outgrown, thus limiting her ability to actively move her right arm at the shoulder and interfering with her visual field. Her new seating system has numerous modifications, but is less restrictive. Joint ROM motion is mildly to moderately limited at most joints and has been maintained for several years. Betty has learned to relax during transfers, avoiding an extensor thrust that previously contributed to difficulty in transfers and correct positioning and was a safety hazard for herself and those lifting her. She has also learned to maintain relaxation in her right arm to keep her forearm and hand on her wheelchair tray in position to access a switch that activates various pieces of equipment.

Betty's new chair is equipped with extensive modifications for support of her head, trunk, hips, legs, and feet. She does not speak, but is skilled at signaling via facial expression. She is dependent on two-person lifts for transfers to and from her chair. She is dependent and cooperative for all personal care and for feeding. She is diapered, but uses a commode for bowel movements. She is bathed on a bed.

The county has several questions as the IEP and ITP for the last year in school are being developed, questions relating to Betty's needs if she should move away from her parents. These are

1.   Can Betty be successfully transferred by one person from chair to bed and/or commode using a mechanical lifting device? The answer is crucial when considering the cost of providing caretaker services outside the institution.

2. Can Betty be bathed in a tub or shower? The answer will have an impact of the availability of alternative living sites.

3. Will Betty have ongoing therapy needs after she leaves school? The answer raises cost and service availability concerns.

4. What other considerations must be planned for?

Along with the teacher, the school-based therapist and a community-based therapist developed the following plan to provide the answers to the county's questions:

1. The use of a Hoyer lift will be evaluated at school as part of the daily routine of lifting. The end product will be a decision as to the practicality of use and a protocol that can be used by future caretakers. Betty will become accustomed to being lifted with the Hoyer rather than a two-person lift.

2. During a home visit, the community-based therapist will evaluate the possibility of one-person care for bathing and shower–chair transfers.

3. The therapist, with the parents and physician, will come to a joint decision on the question of ongoing therapy. The major concerns relate to ongoing monitoring of orthopedic status and the need for routine range of motion exercises. If the caretaker is to be responsible for the range of motion exercise program, he or she will require training with periodic monitoring.

4. Betty's accessibility requirements will be defined for the selected housing relating to amount and arrangement of space, type of bathroom layout, and access to the outside. Also identified is a need for specialized transportation and for access to repair services. The county case manager will evaluate local availability of needed services.

Third-Party Payers

School districts are serving more and more students with very serious health care needs. As costs of meeting those needs continue to rise, the districts are looking for ways to help meet their obligations to the students.[78] Recently, they have initiated use of Medicaid (also known as Title XIX) or other third-party payer funds to pay in part for school-based physical therapy services (and occupational therapy, nursing, audiology, and speech and language services).

Some legislative activity and court decisions relative to this funding approach have occurred. The fact that the school districts are obligated to provide a free and appropriate public education does not cancel the responsibility of other agencies to meet their valid obligations. In 1988, the Supreme Court ruled that Medicaid could be used for these services. Also in 1988, Congress passed the Medicare Catastrophic Coverage Act, which provides that state Medicaid programs cannot refuse payment for a service just because it was contained in a student's IEP or in an individualized family service plan as required in PL 99-457.[79–81]

Billing Medicaid or other insurers for services is not a simple process. Families must voluntarily agree to give the school administration the necessary permissions and information. Provider numbers must be obtained for those giving the service. The school district is responsible for any copayments. Caps (limits on the amount of service found in some insurance contracts) cannot be considered when determining the service plan for a student. For insurances other than Medicaid, the use of the policy cannot result in an increase in the premium cost of the insurance. Since Medicaid is the last payer if an individual also has private insurance, the private insurers must also be billed for the service. Decisions are still being made as to how receiving third-party payments will affect the categoric state aids that now, in combination with local district monies, pay for special education costs.[78]

The introduction of third-party payers as a means of funding therapy will do more than simply alter the source of the money. Therapists will become involved in another type of documentation and justification for the provision of services. Districts will have to develop enabling mechanisms. Many therapy services provided to enhance educational opportunities for a student will not meet the medically based criteria for service in third-party payment regulations. On the other hand, it may provide a way to allow in-school clinical service in the difficult situation when a child is clearly in need of therapy, but is not eligible for related services because of not being handicapped according to educational definitions.

SUMMARY

As the laws and rules governing the education of handicapped children are implemented, the manner in which physical therapists provide service to children in schools has changed substantially. It is essential that therapists look beyond the narrowly defined scope of practice, with its emphasis on normal movement patterns and motor development, to a larger focus on the improvement of function.[82,83] Unlike medically based therapists, school therapists have the opportunity to work with children in their "real" world. The school therapist has the further opportunity to work closely with families and other people of importance in the child's daily life. Our profession has long recognized and is beginning to study the child's relationships to family, school, and community as they affect overall development.[82,83] It is essential that a child feel competent. It is equally important to assist a family and others to see the child as competent. Therapists can enable this process by using their knowledge to enhance the child's abilities. This may well be more important than the traditional approach of primarily working to remediate disabilities.[82,83]

REFERENCES

1. Martin KD (ed): Physical Therapy Practice in Educational Environments: Policies and Guidelines. American Physical Therapy Association, Alexandria, VA, 1990
2. Parks JL: The crippled child. Phys Ther Rev 15:230, 1935

3. Vacha VB: History of the development of special schools and classes for crippled children in Chicago. Phys Ther Rev 13:21, 1933
4. Sever JW: Physical therapy in schools for crippled children. Phys Ther Rev 18:298, 1938
5. Gantzer AV: Physical therapy in schools for crippled children. Phys Ther Rev 28:14, 1948
6. Mulcahey A: Detroit schools for crippled children. Phys Ther Rev 16:63, 1936
7. Ingram ML: The program of Wisconsin's crippled children's division. Phys Ther Rev 15:223, 1935
8. Beard G: A review of the first forty years in terms of education, practice and research. Phys Ther Rev 41:843, 1961
9. Elson M: Editorial: the crippled child. Phys Ther Rev 16:246, 1936
10. A visit to the Spalding. Phys Ther Rev 10:311, 1930
11. Lison ML: Orthopedic schools. Phys Ther Rev 10:444, 1930
12. Hilleboe HE, Harrison ER: Minnesota's services for crippled children. Phys Ther Rev 17:16, 1937
13. Ingram ML: Recent expansion in Wisconsin's program for care and education of crippled children. Phys Ther Rev 17:21, 1937
14. Hood RC: Social security for crippled children in the United States. Phys Ther Rev 16:149, 1936
15. Schipper W: Financial and administrative considerations. J Sch Health 50:288, 1980
16. Weintraub FJ, Abeson A, Ballard J et al (eds): p. 9. Public Policy and the Education of Exceptional Children. The Council for Exceptional Children, Reston, VA, 1976
17. Rehabilitation Act of 1973. PL 93-112, Section 504, 1973
18. Rehabilitation Act Amendments of 1974, PL 93-516, Section III(a), 1974
19. US Department of Health, Education, and Welfare: Nondiscrimination on the basis of handicap in programs and activities receiving or benefiting from federal financial assistance. Fed Regis 45:22676, 1977
20. Education of All Handicapped Children Act of 1975, PL 94-142, 1975
21. Education of the Handicapped Act Amendments of 1986, PL 99-457, 1986
22. Title 34 CRF Ch. III (7-1-88 Ed.): Education Subpart A: General (Purpose, Applicability, and General Provisions Regulations), 1988
23. Title 34 CRF Ch. III (7-1-88 Ed.): Subpart B: State Annual Program Plans and Local Application (Public Participation), 1988
24. Title 34 CRF Ch. III (7-1-88 Ed.): Subpart C: Services, 1988
25. Title 34 CRF Ch. III (7-1-88 Ed.): Subpart E: Procedural Safeguards Due Process Procedures for Parents and Children, 1988
26. Title 34 CRF App. C: Notice of Interpretation, 1988
27. Rourk JD, Andrews J, Dunn W et al: p. 6. Guidelines for Occupational Therapy Services in School Systems. American Occupational Therapy Association, Rockville, MD, 1987
28. York J, Nietupski J, Hamre-Nietupski S: A decision-making process for using microswitches. Journal of the Association for the Severely Handicapped 10:214, 1985
29. Mullins J: New challenges for physical therapy in educational settings. Phys Ther 61:496, 1981
30. Gavin SE, Graff JL: Waukesha Delivery Model: Providing Occupational/Physical Therapy Services to Special Education Students. Wisconsin Department of Public Instruction, Madison, WI, 1982
31. Falconer A, Hanson M, Messina R et al: Occupational and Physical Therapy in

the Public Schools: Philosophy and Service Delivery Concepts. Madison Metropolitan School District, Madison, WI, 1982

32. Lindsey D, O'Neal J, Haas K et al: Physical therapy services in North Carolina's schools. Clin Man Phys Ther 4(6):40, 1984

33. Martin KD: Current status of physical therapists in school settings. Totline 14(3):18, 1988

34. Physical Therapy Practice in Educational Environments: Policies, Guidelines, and Background Information. American Physical Therapy Association, Alexandria, VA, 1980

35. Martin KD (ed): p. 3.2. Physical Therapy Practice in Educational Environments: Policies and Guidelines, American Physical Therapy Association, Alexandria, VA, 1990

36. Campbell PH, McInerney WF, Cooper MA: Therapeutic programming for students with severe handicaps. Am J Occup Ther 38:594, 1984

37. Roberts PL: Effectiveness outcomes of physical therapy in schools. Totline 14(3):31, 1988

38. Harris SR, Atwater SW, Crowe TK: Accepted and controversial neuromotor therapies for infants at high risk for cerebral palsy. J Perinatol 8:3, 1988

39. Jenkins JR, Sells CJ, Brady D et al: Effects of developmental therapy on motor impaired children. Phys Occup Ther Pediatr 2:4, 1982

40. Jenkins JR, Sells CJ: Physical and occupational therapy: effects related to treatment, frequency, and motor delay. J Learn Disabil 17(2):89, 1984

41. O'Neill D, Harris SR: Developing goals and objectives for handicapped children. Phys Ther 62:295, 1982

42. Rainforth B, York J: Integrating related services in community instruction. Journal of the Association for the Severely Handicapped 12:190, 1987

43. Ottenbacher K, York J: Strategies for evaluating clinical change: implications for practice and research. Am J Occup Ther 38:647, 1984

44. Harris SR: Research techniques for the clinician. p. 117. In Connolly B, Montgomery PC (eds): Therapeutic Exercise in Developmental Disabilities. Chattanooga Corporation, Chattanooga, TN, 1987

45. Atwater SW, McEwen IR, McMillan J: Assessment of the reliability of pediatric screening: a tool for occupational or physical therapists. Phys Ther 62:1265, 1982

46. Sommerfeld D, Fraser BA, Hensinger RN et al: Evaluation of physical therapy service for mentally impaired students with cerebral palsy. Phys Ther 61:338, 1981

47. Martin JE, Epstein LH: Evaluating treatment effectiveness in physical therapy: single subject designs. Phys Ther 56:285, 1976

48. Rosenbaum PL, Russell DJ, Cadman DT et al: Issues in measuring change in motor function in children with cerebral palsy: a special communication. Phys Ther 70:125, 1990

49. Giangreco MF: Effects of integrated therapy: a pilot study. Journal of the Association for the Severely Handicapped 11(3):205, 1986

50. Asher IE: An Annotated Index of Occupational Therapy Evaluation Tools. America Occupational Therapy Association, Rockville, MD, 1989

51. Giangreco MF, York J, Rainforth B: Providing related services to learners with severe handicaps in educational settings: pursuing the least restrictive option. Pediatr Phys Ther 1:55, 1989

52. Lins J: New challenges for physical therapy practitioners in educational settings. Phys Ther 61:496, 1981

53. Sternat J, Messina R, Nietupski J et al: Occupational and physical therapy services for severely handicapped students: toward a naturalized public school service delivery model. p. 263. In Sontag E, Smith J, Certo N (eds): Educational Programming for the Severely and Profoundly Handicapped. Council for Exceptional Children— Division of Mental Retardation, Reston, VA, 1977

54. Tada WL, Harris SR: Physical therapy in the educational environment. p. 105. In Connolly BH, Montgomery PC (eds): Therapeutic Exercise in Developmental Disabilities. Chattanooga Corporation, Chattanooga, TN, 1987

55. Effgen S: Physical therapy in the schools. p. 287. In Tecklin J (ed): Pediatric Physical Therapy. JB Lippincott, Philadelphia, 1990

56. Hardy DD, Roberts PL: The educational needs assessment on physical therapy for special educators: enhancing in-service programming and physical therapy services in public schools. Pediatr Phys Ther 1:109, 1989

57. Sears CJ: The transdisciplinary approach: a process for compliance with public law 94-142. Journal of the Association of the Severely Handicapped 6:248, 1981

58. Wolery M, Dyk L: Arena assessment: description and preliminary social validity data. Journal of the Association for the Severely Handicapped 9:231, 1984

59. Giangreco MF: Delivery of therapeutic services in special education programs for learners with severe handicaps. Phys Occup Ther Pediatr 6(2):5, 1986

60. Sparling JW: The transdisciplinary approach with the developmentally delayed child. Phys Occup Ther Pediatr 1(2):3, 1980

61. Lyon S, Lyon G: Team functioning and staff development: a role release approach to providing integrated educational services for severely handicapped students. Journal of the Association for the Severely Handicapped 5:250, 1980

62. Campbell PH: The integrated programming team: an approach for coordinating professionals of various disciplines in programs for students with severe and multiple handicaps. Journal of the Association for the Severely Handicapped 12:107, 1987

63. York J, Rainforth B, Giangreco MF: Transdisciplinary teamwork and integrated therapy: clarifying the misconceptions. Pediatr Phys Ther 2:73, 1990

64. Forest M, Lusthaus E: Promoting educational equality for all students. p. 43. In Stainback S, Stainback W, Forest M (eds): Educating All Students in the Mainstream of Regular Education. Paul H Brookes Publishing, Baltimore, MD 1989

65. Geiger WL, Bradley RH, Rock SL et al: Commentary on Giangreco MF: Delivery of therapeutic services in special education programs for learners with severe handicaps. Phys Occup Ther Pediatr 6(2):5, 1986

66. Ottenbacher K: Transdisciplinary service delivery in school environments: some limitations. Phys Occup Ther Pediatr 3(4):9, 1983

67. McLaurin S: Preparation of physical therapists for employment in public schools. Phys Ther 64:674, 1984

68. Gordon J: Assumptions underlying physical therapy intervention: theoretical and historical perspectives. p. 1. In Carr JH, Shepherd RB, Gordon J et al (eds): Movement Science: Foundations for Physical Therapy in Rehabilitation. Aspen Publishers, Rockville, MD, 1987

69. Harris SR: Functional abilities in context. In Lister MJ (ed): Contemporary Concepts in Management of Motor Control Problems. Williams & Wilkins, Baltimore (In press)

70. Lister MJ (ed): Contemporary Concepts in Management of Motor Control Problems. Williams & Wilkins, Baltimore (In press)

71. Representative: Professional Relations Department. American Physical Therapy Association, Alexandria, VA, 1990
72. Peacock IW: Physical therapy in the public schools. JAPTA 42:172, 1962
73. Waddell JF: The physical therapist in the school. Phys Ther Rev 37:744, 1957
74. Education of the Handicapped Act Amendments of 1986, PL 99-457, Sect. 626(a), 1986
75. The Education of Students With Disabilities: Where Do We Stand? National Council on Disability, Washington, DC, 1990
76. Stowitschek JJ, Kelso CA: Are we in danger of making the same mistakes with ITPs as were made with IEPs? CDEI 12(2):139, 1989
77. Transition From School to Post School Services: Process and Plan. Madison Metropolitan School District, Madison, WI, 1990
78. Exceptional education information update: third party payment for certain related services: bull. no. 90.4. Wisconsin Department of Public Instruction, Division for Handicapped Children and Pupil Services, Madison, WI, 1990
79. Title V of the Social Security Act: Maternal and Child Health. 20 USC 11413(e)
80. Title XIX of the Social Security Act: Medical. 20 USC 11413(e)
81. Medicare Catastrophic Coverage Act of 1988, PL100-360, 1988
82. Harris SR: Efficacy of physical therapy in promoting family functioning and functional independence for children with cerebral palsy. Pediatr Phys Ther 2:160, 1990
83. Proceedings of the consensus conference on the efficacy of physical therapy in the management of cerebral palsy: consensus statements. Pediatr Phys Ther 2:175, 1990

APPENDIX 11-1. Functional Playskill Analysis:
Tire Swing

Name_____ Date_____

Birthdate_____ Evaluator_____

Key:
5—Independent
4—Indirect verbal cue/problem-solving question: "What do you need to do?"
3—Verbal cue statement: "You need to do _____."
2—Prompt: needs slight assistance
1—Prime: needs maximal assistance
0—Does not attempt

_____Positions body in preparation for climbing
_____Holds chains and lifts leg to climb
_____Sits on tire holding chains
  _____Maintains sitting balance
  _____Maintains sitting balance when pushed one or two times
  _____Maintains sitting balance when pushed repeatedly (swinging)
  _____Swings on own
  _____Swings with a partner

_____Stands up on tire swing holding chains
  _____Maintains standing balance
  _____Maintains standing balance when pushed one or two times
  _____Maintains standing balance when pushed repeatedly (swinging)
  _____Swings on own
  _____Swings with partner

_____Sits back down on swing holding chains
_____Stops swing with feet
_____Climbs off swing

Comments: Is activity motivating? Does behavior interfere? Will student play
with peers? What is quality of movement? Other?

12 | Family-Focused Early Intervention

Thubi H. A. Kolobe

The family is the most effective and economic system for fostering and sustaining the development of the child, and there is evidence that involvement of the child's family members as active participants is critical to the success of any intervention program.[1] This chapter will provide a historic and contemporary overview of the role of the family in early intervention, new concepts of family-focused intervention, and the role of the physical therapist.

HISTORICAL OVERVIEW

Practice and research in the area of parent involvement in the intervention of children with disabilities in the 1970s reflected a conceptual framework that regarded parents as valuable and capable resources. During the late 1970s, awareness of the impact of the quality of parent–child interaction on the child's development expanded the roles of professionals providing intervention services for children. Expanded roles included teaching parents developmental principles and specific therapy activities for their children. During the 1980s, environmental factors, which include a variety of social systems, became recognized as having a significant impact on the child's development and family adjustment. This comprehensive view of the child has suggested a shift in focus and theoretic perspectives on parent involvement in early intervention of infants and young children with disabilities. The shift in focus involves enhancing the ability of the caregiving environment to better meet the needs of the child. The passage of the Education of the Handicapped Amendment Act of 1986 (Public Law [PL] 99-457) also reflected this perspective.

Rationale for Family-Focused Intervention

The shift toward family-focused intervention and the increased emphasis on families is attributable to recognition of several factors and findings about children with disabilities and their families, as discussed below.

The Transactional Model of Development

The family and environment have a major impact on the child's development.[2-5] Infants born prematurely without biologic complications have been observed to develop severe social and cognitive deficits later in life when they grow up in socioeconomically disadvantaged environments.[4] Sameroff and Chandler[4] presented a new perspective, the transactional model of development, which emphasizes the active role of the child interacting with the environment. The family and its resources affect the child, and the child affects the family dynamics; hence, there is continual interplay between the child and the environment. Research also indicates that the characteristics of the child's caregiving context, rather than specific characteristics of the child, best predict a broad range of developmental outcomes.[6] Bronfenbrenner's view of the family as one system embedded within a larger ecologic framework of social systems[1] complements the transactional model and emphasizes the significant contribution of the child's caregiving environment to his or her development. Within the transactional model context, the environment is crucial to the child's ultimate development.

Family Systems Theory

Systems theory views the interaction patterns among the child, parents, and environment as dynamic and circular, as opposed to linear.[7-9] The family systems approach emphasizes the importance of interactions among various components of the family system: the child influences the parents, the parents influence one another and the child—the child is linked to the family system.[9] Factors such as relationships among members of the family, resources available to the family, cultural background, and the family's life cycle play an important role in shaping transactional patterns of interactions. The family systems approach emphasizes that (1) both the child and family dyads should be viewed within their environmental context, (2) each family is unique, and (3) families undergo changes that affect all members. Within the last decade, the systems perspective in family theory and family therapy has further advanced the transactional model and family systems approach for early intervention.[10,11]

Outcome Measures of Early Intervention

An increasing number of early intervention studies that have focused on the child and family reported favorable outcomes.[12-17] A meta-analysis of 30 studies of early intervention conducted by Shonkoff and Hauser-Cram[15] revealed that those programs that adopted a joint focus on the child and the family were the most effective in achieving their goals. The analysis also suggested that parent participation might have a greater impact on child outcomes for children younger than 3 years of age who had disabilities compared with children over 5 years of age whose developmental vulnerability was defined by either environment or biology. Favorable outcomes were reported, mostly in areas such as parent–child interaction, cognitive and social development, parental compliance, and family coping skills.

Increasing Parental Involvement

Parental recognition of the need for early intervention services and advocacy by parents on behalf of their families has increased over the last decade.[18–21] Parents generally are becoming more knowledgeable consumers of services for their children and about the dimensions of services they and their children require.[22] Families have also played a major role in formulating public policy to benefit their family members with disabilities by influencing legislative and administrative action.[23] This has been evidenced by parents' input into the formulation of the Education of the Handicapped Children Act (PL 94-142) and PL-99-457, which expanded parents' involvement to virtually all aspects of early intervention with their infants and toddlers.

Professionals' Recommendations of Parent Participation

Professionals working with infants and toddlers with handicaps have expressed the need to extend the focus of intervention beyond the infant.[24–26] These professionals stressed that parent participation in therapy is a crucial variable in increasing the likelihood of obtaining improved performances in children with physical handicaps.

Public Law 99-457 Mandate

The recent laws passed to assist children with disabilities (PL 94-142 and PL 99-457) have mandated the family's participation in program planning. Public Law 99-457 emphasizes the essential role of families in facilitating development of their infants and toddlers with handicaps; it mandates assessment of the family's strengths and needs and formulation of the Individualized Family Service Plan (IFSP).[27] This law contains numerous provisions designed to increase family involvement in early intervention services, including membership on each State Interagency Coordinating Council.

Implications of Public Law 99-457. Public Law 99-457 shifts the emphasis of early intervention from teaching the family to change the child toward adapting the environment to increase the likelihood that the family will be able to meet the child's special needs. The family is viewed as an important target of intervention in its own right.[22] Because of the comprehensive nature of the services, a multidisciplinary approach to service provision is recommended. The law also provides guidelines regarding primary developmental services that should be provided: audiology; case management services; family training, counseling, and home visits; health services; nursing; nutrition; occupational therapy; physical therapy; psychological services; social work; transportation; special education; and speech therapy. Physical therapy is considered one of the primary developmental services under PL 99-457. This implies that:

1. physical therapy is not considered a related service supporting special education, as is the case under PL 94-142, and
2. physical therapists can be expected to be active participants in all three general roles listed under the law for provision of services.

Listed in the final rules and regulations regarding PL 99-457 are three general roles to be performed by the primary service providers (Fig. 12-1). Because of the commonality of the roles, a degree of overlap among service providers can be expected. The first two roles have been implemented since the enactment of PL 91-230, The Education of the Handicapped Act (EHA), particularly after 1975, when Part B of EHA, commonly known as PL 94-142, was enacted (see Ch. 11). The third role represents the newest and most far-reaching provision for services to infants and toddlers with disability and their families.

DIFFERENCES BETWEEN CHILD- AND FAMILY-FOCUSED INTERVENTION

Therapists need to be aware that there is no clear division between child- and family-focused intervention. It is conceptually and practically difficult to design intervention targeted exclusively at either parents or their children. The transactional and family systems models imply that there are circumstances in which interventions directed toward the child may result in changes in the parents.[5] There are instances in which interventions directed toward altering the parents' perceptions may result in better caregiving practices.[28,29] An example used to illustrate direct child-focused intervention is feeding problems in newborn premature infants. The premise is that improvement in the infant's feeding will result in more optimal caregiving by the parents. Most children, however, present with multiple problems that may require different types of services. For example, the child's cognitive limitations may interfere with the ability to use movement or language effectively, and vice versa. Parents sometimes may be more able to meet the early educational needs of the child (e.g., infant stimulation with age-appropriate toys), but have difficulty in meeting therapeutic needs (e.g., teaching the child activities to improve balance in sit-

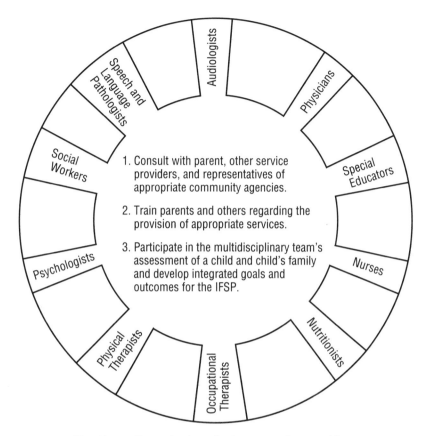

Fig. 12-1. General roles of primary service providers.

ting). In other instances, a child who has mild handicaps may live in a non-stimulating restricted environment, or working parents may have child-care problems. Management of such children must be expanded to include the family if it is to be effective.

In essence, family-focused intervention is an expansion of child-focused intervention, and they are not mutually exclusive. In child-focused intervention, treatment activities are designed for the child while the parent's role is peripheral. Parents may either be used as cotherapists or may assume a passive role, and the outcomes of child-focused intervention are based only on child characteristics. In family-focused intervention, treatment programs are designed for either the family or the child, or for both conjointly.[22] Individual families are either participants in the service provision or are consumers of the services;[23] Table 12-1 depicts levels of family involvement in intervention. The

Table 12-1. Hierarchial Dimensions of Family Involvement in Early Intervention: Family and Interventionist Roles

Level	Dimensions of Involvement	Family Role	Interventionist Role
0	Elective noninvolvement	Rejects available services	Informs and offers available services
I	Passive involvement	Acknowledges but does not use services	Monitors and advises families
II	Consumer involvement	Consumer of child-related services	Provider or broker of child-related services
III	Involvement focusing on informational and skill needs	Information seeking; acquiring teaching and management skills	Consultant and teacher roles in information sharing
IV	Personal involvement to secure or extend personal or social support	Seeking support to build or strengthen formal or informal recourses	Advocacy and relationship building
V	Behavioral involvement to define and deal with reality burdens	Partnership to identify, prioritize, and implement intervention	Goal setting to develop interventions
VI	Psychological involvement to define and deal with value conflicts	Client role in seeking psychological change at family or personal level	Therapist or counselor role to help with psychological or existential issues

(Adapted from Simeonsson and Bailey,[22] with permission.)

outcomes of family-focused intervention are based on change in both family and child variables.

For physical therapists, the major distinction between child- and family-focused intervention is in family assessment and strategies for intervention. Unlike child-focused therapy, in family-focused intervention the physical therapist must include family assessment and interview information in addition to the child's evaluation findings when planning and implementing treatment. If information on the family's strengths and needs is not available, the therapist has the responsibility to solicit it from the parents. Therapy goals should be geared toward enabling the parents and the immediate environment to enhance the child's development, not vice versa. Consequently, there will be times when working with the parents will be more beneficial to the family than hands-on therapy with the child. Similarly, adjustments in the frequency and duration of therapy sessions should reflect the extent to which the family is able to meet the needs of the child.

The overall assumption of family-focused intervention is based on the systems and ecologic view of family functioning and the child's needs. An assumption underlying family-focused intervention is that intervention strategies can be structured in such a way that the interaction or transaction among the child, the child's caregivers, and the caregiving environment are enhanced,[5,29,30] thus maximizing the functional potential of infants and toddlers with disabilities.

Several factors appear to be crucial to the success of family-focused intervention:

1. understanding of families and family dynamics,
2. working knowledge of families of infants and toddlers with disabilities;
3. awareness of methods of assessing families' strengths and needs;
4. ability to effectively communicate with families with diverse cultural backgrounds and with members of other disciplines;
5. comprehensive, up-to-date knowledge of infant development, assessment, and intervention techniques; and
6. ability to integrate information about the family and child in the development of the IFSP.

The physical therapist's ability to implement family-focused intervention effectively with infants, toddlers, and their families, will depend on the therapist's skills in these areas. The purpose of this chapter is to discuss pertinent findings and concepts of family dynamics and functioning, factors influencing interaction patterns of families who have children with disabilities, and how these concepts and theories relate to family-focused intervention and to the PL 99-457 mandate. The role of physical therapy will also be discussed.

FAMILY DYNAMICS AND FAMILY FUNCTIONING

A family is equated to a system embedded in the larger ecologic framework, having organized patterns of interactions that are circular rather than linear in form[10,11]. The child and the child's caretaking environment tend mutually to alter one another, thus creating interactive systems. (Fig. 12-2).[4,5] Similarly, within a family, the action of any member affects all other members, producing reactions, adjustment, and adaptations in the family structure and modifications in roles and functioning.[7,8] This transactional and systemic view of family functioning implies that the family is an open system, subject to inner pressure coming from developmental changes of its own members and to outer pressure comming from demands to accommodate to significant social and environmental factors.[7,8,10] According to Minuchin,[7] responding to demands (from within and without) requires a constant transformation of position of family members in relation to one another, so that they can grow while the family system maintains continuity. Periods of stability and change are considered to be part of the same process moving through time.[8,10] In systems theory, a

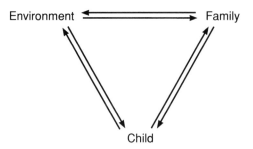

Fig. 12-2.   Transactional family process.

functional family is considered to be one that has the capacity to change, re-organize, and adapt when internal and external (environmental) conditions demand restructuring.[7] Within this context, a dysfunctional family is one that is either rigid or is constantly changing and therefore unable to adapt.[7,31]

Research on families suggests that family dynamics and functioning are complex; families react differently, even to *similar* events. The reaction of the family to an event is believed to be instigated by the family's perception of the significance of the event, the timing of the event in relation to the family's life cycle,[32,33] and the family's past experiences.[7] From observations of more than 200 normal or average families, Haley[34] found patterns of functioning and interactions to be so diverse that he cautioned against stereotyping families as normal or dysfunctional.

FAMILIES OF CHILDREN WITH HANDICAPS

Research suggests that, in general, family dynamics in families caring for children with disabilities are similar to those of families caring for children with no disabilities, except in a few specific aspects, which will be highlighted and discussed below. The reader is cautioned that although a comparison is made in this chapter between families of children with and without disabilities, the former group is not homogeneous; differences also exist within the group of parents of children with disabilities.[32,35,36] Major differences between families or parents of children with and without disabilities have been observed in their parent–child interaction styles,[29,37,38] parents' stress levels and coping skills,[39–42] reactions of siblings,[13,19,43] and some aspects of child-rearing practices, such as discipline.[2,44] All of the factors listed above have also been found to be closely related to the quality of caregiving in families and are assumed to contribute significantly to the outcome of the child's development.

Caregiver–Child Interaction

Much has been written about interaction patterns between parents and their infants with disabilities[45] and how parent–child interaction patterns influence caregiving and the infant's subsequent development.[29] Of significance are findings indicating that interaction patterns between mothers and their infants during early stages are characterized by asynchrony.[19,38,45–49] The caregiver's inability to recognize the infant's signaling abilities[38] and the less competent and rewarding interaction responses displayed by infants with disabilities[50] appeared to contribute to interactional problems. The caregivers' responses have been observed to vary from overstimulation to indifference. Based on an analysis of studies on parent–child interaction, Rosenberg and Robinson[38] concluded that mothers of infants with handicaps were as competent as mothers of nondisabled infants, but had to initiate more interactions and also received less gratifying responses from their infants. Parents also varied in providing contingent and appropriate responses to their infants' signals.

Differences in the interaction patterns with cohorts of infants with disabilities and their families also appear to be a function of the child's cognitive levels; duration of observation of interaction; whether interaction was observed at home, in the nursery, or at a developmental center; and the caregiver's perceptions and knowledge about the child and development. For example, Parke and Tinsely[29] noted that the presence of another member, father, mother, or extended family members, appeared to influence the interactional patterns.

Follow-up studies investigating long-term outcome of children with disabilities with various styles of caregiver–child interactions are sparse. Consequently, the ability to determine the relationship between the variables listed above and the outcome of the child's development is limited. Physical therapy entails dyadic interaction between infants and caregivers through handling, positioning, and feeding techniques. The success of physical therapy in family-focused intervention will therefore depend on the physical therapist's sensitivity to interactional processes between family members and child, the therapist's awareness of how intervention interacts with the observed interaction styles, and what modification will be necessary to meet the needs of the child and family. Because of the diversity of interactional styles, therapists will do well not to make assumptions about infants and caregivers without individualized observations.

Stress

A common finding of studies of families of disabled children is that these families experience more stress than families of nondisabled children.[39–42, 51–54] Stress observed or reported by parents, particularly mothers of children with disabilities, appears to be related to numerous factors: the care required by the child with disability, the age of the child (the older the child, the higher the stress level), and the extent to which the child is dependent on the caregiver. Mothers of children who were severely disabled showed increased stress levels.[40,42,55-58] Single mothers of children with disabilities have also been reported to experience more stress than mothers in two-parent families.[56] The stress for single parents, however, has also been associated with the fact that these parents are both primary caregivers and primary wage earners.[59] An association between the quality and quantity of resources available to the family and stress has also been reported.[39,60] Transitional periods such as initial diagnosis, seeking early intervention services, and transition of infants into preschools were found to produce stress in parents.[61] Bernheimer and associates[60] found that certain aspects of professionals' attitudes, such as insensitivity, use of jargon, professional's lack of knowledge of available resources, inadequate information given by professionals, and inadequate guidance during transition into preschool, were among variables cited by parents as stressful.

Demoralization, which relates to stress, was also reported in a group of mothers of children with disabilities.[61] Demoralization was defined as a complex of negative affect and somatic complaints that is characteristic of many people who are exposed to persistent stressors such as chronic illness or poverty.[61] Demoralization lowers parental feelings of competence, self-esteem, and ability to cope with the demands of caring for chronically ill children.

However, not all parents of disabled children reported being stressed by caring for their disabled children.[42,55,58,62] Breslau and associates[58] found that only two-thirds of the mothers in their sample experienced stress. Parents in Abbot and Meredith's study[62] reported positive contributions to the family by their children with disability. In addition, McKinney and Peterson[42] did not find significant differences in stress response on the Parenting Stress Index (PSI) when parents of children with handicaps were compared with the population on which the test was standardized.

Perception, including the meaning a family attaches to a stressful situation, appears to be a crucial factor determining the severity or the impact of the stressor, i.e., whether the family will experience a crisis.[63] Each family's transitional stage in its life cycle will also determine the extent to which a family attaches meaning or responds to a stressful situation. Therefore, a stressor affects each family differently at different times.

The impact of acute stress versus chronic stress has not been fully explored. Contemporary theories propose that interventionists should be most concerned when a family already experiencing chronic stress encounters an additional acute stress.[54,64]

Stress should be examined in terms of family dynamics and functioning. This will require longitudinal studies of families as opposed to cross-sectional studies because the cross-sectional approach may not be appropriate for capturing the family's reorganization and adaptation process. Physical therapists are in a position to collect this information as they see these families on a regular basis over extended periods. Physical therapists' awareness and sen-

sitivity to the stress-related factors described above can also be used prophylactically to lessen stress in these families.

Coping Skills

The tremendous interest in investigating the impact of stress associated
with caring for a child with disabilities overshadows coping skills often exhibited by families of these children. Stress and coping go hand in hand.[64] Researchers found that coping parents seemed to use three coping patterns: maintaining family integration; maintaining social support, self-esteem, and
psychological stability; and understanding the medical situation through communication with other parents and consultation with staff. Although these families experienced stress, they also displayed areas of strength as observed in
adaptability and nondysfunctional patterns of interaction.[35,39,65,66] Beavers and
associates[32] found that 22 of 40 families in their study adjusted to the child's
presence and needs and functioned well. These investigators isolated factors
that may contribute to coping in families, such as

1. the family's values—what they have been told about the child and how
they view disability;
2. the family's feelings—whether negative feelings and frustrations are
recognized and permitted by the family; and
3. the relative power of the handicapped child in the family system.

These factors may dictate the extent to which a stressor leads to a crisis for
an individual family, which in turn will affect its coping style. The power of
the child with disability is seen in the degree to which the family's life or
behavior is organized around the child. Members of more adaptive families can
be attuned to the needs of the child, but still have energy and concern for
interest and satisfaction in other family relationships and activities.

Other coping skills that differentiated successfully coping families from
those not successful were

1. the family's ability to focus on small gains and positive contributions
made by the child[62];
2. being well informed about the functioning capacity of the retarded
child[60];
3. if there were two or more adults caring for the child[55,59]; and
4. having family system resources, such as the extended family, social
networks, and financial support.[7,32,36,39,40,67]

Although families of children with disabilities were found to be more socially
isolated than families of children with no disabilities, Kazak and Wilcox,[36]
suggested that it may not be social isolation that differentiates these families,
but underdevelopment of particular types of relationships.

Stress may be difficult to prevent; however, coping skills can be taught.[68] Coping skills such as relaxation, communication, assertiveness, and increasing pleasurable events have been proved to alleviate stress, including depression.[69] For more information on this topic, the reader is referred to Summers et al.[70] and McCubbin and Patterson,[64] who provide a comprehensive discussion of stress, positive adaptation, and coping strengths in families who have children with disabilities. Attempts to isolate other factors that may contribute to successful coping in families continues.[62,64,71] Knowledge of such factors will enable professionals to develop intervention strategies to enhance those factors, thereby encouraging positive adaptation of the family.

Marital Relationships

Another source of stress and disruption to family functioning frequently cited in the literature is marital discord.[40,72–74] A conjecture put forward by some is that a child with handicaps attacks the matrix of marriage, particularly in child-rearing practices such as discipline and decision making. Marital discord has also been linked to problematic parenting behavior.[75] Unfortunately, the findings on marital discord are inconclusive. Kazak[40] found that although mothers of children with disability experienced higher levels of stress than mothers in a matched-comparison group, there were no group differences with respect to marital satisfaction.

Findings on divorce rates are also conflicting. Gath[72] reported that families with children who had severe disabilities had higher divorce rates than those with less involved children. On the other hand, Williams and McKenny[73] found no differences in divorce rates. Differences between divorce rates of parents of nondisabled children and those of parents of children with developmental disabilities were found to be insignificant when social class was held constant.[74,76,77]

The findings on marital relationships suggest the importance of looking beyond the nuclear family for understanding parental behavior and caring for a child with disabilities. The findings of Kazak[40] and Goldberg and Easterbrooks[78] imply that other sources besides the child's disabilities may contribute to marital discord. Physical therapists should concern themselves with how marital discord affects the family's ability to care for the child rather than whether the child causes the discord.

Siblings of the Child with Disabilities

Siblings of children with disabilities have frequently been excluded from studies that examined parent–child interaction and developmental outcomes. Recently, increased interest in the dynamic and transactional interactions among the child, the family, and the environment has drawn attention to the siblings' role.[13,14,43,79–82] Siblings of children with mental and behavioral handicaps have been the major focus of observation. Few studies have included children with physical disabilities. The general finding, however, is that siblings of children with disabilities may be at risk for emotional problems and experience increased demands and expectations from their parents and themselves. Siblings of children with disabilities were more sensitive than those of nondisabled children to differences in the parents' behavior toward each of them,[83] and the parents' feelings about the child with disabilities were found to be the strongest factor affecting the normal siblings.[43] Sisters of children with disabilities appeared to be most vulnerable to emotional distress.[13,43] An earlier study by Grossman[43] also reported that sisters were more involved in their sibling's care than brothers.

Not all siblings reported negative feelings. Some brothers and sisters reported that they benefited from the experience of having a sibling with disabilities.[84] Adjustment of the siblings was found to be related to the parents' communication about the capacity and needs of their disabled sibling. Those siblings that were fully informed exhibited positive behaviors toward their disabled siblings and toward their parents.[19,81,83–85] Including the siblings in family decision-making processes was also reported to enhance their self-esteem.[19] Siblings should therefore be included in assessment and intervention processes as often as possible.

Child-Rearing Practices

Discipline

Discipline is a child-rearing transaction that distinguishes families of children with disabilities from those without.[13,31,32,86] Uncertainty as to how much discipline to use with a child who has limited capacity to respond, both mentally and physically, has been apparent in the former groups of families.[32] According to Beavers and associates,[32] some parents also may not comprehend the demands they are making on the child's cognitive capacity. Research findings have shown that parents of children with mental handicaps tend to withhold discipline.[13] When discipline is withheld, or is inconsistent, the child may develop low tolerance for frustration, may not learn to differentiate good and bad,[87] and problems with siblings may ensue. The child may also be treated as the youngest sibling despite birth order or chronologic age.[88]

Marital discord is related to problems in disciplining children, both nondisabled[89] and disabled,[19] and predicts the child's behavior problems at a subsequent point in development.[90] Featherstone[19] suggested that repeated arguments between parents about child-rearing practices may stress the parents' relationship and lead to marital discord; therefore, the child's behavior and discipline issues should be assessed in all children eligible for family-focused intervention. Strategies for behavior modification should be worked out with parents when necessary.

Because disciplinary practices are culture bound, professionals need to exercise caution when suggesting a behavior modification program. Behaviors that are intolerable in the professional's culture may be acceptable within the family's. Therapists need to ask parents about how the family feels about the child's behavior, how the behavior has been handled in the past, and if the family has expectations of therapists regarding discipline.

CULTURAL DIVERSITY IN FAMILIES

Culture is one dimension that conditions family life and has a significant impact on family functioning. Child-rearing practices are embedded in a sociocultural content.[90-92] An understanding of cultural diversity in families; therefore, is crucial to effective family-focused intervention. The concept of what constitutes a family differs from culture to culture. In some cultures, an "extended" family is included in the definition of family since they may be part of the same household. Extended family members in such cultures, e.g., grandparents, may have a greater influence on children's upbringing than in others.[93] In such cultures, grandparents are widely accepted and respected primary caretakers and are the family's most important support system.[94] In other cultures, there is a system of shared child care; individuals within such family structures, including mothers, may be expected to adapt their child-rearing practices to traditional expectations, regardless of outside intervention. Mothers from such cultures may not display stress from caregiving, but from other cultural expectations.

According to Green,[95] there is often a misconception about the meaning of *culture*. Concepts such as race or minority status are often used interchangeably with culture. Green points out that "race is a social concept and exists only to the degree that differentiations could be made to phenotypic characteristics of individuals, such as skin color or hair form, while minority refers to the power given to numbers.[11] To ascribe cultural differences in terms of race will therefore not only be misleading, but will greatly affect professionals' potential to work effectively with families and their children with disabilities.

Any culture provides a repertoire of explanations for problems, explanations related to etiology of diseases, and expectations of treatment outcomes and values about the illness.[95] In some cultures, the birth of a child with disability may be regarded as a punishment for the mother's wrongdoing.[96] Such explanations or beliefs contribute significantly to child-rearing practices and are highly related to child behaviors that will be encouraged or tolerated. According to Werner and Smith,[2] when family cultural practices and beliefs hinder development, even infants without biologic complications have developed severe social and cognitive deficits later in life.

Cultural issues are also present in the family's interactions with other organizations.[95] Families in some cultures tend to rely on professionals, particularly in areas where they feel uncertain, such as therapeutic, educational, and medical needs of their children with handicaps.[93] Some families may rely more on their cultural values and beliefs, choosing to engage in other forms of treatment for their child, such as massage or interventions prescribed by spiritual or traditional healers or herbalists who may give recommendations to the parents that are in contradiction with therapy goals. For example, they might advise the parents of a child with no head control to support the head and massage the neck, while the physical therapist advocates minimal head support to facilitate head control. Conflicting opinions may thus lead to communication problems.

Two factors are considered to be critical to effective interaction with culturally distinctive families: the professional's understanding and knowledge of the family's culture, and the professional's own cultural beliefs and values.[44, 93,95,97] It is commonly suggested that health care providers working with culturally distinctive clients should establish rapport and develop empathic relationships to further treatment objectives. In family-focused intervention, in which the family's articulation of their needs and decisions regarding their handicapped child form the basis of long-term therapy and of the IFSP, empathy will not always be sufficient. According to Taft,[97] to understand members of other cultures, one must learn what members of that culture know: their beliefs, values, ideology, and how they judge their relationships to the world. Taft proposes two levels of learning about culture:

1. cognitive—by listening and reading about how members of the culture act and what they believe to be appropriate, and
2. affective—by observing how they express feelings and interpret emotions or behaviors.

Health professionals are also culture bound.[98] When interacting with families, the health professional uses a point of view that is central to his or her own cultural beliefs and values. There is therefore a danger of the therapist underestimating the impact of culture and incorrectly judging as abnormal behaviors that are considered normal in the family's culture. Therapists may also overestimate the importance of culture at the expense of failing to recognize dysfunctional interaction patterns, or unknowingly impose his or her own values on the family's belief systems.

Language

Language is one of the most significant symbols of a culture or subculture.[95] Language within a cultural context can be used for numerous purposes, such as communicating and shaping the caregiving environment, expressing needs and achievements, and building boundaries around family units, just to name a few. Body language such as eye contact is used by some cultures to show authority or respect. A child may be considered disrespectful if he or she maintains prolonged eye contact with an authority figure.[93] Similarly, some families may not maintain eye contact when interacting with professionals. In other cultures, spontaneity and impulsiveness as a form of expression in children may be discouraged. Such cultural communication patterns can create barriers between the family and health professionals. The therapist's understanding of the language and culture of the families with whom he or she works will be an added asset in family-focused intervention.

Early intervention programs serving infants and families under Part H of PL 99-457 are required to conduct the IFSP "in the native language of the family or other mode of communication used by the family, unless it is clearly not feasible to do so" (p. 26321). Therapists therefore have a responsibility to ensure that channels of communication exist between them and the families with whom they work. Although the use of translators has offered expediency and comfort for the family and therapists, therapists need to be aware of some of the disadvantages outlined by Lappin,[99] who asserts that using translators

1. puts the family in the one-down position at a time when they need to be one-up;
2. results in communication *through* not *to* someone, thereby diminishing the intensity of any possible cross-cultural dyadic interactions;
3. puts the translator as the central figure in the communication, as opposed to the family or the child;
4. creates uncertainties in the therapist and family, as each cannot always be sure of the clarity of the message or how distorted the information may be; and
5. dilutes the richness of cross-cultural experience for both therapist and family.

Therapists will do well, therefore, to choose a translator who not only knows the language, but understands the culture. Some parents tend to bring their own translators to therapy and should be encouraged to do so. According to PL 99-457, "other family members, as requested by the parent"(p. 26321) may participate in IFSP meetings.

Perhaps one way of dealing with this complex situation can be found in Lappin's[99] suggestion that "in order to go home, one must know how to get there." Therapists should be aware of their own cultural biases. A few ways may be to talk openly to other professionals about their own experiences or beliefs regarding the issue causing a conflict, share their views with the parents without being judgmental, and listen carefully to the family's response to suggestions made by other professionals.

THE ROLE OF PHYSICAL THERAPY IN FAMILY-FOCUSED INTERVENTION

If physical therapists accept that family functioning is important to the success of infant and child development, they must identify the skills of the family and child that can be enhanced through physical therapy and incorporate development of those skills into their intervention programs. In the past, physical therapists have relied heavily on the primary caregiver to follow through with intervention activities at home, as evidenced by the use of home programs. The emphasis has been on parent training and on parents acting as cotherapists. Family "assessment" often was limited to obtaining demographic data and the child's developmental history. The therapy program was highly individualized, based on the child's functional limitations and needs rather than the needs of the family. Based on the transactional model of development, this approach may be limited in its capacity to improve the family's ability to meet the needs of the child.[100] The interaction of parent or family variables with intervention approaches used by physical therapists has not been fully explored.

Physical therapy as defined in PL 99-457 includes "screening infants and toddlers to identify movement dysfunction; obtaining, interpreting and integrating information appropriate to program planning; preventing or alleviating movement dysfunction and related functional problems; and providing services to prevent or alleviate movement dysfunction and related functional problems" (p. 26312). In addition, the physical therapist, like members of other disciplines, is responsible for assuming the roles listed in Figure 12-1 as well as being a case manager when needed. The development of specific physical therapy competencies in early intervention is in progress. To appropriately serve children with handicapping conditions, physical therapists must

1. develop skillful use of methods to assess and evaluate infants;
2. possess the skills to identify family strengths that may enhance the child's development, particularly motor development;
3. possess the ability to identify specific needs of the child and caregiving environment that should be targeted in intervention; and
4. possess the skill to integrate physical therapy goals and activities with those of other disciplines.

ASSESSMENT

Public Law 99-457 makes a distinction between *assessment* and *evaluation*. *Evaluation* is defined in the law as "the procedures used by appropriate qualified personnel to determine a child's initial and continuing eligibility under Part H . . . including determining the status of the child in each of the developmental areas." *Assessment*, on the other hand, is defined as "the ongoing procedures used by appropriate qualified personnel throughout the period of a child's eligibility under Part H to identify: a) the child's unique needs; b) the family's strengths and needs related to development of the child; and c) the nature and extent of early intervention services that are needed by the child and the child's family to meet the child's needs" (p. 26320). Based on the law, both an evaluation and an assessment of the child must be conducted; for the family, only an assessment must be done.

According to PL 99-457, the evaluation and assessment of each child must be conducted by personnel trained to use appropriate methods and procedures and be based on informed clinical opinion.

Physical Therapy Assessment and Evaluation of the Child

To determine the functional levels of the child, physical therapists working with infants and toddlers must know how to administer standardized tests that assess functional skills in this population. Each state is required to select one standardized test to be used to assess the needs of all eligible children whose services will be covered under Part H of PL 99-457 and to determine eligibility criteria. Physical therapists will have to become proficient in administering and scoring the test, and interpreting the results. Occasionally, a child may require physical therapy and case management only. In such cases, the referring physician, the case manager, and the physical therapist will be responsible for conducting the multidisciplinary assessment. Physical therapists, therefore, should possess some basic knowledge of other areas of development, such as language, cognition, and psychosocial development, in order to make appropriate recommendations.

The law also specifies that each discipline may also conduct an evaluation based on clinical observation. In conducting such an evaluation, physical therapists must possess a comprehensive knowledge of motor development and how movement dysfunction affects other areas of the child's development. This information is presented in various chapters of this volume and will therefore not be addressed in this chapter. Family-focused evaluation should include an evaluation of how the child uses movement to interact with his or her caregivers and to function in and explore the environment. This will entail observations (structured or unstructured) across a variety of situations and tasks, in addition to handling, and should include parent–child interaction as part of the evaluation process. If interdisciplinary or transdisciplinary "arena-type" evaluations are used, the physical therapist can observe the child during parent–child or sibling–parent–child interactions, during free play, and during feeding or snack time. Caution should be exercised when interpreting the results because behaviors observed in simulated situations may not accurately reflect the true dynamic nature of interactions in the home. The therapist may also want to confirm the findings by asking the parent if the child's responses and movement patterns were typical of those displayed at home.

Family Assessment

Traditionally, assessment of families has been conducted by social workers, case managers, and psychologists. Family assessment often focused on the family's needs as opposed to child assessment. Child-focused assessment was performed by members of other disciplines, including physical therapists.

Unless well coordinated, this approach may lead to information gaps. Child-focused assessments often fail to adequately address the child's caregiving environment and family assessments may overlook the dynamic contribution of the child to family functioning. With the family-focused approach, all professionals listed in Figure 12-1 have the responsibility to participate in the assessment of the family's strengths and needs. In other words, family assessment can be conducted by social workers and psychologists as members of a team, or by physical therapists when appropriate.

As noted earlier, the objective of family assessment must be to determine the "family's strengths and needs related to enhancing the child's development" (PL 99-457, p. 26320), and not to diagnose functional or dysfunctional patterns in families. Family assessment must be voluntary on the part of parent, and assessments should be coordinated so that the family does not have to repeat information for several professionals. Therapists should ensure that the information is not available elsewhere before asking the parents.

The extent of physical therapist participation in family assessment will vary from program to program. In most programs, information on families is available before the family comes in for comprehensive child evaluation; in some, it is not. In the latter situation, the physical therapist should also use the child's motor development as a framework within which to assess the family's strengths and needs. The therapist must select motoric behaviors in the child that are likely to affect caregiving and attempt to solicit the parents' perception and responses to them.

Methods of Assessing Families' Strengths and Needs

Physical therapists can use observations, interviews, and questionnaires to assess family strengths and needs, but need to be cognizant of the advantages, disadvantages, and limitations of each method before using it. One of the advantages of observation is that it provides the observer a full view of dynamic transactions and interactions. One limitation of this method is that observation focuses on an external behavior; the observer cannot know what is happening inside those being observed. An interview, on the other hand, may allow the interviewer to gain insight into the interviewee's feelings or thoughts, but there are limitations: (1) reactivity of the interviewee to the interviewer, (2) self-serving responses on the part of the interviewee, and (3) the fact that the interviewee reports his or her perceptions and perspectives, which are subject to distortion due to personal bias, anger, anxiety, politics, and simple lack of awareness.[101] Interviewing also requires good listening skills.[44] Questionnaires are perhaps the simplest form of getting information from families; they do not always require experience or training to administer. Questionnaires, however, do not capture interactional patterns, often reflect the author's point of view or bias, often address a specific area of inquiry, and can be viewed as impersonal. Questionnaires such as the Parenting Stress Index or Questionnaire on Resources and Stress can be useful in assessing resources available to the family or quantifying individual family members' feelings or emotional well being.

Patton[101] outlined a few suggestions on how to improve interviewing and observation skills, which physical therapists may find useful:

1. Gather a variety of information from different perspectives and multiple sources if you can (e.g., siblings, father, or mother).
2. Be careful to be descriptive in taking notes or reporting.
3. Separate description from interpretation.

The manner in which questions are phrased may either be threatening or encouraging to the family.[20] An example of questions that may encourage the family to be "open" and less threatened are presented below in no specific order.

Have you and your family members encountered problems related to muscles and joints in caring for your infant? How have you dealt with them?

In what ways does your infant assist you and your family in caring for him?

What are some of the things you and your family have done that seem to help your child?

What are some of the things that your infant does best with his body, arms, legs, etc? How important is that to you and your family?

In what way do you think therapy will change your child's movement? Why is your child's ability to sit or stand or walk important to you and your family?

What are your family's and relatives' expectations about your child? What are yours?

How much time do you usually spend alone with your child? How much time do other members of your family spend with him? What are some of the things you or your family members do with him/her during that time?

What is your child's favorite play activity?

These questions may help parents delineate problematic areas related to the infant's motor function and assist the therapist and family to develop a treatment plan that addresses those needs. For example, if the parents do not feel that their child's movement problems have interfered with family functioning and yet fail to identify things that the child does best with his or her arms, legs, body, etc., the therapist should ascertain the family's expectations of the child and therapy. On the other hand, the parents may respond that they have not been able to spend much time alone with the child and may explain why. This information should be a warning sign that parent training and home programs may be inappropriate options for physical therapy until the case manager has explored the situation further.

In using observations, an inexperienced physical therapist may choose to limit the scope of observations to play or turn-taking behaviors between the child and parents. On the other hand, an experienced therapist may want to address other behaviors that may affect parent training or the child's exploration of the environment. Useful observations include persistence on the part of both the parents and the child, the level of instruction used by the parents with the child, use of eye contact as a way to engage a child in an activity or redirect the child, how the parents pace tasks the child may be engaged in, and the parents' energy levels. Physical therapists can also use the Nursing Child Assessment Feeding and Teaching Scales.[102]

Inexperience may also lead the therapist to make premature judgments regarding the family based on limited understanding of families. Furthermore, it is important to understand the context within which the family operates in order to gain a holistic perspective.

Ongoing Assessment

Just as physical therapists have traditionally performed ongoing assessment of the child's performance or the caregiver's compliance, the therapist should use ongoing assessment to monitor changes in the family's ability to continue to meet the needs of their child in therapy and make accompanying program modifications. Parents tend to develop a close relationship with their child's therapist over time. Some relationships may be in the form of mentor, friend, consultant, or confidante. The disadvantages of such relationships have been pointed out before (e.g., dependency roles on the part of the family and rescuer roles on the part of the therapist). The advantage is that therapists can use the relationships to continually monitor or assess the family's response, not only to therapy or the early intervention program, but to other external demands.

Families are dynamic, and family roles change in response to developmental events within the family and environment.[7] When intervention is initiated, the family has no way of knowing how therapy will disrupt or enhance its functioning. Because the social workers in most early intervention programs are not in contact with the family as often as therapists are, it is the responsibility of the physical therapist and other professionals to be sensitive to the family's needs. Hence, the physical therapist must have a good working knowledge of family dynamics and functioning.

FAMILY-FOCUSED PHYSICAL THERAPY

Family-focused intervention is fairly new, and there is a paucity of literature on effective models of intervention. Studies conducted by other disciplines reporting on motor outcome together with other areas of the child's development are also sparse. Those studies that assessed motor development did so following a general rather than specific intervention package, and the results have been conflicting.[103,104] Heavy emphasis in these studies was placed on specific aspects of the quality of mother–child interaction, and intervention was not clearly defined.

In the preceding sections, ways in which physical therapy can enhance parents' capacity to meet the needs of their child with handicaps have been alluded to. In the absence of information about specific family or child variables that have consistently predicted good or poor developmental outcome, physical therapists are challenged to select or develop strategies that can be adapted to meet the family and child's needs. This situation is compounded by the fact that the needs of children with handicaps and their families are as varied as the problems they and their families must overcome. After reviewing studies of family-focused intervention, Meisels concluded that no single formula or prescription can be applied to this diverse population; intervention requires services from a variety of professionals.[105] To be effective, physical therapists must recognize the contribution of other disciplines and integrate their intervention goals and activities with those of other services in an interdisciplinary, multidisciplinary or transdisciplinary approach.

This section will focus on how physical therapy can be expanded to enhance the family's ability to care for their handicapped infant and to meet the mandate of PL 99-457. Therapeutic techniques focusing on the specific needs of children with various disabilities are addressed in other chapters in this volume.

General Goals of Family-Focused Intervention

The goals for physical therapy should be consistent with and may in some cases overlap those of other disciplines. General goals for family-focused intervention are listed in PL 99-457 rules and regulations, and some have been presented by various authors.[106,107] Early intervention has its foundations in several premises and assumptions.[100,108] Some of the assumptions form the basis for the physical therapist's perspective and formulation of goals for the provision of services for children and their families. Formulating general goals helps to (1) define the scope within which outcomes of family-focused physical therapy can be expected, (2) delineate areas that are unique to physical therapists and those overlapping with other disciplines, and (3) determine competencies needed by physical therapists to serve developmentally delayed children and their families. General goals should not be confused with specific therapy goals. Specific therapy goals must be based on the outcome of each child's evaluation and family assessment, the parent's goals, and those of other disciplines involved with the child. According to PL 99-457, therapy goals must be determined during the development of the IFSP in collaboration with the parents.

The general physical therapy goals listed below incorporate those listed under PL 99-457.

1. To enhance functional independence in children with disabilities or developmental delays.

2. To help parents understand their infants' and toddlers' disabling conditions and the implications of those conditions.

3. To enhance or teach specific skills and knowledge that will enable families to cope with the unique needs of their infants and toddlers with movement disorders.

4. To assist families in making decisions regarding evaluations and treatment plans for their infants and toddlers with handicaps.

5. To promote appropriate and stimulating family–parent–child and sibling–child interactions that are mutually enjoyable.

6. To assist families to gain access to relevant community services and to make smooth transitions into preschool programs.

7. To advise parents concerning environmental and home adaptations or modifications.

PHYSICAL THERAPY INTERVENTION STRATEGIES

Suggestions for how physical therapists can use information on family systems theory and family dynamics and functioning to meet some of the goals listed above are outlined below.

Helping Parents Understand Their Infant's Developmental Capabilities and Limitations

The need for information about the child and available services is a high priority among families participating in early intervention.[109] Limited understanding of their children's capabilities has been reported to be related to increased levels of stress in mothers,[28,110] particularly those mothers whose infants were born prematurely or were cared for in special care nurseries. Physical therapists working in newborn nurseries and neonatal intensive care units have several opportunities to educate the family or parents about their infant. They are often among the first early intervention providers to come into contact with the family and their infant with handicaps or at risk for developmental delay. Also, therapists work one-on-one with infants and their families. To address the goal of educating the family, therapists should, whenever feasible, perform infant assessments in the presence of the family. Similarly, in neonatal follow-up clinics, physical therapists can "talk" the parents through developmental or screening tests and clinical assessments, highlighting the positive aspects of the infant's development and performance and providing anticipatory guidance. Teaching handling and positioning skills may or may not be part of the educational process at this time. Some parents may not yet be ready to be actively involved with the infant's care,[57,108] but may be content to observe.

Allowing parents to be observers may seem unusual to physical therapists who are used to teaching parents how to facilitate the child's development through handling. In family-focused intervention, however, the therapist has to make sure that parents are ready to assume new roles. Fear of attachment has been reported to be an emotional reaction of some parents of ill, premature infants,[57] while desire for strong parental attachment has been reported by others.[111] Therapists must be sensitive to these diverse reactions.

With help in understanding their infant's developmental capabilities, the family will be encouraged to engage in a dialogue with their other children about their sibling with handicaps and include them in decision-making processes. Siblings have been reported to feel positive about the child with handicaps after their parents communicated their sibling's capabilities and limitations to them.[19] Parent education within the context described above fits also into the category of preventive family-focused therapy.

The general question often raised by professionals regarding giving families information is, "How much and how soon?" It is often argued that too much too soon causes the family undue stress, while too little too late may lead to frustrations and resentment.[60] No guidelines have been specified in the literature. The therapist has to rely on using the number and depth of the family's questions as a crude estimation of how much information the family can handle. The family's expectations of physical therapy can also be used as an indication of the family's understanding of their child's capabilities. In addition, therapists can create linkages among parents that can be of mutual benefit. Families can be matched in many ways: according to the children's disabilities, an older with a younger child, newer families with those who have been in therapy for a while, etc. Other parents can also be used as resources to families.

Enhancing Family Skills and Knowledge of How to Enhance the Child's Development

Parent training has been a widely used and accepted form of parent involvement in early intervention. Studies examining the effects of parent training are among those reporting significant improvement in parenting skills.[28,105,112,113] Literature on the effectiveness of parent training by physical therapists, however, is sparse.[24,114] The objectives of parent training have varied, from improving parent–child interaction, to ensuring carry over of therapy activities, to enhancing caregiving practices. Parents are encouraged to carry out therapeutic or educational activities with their child who has handicaps and to act as cotherapists. In most instances, the therapist or educator decides which activities are important for the child to learn, with little parental input.

Parent training used in the family-focused context entails mutual agreement between the parents and therapists on activities that parents feel are important to practice at home with the child. It also implies that if a technique, procedure, or piece of equipment has been successful in encouraging desirable responses from the child, that procedure should be taught to the parents or the equipment should be made available to the family. Taken a step further, no family should be denied access to procedures or equipment that have been found successful in enhancing the child's development. Under PL 99-457, each state will decide how the cost of such procedures or equipment will be covered.

Suggestions for enhancing the parents' knowledge and skills include (1) teaching parents only those activities that are related to day-to-day caregiving (e.g., range of motion during dressing or diaper changing),[24] (2) providing activities that allow the whole family to participate in the treatment program,[115] (3) asking parents to choose activities they feel will be feasible to teach other members of the family, thus providing respite for the primary caretaker,[116] and (4) if the child receives day-care services, the therapist and parents jointly teaching activities to the staff at the day care center or the primary caretaker when parents are at work. The Nursing Child Assessment Teaching Scale[102] could be used to guide and evaluate parent teaching.

Several authors have warned against excessive dependency on parents to carry out educational and therapy activities for their children.[22,100, 116–118] The concern is that this practice may place unreasonable demands on the family's schedules and disrupt relationships between parents and their children (clashes of wills). The assertion of other researchers is that the parents' success at developing therapy skills at home may jeopardize normalized parenting interactions.[119] Some parents may become overinvolved with the child's therapy with the hope of immediate pay-offs and become frustrated in the process. Using parents as therapists may also lead to the child becoming the center of family functioning, which imparts undue power to the child. The relative power of the handicapped child in the family has been cited to be a useful indication of the family's overall adaptation; families that displayed poor coping behaviors were found to organize their behaviors around the child.[32] An alternative "consumer model," which allows parents to actively decide on their level of involvement, has been proposed.[44] The problem with this model is that it provides no guidelines for monitoring parent's cooperation and compliance.

Encouraging and Assisting the Family in Making Decisions

Family-focused intervention is as new to most parents of infants with disabilities as it is to professionals. Making decisions regarding the child's therapy or educational placement will be more difficult for some parents and less for others. On the whole, parents are responsible for decisions that accommodate the needs of any child in the family and they decide the family's priorities.[119] Physical therapists, on the other hand, possess technical knowledge and expertise in motor development and intervention. Parents need the professional's evaluation of the child to make informed decisions about therapy, day-care arrangements, or the parents' current job situations; to determine how their decisions will affect other members of the family; and to solicit advice from extended family members or friends.[19]

Therapists can facilitate the above process by making sure that the family is given a full report of the child's evaluation several days or weeks before the IFSP meeting. Depending on procedures followed in each early intervention program, this may entail the evaluation team going over the results of the evaluation with the family members, addressing the questions they might have, and not sharing recommendations that may bias the family's decision until they have had time to think about alternatives on their own. Therapists must resist the urge to influence the parents' decisions by sharing goals for the child with the parents and recommending services without first soliciting the parents' point of view. Collaborating with the parents on the IFSP entails full partnership.

Recently, some early intervention programs have adapted their service to families by offering day-care for children with handicaps and providing supervised sibling rooms for those siblings who are not able to participate in the child's therapy sessions. (Whenever possible, siblings should be allowed to observe therapy or educational sessions.) Other programs offer home-based intervention. Therapists should give parents the option of these services and allow them to choose a program that will be least disruptive to the family's coping strategies.

Promoting Parent–Child and Sibling–Child Interaction

Teaching parents how to engage in social interactions with their infants has been shown to result in significant improvement in mothers' parenting skills and increased child interest in interaction with their parents.[112] Physical therapists have always acknowledged the importance of parent–child interaction to the development of healthy relationships between the infant and caregivers (see Ch. 4). Physical therapy involves physical contact and turn-taking behaviors between the child and caregiver. For neonates and infants who have disabilities, or who are at risk for developmental delays, and whose parents exhibit parent–child interaction difficulties, physical therapy may be one of the most effective interventions.

Detecting atypical interaction patterns between parent and child during the early stages of infant development requires skill and systematic observation on the part of the therapist. Interaction patterns may change if the parents know they are being observed or if other members of the family are present.[57] Sometimes it may be important to disclose the purpose of the observation to the parents, particularly if the goal is to help the family improve their interaction or teaching skills. Play can be used to assess interaction between the parents and child. Based on observational data, the therapist may choose activities with which to engage the child and the parents. If the parents appear intense and dominating during interaction, the therapist may, for example, select activities that elicit more spontaneity on the part of the parents and child, such as ball activities. If negative behaviors persist, the therapist may need to allow the child and caregiver to reorganize, talk to the caregiver about them, temporarily suspend home programs, or consult with other team members, especially the case manager or family counselor.

The duration and frequency of treatment should reflect family and child individuality. Many programs tend to provide treatments once or twice a week for 45 to 60 minutes. These times and frequencies are often arbitrarily decided by therapists or referring physicians, or are based on reimbursement policies. Although schedule times may be flexible, families are nonetheless expected to "fit" the programs' policies. Where reimbursement issues allow and the duration and frequency are not prescribed by a physician, therapy schedules should reflect the family's needs, structure, and level of competency in their child's home program.

TEAM APPROACH TO FAMILY-FOCUSED INTERVENTION

At the core of family-focused intervention is the belief that all aspects of a child's development and the caregiving environment are interrelated. This approach emphasizes a multidisciplinary or interdisciplinary team approach to the assessment and treatment of children with disabilities and their families. Public Law 99-457 also mandates that assessment of family strengths and needs of the child be conducted by two or more disciplines. The effectiveness of teams lies in the realization that no area of the child or family's functioning is an exclusive concern of any single discipline.[120] The purpose of assigning professionals to a team is to obtain the contribution of specific expertise.[120] Professionals working in teams serving infants and toddlers with disabilities and their families should be able to appreciate the contribution made by other team members, and each member should possess the necessary up-to-date skills and knowledge of their own discipline.

The level of experience and knowledge of physical therapists involved in family-focused intervention will be crucial to the success of the role of physical therapy in the team approach to early intervention in general and in meeting the provisions of PL 99-457 in particular. A physical therapy service provider who lacks experience and adequate knowledge of family functioning or understanding of the environmental context within which the child with disabilities develops or lacks methods of assessing the child's functional abilities will be ineffective in implementing the appropriate team-based, family-focused physical therapy program. These insufficiencies will greatly limit the contribution of physical therapy and its potential impact on team decision-making processes. The success of family-focused intervention and effectiveness of physical therapy will also depend on the physical therapist possessing the essential teaming knowledge and skills.

DEVELOPING THE INDIVIDUALIZED FAMILY SERVICE PLAN

The IFSP is a "written plan for providing early intervention services to a child eligible under Part H and the child's family" (Federal Register, 1989, p. 26320). The law specified three major requirements regarding the IFSP and states that persons directly involved in conducting the evaluations and assessments must participate in the initial and annual IFSP meetings. Certain early intervention programs, because of the shortage of physical therapists and the small number of hours that physical therapy is available, tend to exclude them from IFSP meetings. Details of who should attend the meeting should be of significance to physical therapists, particularly those who provide contracting services. Therapists providing services to infants and toddlers under PL 99-457 must familiarize themselves with what should be contained in the IFSP.

How the IFSP meetings are conducted vary from program to program. No single formula exists for conducting IFSP meetings.[121] Most programs are still experimenting with several ways of making the meetings effective and beneficial to all involved parties. Professionals need to acknowledge that parents bring a comprehensive knowledge about the child's environment, cultural traditions, and values. Professionals bring comprehensive knowledge about the child's developmental status, formal support systems, and family systems. Professionals usually have the information about the child and family long before the meeting. The family should be given information about the child in advance in order for the family to make informed decisions and to be active partners in the development of the IFSP. An appropriate IFSP will be one that blends this information into intervention goals and strategies mutually agreed on by the family and professionals. Johnson and colleagues provide examples of IFSPs.[121]

PERSONNEL PREPARATION

Family-focused intervention, as mandated by the law, requires not only a shift in focus, but additional knowledge in working with families. Key competencies identified by physical therapists as areas in which they require training are assessing, understanding, and communicating with families as well as how to recognize cultural and social family parameters. As one of the primary providers of services to infants and toddlers under PL 99-457, physical therapists are expected to assume roles for which they have not been adequately trained, at least at preservice level. Furthermore, the shortage of physical therapists has led to a situation in which physical therapists involved in early intervention are used primarily in consultative capacities as opposed to providing therapy directly to the children and working with families.

Each profession is responsible for not only defining the standards and levels of competence needed, but also ensuring that qualified members of its profession provide comprehensive and effective services to children. According to PL 99-457, a qualified person means that the person has met state-recognized certification, licensing, registration, or other comparable requirements that apply to the area in which the person is providing early intervention services. The American Physical Therapy Association (APTA) is currently responsible for accreditation of all physical therapy preservice programs. It is, therefore, the APTA's responsibility to ensure that the curriculum that prepares physical therapists includes basic information on families and family-focused intervention to reflect this shift in focus. The Section on Pediatrics of the APTA supports the active participation by physical therapists trained in pediatrics in providing early intervention services to infants, toddlers, preschoolers, and their families.[109]

Therapists already working in early intervention must take the initiative to develop skills in the needed areas through continuing education and graduate level pediatric courses. Most states also provide a series of personnel preparation workshops to upgrade the skills of service providers.

RESEARCH IN FAMILY-FOCUSED PHYSICAL THERAPY

Despite the increasing acceptance of the family-focused approach to early intervention, there are still no well-established models.[100,106] The types of programs reporting successful outcomes vary widely,[18,24,30,105] thus making it difficult to determine which programs promote greater progress for certain subgroups of children.[16,100] In studies showing parental gains, questions remain regarding which factors were responsible. The literature demonstrates ambiguity on the part of clinicians regarding what aspects of the family should be measured and what tools are appropriate.[15] Development of successful and effective family-focused physical therapy will require clinical studies and systematic documentation in collaboration with other disciplines.

When developmental outcomes are the results of an intervention program using the transactional model of infant development or the systems theory model, a single measure of child behavior will be insufficient. Physical therapists need to look beyond gross motor performance when assessing the outcome of physical therapy. A gross motor program of physical therapy also affects other areas of the child's development, such as cognition, psychosocial and language development, and self-help skills. Parent–child interaction may also be enhanced. For example, in an activity such as teaching a child to shift weight onto the left leg, the child may be seated on a bolster and instructed to reach out to the puzzle pieces placed on the right side, identify their shapes as he or she picks one up, and reach across to the left side to place it in the appropriate hole on the form-board. Applause from the mother and therapist (or even from the child) follows a successful attempt. Such an activity stimulates cognition, receptive (and expressive) language, and fine and gross motor development; therefore, studies investigating the effectiveness of family-focused physical therapy should begin using multivariate designs. Outcome measures must at least include parent, sibling, and child variables.

One of the questions that needs to be addressed by physical therapists providing early intervention under the provisions of PL 99-457 is, "Does educating the family on the functional abilities of the child, involving other family members in therapy, providing respite care for the family, increasing or decreasing the number of activities the family is expected to perform at home, varying the frequency of intervention and allowing the primary caregiver the choice of intervention activities to practice at home enhance the child's motor performance and increase the family's coping skills?''

At the heart of the problems related to assessment of the effectiveness of family-focused intervention is the availability of measurement tools.[9,16] The dynamic nature of families and family functioning is complex and difficult to capture with linear models of intervention and assessments. Methods of assessing the dynamic component of family functioning are still in their embryonic stages.[11] Therapists and other team members need to agree on the nature of successful outcomes and the most appropriate measurement tools to use.

Finally, the dynamics of the family are regulated by a family "clock" monitoring the family's life cycle and transitional periods. This implies that observing the family interaction at one moment in time provides evidence or observation of only a fraction of functional patterns used by that family in response to internal and external pressures or demands. Through cross-sectional studies of family functioning and family interactions, professionals can gain an understanding of the families and children with whom they work. More longitudinal studies, however, are needed to document changes and reorganization and adaptation processes that these families use to maintain stability across time. The relationship between the child's age, severity of the disability, and family functioning also needs further exploration.

ACKNOWLEDGMENT

The author wishes to thank Cathy Franks and Dianne Cherry for their editorial assistance.

REFERENCES

1. Bronfenbrenner U: The Ecology of Human Development: Experiments by Nature and Design. Harvard University Press, Cambridge, MA, 1979
2. Werner EE, Smith RS: Vulnerable But Invincible: A Longitudinal Study of Resilient Children and Youth. McGraw-Hill, New York, 1982
3. Cramer BB: Objective and subjective aspects of parent-infant studies and clinical work. p. 1037. In Osofsky JD (ed): Handbook of Infant Development. 2nd Ed. John Wiley & Sons, New York, 1987
4. Sameroff AJ, Chandler MJ: Reproductive risk and the continuum of caretaking casualty. p. 187. In Horowitz F, Hetherington M, Scarr-Salapatek S, Seigel S (eds): Review of Child Development Research. Vol. 4. University of Chicago Press, Chicago, 1975
5. Sameroff AJ, Fiese BH: Transactional regulation and early intervention. p. 119. In Meisel SJ, Shonkoff JP (eds): Handbook of Early Childhood Intervention. Cambridge University Press, New York, 1990
6. Sameroff AJ: Environmental context of child development. J Pediatr 109:192, 1986
7. Minuchin S: Families and Family Therapy. Harvard University Press, Cambridge, MA, 1974

8. Walsh F: Conceptualizations of normal family functioning. p. 3. In F Walsh (ed): Normal Family Processes. Guilford Press, New York, 1982

9. Minuchin P: Families and individual development: provocations from the field of family therapy. Child Dev 56:285, 1985

10. Minuchin P: Relationships within the family: a systems perspective on development. p. 7. In Hinde RA, Stevenson-Hinde J (eds): Relationships Within Families: Mutual Influences. Oxford University Press, New York, 1988

11. Campbell D, Draper R: Applications of Systemic Family Therapy. Grune & Statton, London, 1985

12. Rosenberg S, Robinson C, Beckman P: Teaching Skills Inventory: a measure of parent performance. J Div Early Child 8:107, 1984

13. Vadassy PF, Fewell RR, Meyer DJ, Schell S: Siblings of handicapped children: a developmental perspective on family interactions. Fam Process 23:155, 1984

14. McCollum JA, Stayton UD: Infant/parent interaction: studies and intervention guidelines based on the SIAI Model. J Dev Early Child 9:125, 1985

15. Shonkoff JP, Hauser-Cram P: Early intervention for disabled infants and their families: a quantitative analysis. Pediatrics 80:650, 1987

16. Dunst CJ: Rethinking early intervention. Analysis and Intervention in Dev Dis 6:165, 1985

17. Dunst C, Trivett R, Deal A: Enabling and Empowering Families. Brookline Books, Cambridge, MA, 1988

18. Turnbull AP, Turnbull HR: Parent involvement in the education of handicapped children: a critique. Ment Retard 20:115, 1982

19. Featherstone H: A Difference in the Family: Life With a Disabled Child. Basic Books, New York, 1980

20. Turnbull A, Turnbull H: Parents Speak Out. 2nd Ed. Merrill Publishing, Columbus, OH, 1985

21. Mullins JB: Authentic voices from parents of exceptional children. Fam Rel 36:30, 1987

22. Simeonsson RJ, Bailey DB: Family dimensions in early intervention. p. 428. In Meisels SJ, Shonkoff JP (eds): Handbook of Early Childhood Intervention. Cambridge University Press, New York, 1990

23. Turnbull A, Turnbull HR: Families, Professionals and Exceptionality: A Special Partnership. Charles E Merril, Columbus, OH, 1986

24. Gross AM, Eudy C, Drabmen RS: Training parents to be physical therapists with their physically handicapped child. J Behav Med 5:321, 1982

25. Harris SR: Effects of neurodevelopmental therapy on motor performance of infants with Down syndrome. Dev Med Child Neurol 23:477, 1981

26. Redman-Bentley D: Parent expectations for professionals providing services to their handicapped children. Phys Occup Ther Pediatr 2:13, 1982

27. Education of Handicapped Act Amendments of 1986 (Public Law 99-457), 20 U.S.C. §1400

28. Parke RD: Fathers, families and support systems: their role in the development of at-risk and retarded infants and children. p. 101. In Gallagher J, Vietze P (eds): Families of Handicapped Persons. Paul H Brookes Publishing Co., Baltimore, 1986

29. Parke RD, Tinsley BJ: Family intervention in infancy. p. 579. In Osofsky JD (ed): Handbook of Infant Development: John Wiley & Sons, New York, 1987

30. Dunst CJ, Trivette CM, Gordon NJ, et al: Building and mobilizing informal family support networks. p. 121. In Singer GHS, Irvin LK (eds): Support for Grieving Families: Enabling Positive Adaptation to Disability. Paul H Brookes Publishing Co., Baltimore, 1989

31. Kirschner DA, Kirschner S: Comprehensive Family Therapy: An integration of systemic and psychodynamic treatment models. Brunner/Mazel Publishers, New York, 1985

32. Beavers J, Hampson RB, Hulgus VF, Beavers RW: Coping in families with a retarded child. Fam Process 25:365, 1986

33. Combrinck-Graham L: A developmental model for family systems. Fam Process 24:139, 1985

34. Haley S: Problem-solving Therapy. McGraw-Hill, New York, 1976

35. Longo DC, Bond L: Families of the handicapped child: research and practice. Fam Rel 33:57, 1984

36. Kazak AE, Wilcox BL: The structure and function of social networks in families with handicapped children. Am J Community Psychol 12:67, 1984

37. Waisbren SE: Parents' reactions after the birth of a developmentally disabled child. Am J Ment Defic 84:345, 1980

38. Rosenberg SA, Robinson CC: Interactions of parents with their young handicapped children. p. 159. In Odum SL, Karnes MB (eds): Early Intervention for Infants and Young Children With Handicaps: An Empirical Base. Paul H Brookes Publishing Co., Baltimore, 1988

39. Peterson P, Witkoff RL: Home environment and adjustment in families with handicapped children: a canonical correlation study. Occup Ther J Res 7(2):67, 1987

40. Kazak AE: Families with disabled children: stress and social networks in 2–3 samples. J Abnorm Child Psychol 15:137, 1987

41. Breslau N, Davis GC: Chronic stress and major depression. Arch Gen Psychiatry 43:309, 1986

42. McKinney B, Peterson RA: Predictors of stress in parents of developmentally disabled children. J Pediatr Psychol 12(1):133, 1987

43. Grossman FK: Brothers and Sisters of Retarded Children: An Exploratory Study. Syracuse University Press, Syracuse, NY, 1982

44. Zeenah CH, McDonough S: Clinical approaches to families in early intervention. Semin Perinatol 13(6):513, 1989

45. Hanzlik JR: Interactions between mothers and their infants with developmental disabilities: analysis and review. Phys Occup Ther Pediatr 9(4):33, 1989

46. Bakeman R, Brown J: Assessment of mother–infant interaction. Child Dev 48:195, 1977

47. Emde R, Brown C: Adaptation to the birth of a Down syndrome infant—grieving and maternal attachment. Am Acad Child Psychol 17:299, 1978

48. O'Sullivan SB: Infant-caregiver interaction and the social development of handicapped infants. Phys Occup Ther Pediatr 5(4):1, 1985

49. Brooks-Gunn J, Lewis M: Maternal responsibility in interaction with handicapped infants. Child Dev 55:782, 1984

50. Hanzlik J, Stevenson M: Mother-infant interaction in families with infants who are mentally retarded, retarded with cerebral palsy, or non-retarded infants. Am J Ment Defic 90:513, 1986

51. Friedrich WN, Friedrich WL: Psychosocial aspects of parents of handicapped and non-handicapped children. Am J Ment Defic 85(5):551, 1980

52. Murphy MA: The family with a handicapped child: a review of the literature. J Dev Behav Pediatr 3:73, 1982

53. Gallagher JJ, Beckman P, Cross AH: Families of handicapped children: sources of stress and its amelioration. Except Child 50:10, 1983

54. Cherry DB: Stress and coping in families with ill or disabled children: application of the model to pediatric therapy. Phys Occup Ther Pediatr 9(2):11, 1989

55. Beckman P: Influence of selected child characteristics on stress in families of handicapped infants. Am J Ment Defic 88:150, 1983

56. Holroyd J, Gutline D: Stress in families of children with neuromuscular disease. J Clin Psychol 35(4):734, 1979

57. Parke RD, Tinsley BR: The early environment of the at-risk infant: expanding the social context. p. 153. In Bricker DO (ed): Intervention With At-risk and Handicapped Infants: From Research to Application. University Park Press, Baltimore, 1982

58. Breslau N, Staruch KS, Mortimer EA: Psychological distress in mothers of disabled children. Am J Dis Child 136:682, 1982

59. Wikler L, Haack J, Intagliata J: Bearing the burden alone? Helping divorced mothers of children with developmental disabilities. p. 44. In Hansen JC (ed): Families With Handicapped Members. Aspen Systems, Rockville, MD, 1984.

60. Bernheimer LP, Young MS, Winton PJ: Stress over time: parents with young handicapped children. Dev Behav Pediatr 4(3):177, 1983

61. Depue RA, Monroe SM: Conceptualization and measurement of human disorder in life stress research: the problem of chronic disturbance. Psych Bull 99:36, 1986

62. Abbot DA, Meredith WH: Strengths of parents with retarded children. Fam Rel 35(4):371, 1986

63. McCubbin H, Joy C, Cauble A, et al: Family stress and coping: a decade review. J Marriage Fam 42:855, 1980

64. McCubbin HI, Patterson JM: The family stress process: the double ABCX model of adjustment and adaptation. In McCubbin HI, Sussman MB, Patterson JM (eds): Social Stress and the Family: Advances and Developments in Family Stress Theory and Research. Haworth Press, New York, 1983

65. Summers JA: Family adjustment: issues in research on families with developmentally disabled children. p. 215. In Van Hasselt UB, Strain PS, Hesen M (eds): Handbook of Developmental and Physical Disabilities. Pergamon, Elmsford, NY, 1988

66. McCubbin HI, Patterson JM: Family adaptation to crises. In McCubbin HI, Cauble AE, Patterson JM (eds): Family Stress, Coping and Social Support. Charles C. Thomas, Springfield, IL, 1982

67. Singer SH, Irvin AB, Irvin LK: Expanding the focus of behavioral parent training: a contexual approach. p. 85. In Singer SH, Irvin SL (eds): Support for Caregiving Families: Enabling Positive Adaptation to Disability. Paul H Brookes Publishing Co., Baltimore, 1989

68. Singer SH, Irvin SL: Family caregiving, stress and support. p. 3. In Singer SH, Irvin SL (eds): Support for Caregiving Families: Enabling Positive Adaptation to Disability. Paul H Brookes Publishing Co., Baltimore, 1989

69. Woolfolk RL, Lehrer PM: Principles and Practice of Stress Management. Guilford Press, New York, 1984

70. Summers JA, Behr SK, Turnbull AP: Positive adaptation and coping strengths of families who have children with disabilities. p. 27. In Singer SH, Irvin LK (eds): Support for Caregiving Families: Enabling Positive Adaptation to Disability. Paul H Brookes Publishing Co., Baltimore, 1989

71. Turnbull AO, Summers JA, Bromick SJ, et al: Stress and Coping in Families Having a Member With a Disability. ATA Institute (NARIC Rehabilitation Research Review), Washington, DC, 1986

72. Gath A: The impact of an abnormal child upon the parents. Br J Psychiatry 130:405, 1977

73. Williams RS, McKenny PC: Marital adjustment among parents of mentally retarded children. Fam Perspect 15:175, 1981
74. Kazak AE, Marvin RS: Differences, difficulties and adaptation: stress and social networks in families with a handicapped child. Fam Rel 33:67, 1984
75. Dadds MR, Schwatz S, Sanders MR: Marital discord and treatment outcomes in behavioral treatment of child conduct disorders. J Consult Clin Psychol 55:396, 1987
76. Roesel R, Lawlis GF: Divorce in families of genetically handicapped/mentally retarded individuals. Am J Fam Ther 11:45, 1983
77. Sabbeth R, Leventhal J: Marital adjustment to chronic childhood illness: a critique of the literature. Pediatrics 73:762, 1984
78. Goldberg WA, Easterbrooks MA: The role of marital quality in toddler development. Dev Psychobiol 20:504, 1984
79. Breslau N, Weitzman M, Messenger K: Psychological functioning of siblings of the disabled children. Pediatrics 67:344, 1981
80. Skirtc TM, Summers JA, Brotherson MJ, et al: Severely handicapped children and their brothers and sisters. p. 215. In Blacher J (ed): Severely Handicapped Young Children and Their Families: Research in Review. Academic Press, San Diego, 1983
81. Trevino F: Siblings of handicapped children: identifying those at risk. Soc Casework 60:488, 1979
82. Breslau N, Prabucci K: Siblings of disabled children: effects of chronic stress in the family. Arch Gen Psychiatry 44:1040, 1987
83. Dunn J: Connections between relationships: implications of research on mothers and siblings. p. 168. In Hinde RA, Stevenson-Hinde J (eds): Relationships Within Families: Marital Influences. Oxford University Press, New York, 1988
84. Grossman FK: Brothers and Sisters of Retarded Children: An Exploratory Study. Syracuse University Press, New York, 1972
85. Pearlman L, Scott KA: Raising the Handicapped Child. Prentice Hall, Englewood Cliffs, NJ, 1981
86. Dobson J: Dare to Discipline. Living Books, Wheaton, IL, 1988
87. Patterson SR: Accelerating stimuli for two classes of coercive behaviors. J Abnorm Child Psychol 5:335, 1977
88. Sigel E: Parental Belief Systems: The Psychological Consequences for Children. L Erlbaum, Hillsdale, NJ, 1985
89. Block JH, Block J, Morrison A: Parental agreement-disagreement on child-rearing orientations and gender-related personality correlates in children. Child Dev 52:965, 1981
90. Bernal S, Alverex AI: Culture and class in the study of families. p. 33. In Hansen JC (ed): Cultural Perspectives in Family Therapy. Aspen Systems, Rockville, MD, 1983
91. Fewell RR, Gelb SA: Parenting moderately handicapped persons. p. 175. In Seligman M (ed): The Family With a Handicapped Child: Understanding and Treatment. Grune & Stratton, London, 1983
92. McGoldrick M, Pearce J, Giordano J: Ethnicity and Family Therapy. Guilford Press, New York, 1982
93. Anderson PP, Fenichel ES: Serving Culturally Diverse Families of Infants and Toddlers With Disabilities. National Center for Clinical Infant Programs, Washington, DC, 1989
94. Ogbu J: Cultural influences on plasticity in human development. p. 155. In Gal-

lagher JL, Ramey CT (eds): The Malleability of Children. Paul H Brookes Publishing Co., Baltimore, 1987

95. Green JW: Cultural Awareness in the Human Services: Ethnicity and Social Services. Prentice-Hall, Inglewood Cliffs, NJ, 1982

96. Samora J: Conceptions of health and disease among Spanish Americans. Am Catholic Sociol Rev 22:314, 1978

97. Taft R: Coping with unfamiliar cultures. p. 121. In Warren N (ed): Studies in Cross-Cultural Psychology. Academic Press, San Diego, 1977

98. Falicov CJ: Cultural Perspectives in Family Therapy. Aspen Systems, Rockville, NY, 1983

99. Lappin J: On becoming a culturally conscious family therapist. p. 122. In Hansen JC (ed): Cultural Perspectives in Family Therapy. Aspen Systems, Rockville, MD 1983

100. Gallagher JJ: The family as a focus for intervention. p. 540. In Meisels JP, Shonkoff SJ (eds): Handbook of Early Childhood Intervention. Cambridge University Press, New York, 1990

101. Patton MQ: Qualitative evaluation. SAGE 121, Sage Publications, Newbury Park, CA, 1980

102. Barnard K: Nursing Child Assessment Learning Resource, Manual Feeding and Manual Teaching. NCAST Publications, Seattle, 1979

103. Ross GS: Home intervention for premature infants of low-income families. Am J Orthopsychiatr 54:263, 1984

104. Barrera ME, Rosenbaum PL, Cunningham CE: Early home intervention with low-birth-weight infants and their parents. Child Dev 57:20, 1986

105. Meisels SJ: The efficacy of early intervention and why are we still asking this question? Top Early Child Spec Educ 5:10, 1985

106. Marfo K, Keysela GM: Early intervention with mentally handicapped children: a critical appraisal of applied research. J Pediatr Psychol 10(3):305, 1985

107. Bailey D, Simeonsson R, Winton P et al: Family focused intervention: a functional model for planning, implementing, and evaluating individualized family services in early intervention. J Dev Early Child 10:156, 1986

108. Effgen SK, Bjornson K, Chiarello L et al: Role of physical therapy in early intervention. Pediatr Phys Ther 2(2):97, 1990

109. Bailey DB, Simeonsson RJ: Assessing the needs of families with handicapped infants. J Spec Educ 22:117, 1988

110. Widmayer SM, Field TM: Effects of Brazelton demonstrations for mothers on the development of preterm infants. Pediatrics 67:711, 1981

111. Parmalee AH: Assessment of the infant at risk during the first year. p. 29. In Sell EJ (ed): Follow-up of the High Risk Newborn—A Practical Approach. Charles C Thomas, Springfield, IL, 1980

112. Rosenberg SA, Robinson CC: Enhancement of mother's interactional skills in an infant education program. Educ Training Ment Retard 20:163, 1985

113. Hanson MJ: An analysis of the effects of early intervention services for infants and toddlers with moderate and severe handicaps. Top Early Child Spec Educ 5:36, 1985

114. Dickson JM: A model for the physical therapist in the intensive care nursery. Phys Ther 61:45, 1981

115. Cohen S, Warren R: Respite Care: Principles, Programs, and Policies. Pro-Ed, Austin, TX, 1985

116. Salisbury CL: Parenthood and the need for respite. p. 3. In Salisbury CL, Intagliata

J (eds): Respite Care: Support for Persons With Developmental Disabilities and Their Families. Paul H Brookes Publishing Co., Baltimore, 1986

117. Allen DA, Hudd SS: Are we professionalizing parents? Weighing the benefits and pitfalls. Ment Retard 25:133, 1987

118. Slentz KL, Walker B, Bricker D: Supporting parent involvement in early intervention: a role-taking model. p. 221. In Singer GHS, Irvin LK (eds): Support for Caregiving Families: Enabling Positive Adaptation to Disability. Paul H Brookes Publishing Co., Baltimore, 1989

119. Tyler MB, Kogan KL: Reduction of stress between mothers and their handicapped children. Am J Occup Ther 31:151, 1974

120. Spencer PE, Coye RW: Project BRIDGE: a team approach to decision-making for early services. Infants and Young Children 1(1):82, 1988

121. Johnson BH, McGonigel MJ, Kaufman RK: Guidelines and Recommended Practices for the Individualized Family Service Plan. HEC *TAS, University of North Carolina at Chapel Hill, NC, 1989

Index